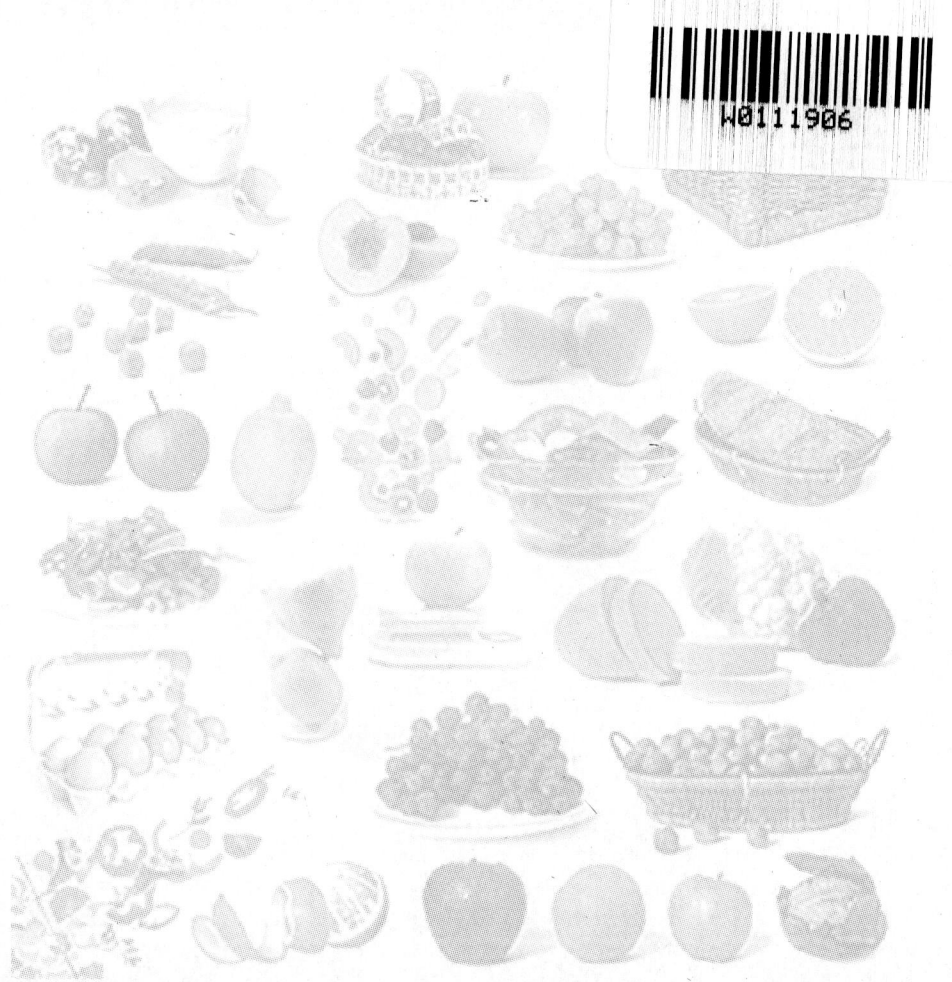

Nutrition Science

Nutrition Science

R. Gajalakshmi
MSc, MPhil

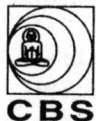

CBS

CBS Publishers & Distributors Pvt Ltd

New Delhi • Bengaluru • Chennai • Kochi • Kolkata • Mumbai
Hyderabad • Jharkhand • Nagpur • Patna • Pune • Uttarakhand

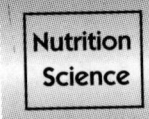

Nutrition
Science

ISBN: 978-81-239-2215-7

First Edition: 2014
Reprint: 2015, 2018

Published by Satish Kumar Jain and produced by Varun Jain for
CBS Publishers & Distributors Pvt Ltd
4819/XI Prahlad Street, 24 Ansari Road, Daryaganj, New Delhi 110 002, India.
Ph: 23289259, 23266861, 23266867   Website: www.cbspd.com
Fax: 011-23243014   e-mail: delhi@cbspd.com; cbspubs@airtelmail.in.
Corporate Office: 204 FIE, Industrial Area, Patparganj, Delhi 110 092
Ph: 4934 4934   Fax: 4934 4935   e-mail: publishing@cbspd.com; publicity@cbspd.com

Branches

- **Bengaluru:** Seema House 2975, 17th Cross, K.R. Road, Banasankari 2nd Stage, Bengaluru 560 070, Karnataka
  Ph: +91-80-26771678/79   Fax: +91-80-26771680   e-mail: bangalore@cbspd.com
- **Chennai:** No. 7, Subbaraya Street, Shenoy Nagar, Chennai 600 030, Tamil Nadu
  Ph: +91-44-26680620, 26681266   Fax: +91-44-42032115   e-mail: chennai@cbspd.com
- **Kochi:** Ashana House, 39/1904, AM Thomas Road, Valanjambalam, Ernakulam 682 016, Kochi, Kerala
  Ph: +91-484-4059061-65,67   Fax: +91-484-4059065   e-mail: kochi@cbspd.com
- **Kolkata:** No. 6/B, Ground Floor, Rameswar Shaw Road, Kolkata-700014 (West Bengal), India
  Ph: +91-33-2289-1126, 2289-1127, 2289-1128   e-mail: kolkata@cbspd.com
- **Mumbai:** 83-C, Dr E Moses Road, Worli, Mumbai-400018, Maharashtra
  Ph: +91-22-24902340/41   Fax: +91-22-24902342   e-mail: mumbai@cbspd.com

Representatives

- **Hyderabad** 0-9885175004
- **Patna** 0-9334159340
- **Jharkhand** 0-9811541605
- **Pune** 0-9623451994
- **Nagpur** 0-9021734563
- **Uttarakhand** 0-9716462459

Printed at India Binding House, Noida, UP

to

my parents

and

the readers

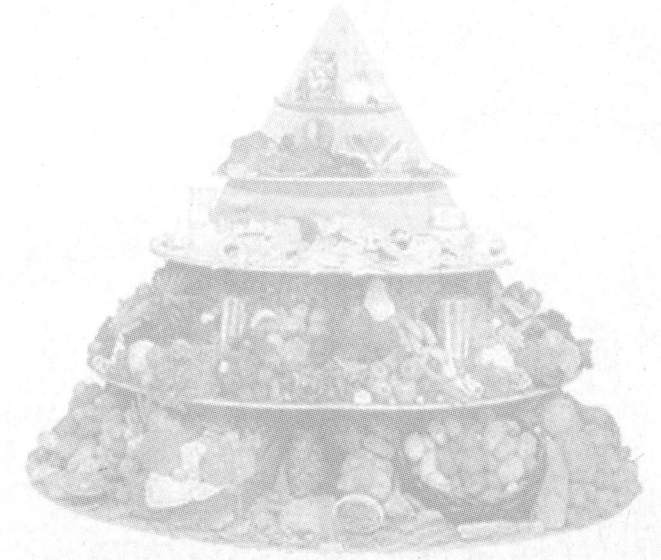

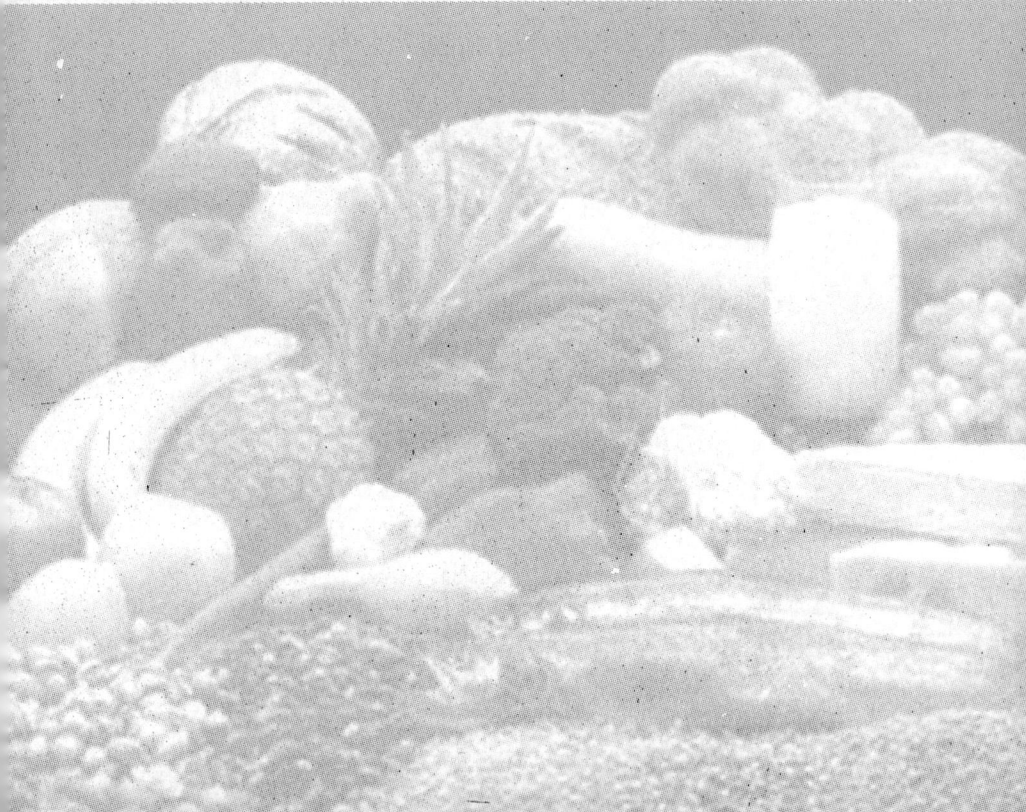

Preface

Nutrition is the study of foods and their effects upon health, development and performance. This textbook on nutrition explains its concepts accurately, clearly and completely in such a way that all students can understand. This book is developed with nutrition and science majors in mind. The chemistry, biochemistry, and physiology presented in the text will take the students with better understanding. I hope that this book will allow all students, even those with a little or no science background, to find the science of nutrition approachable, understandable and useful in their lives.

A request to the teachers and students who use this book : If you find any content needs more consideration, please feel free to contact me through e-mail.

I extend my best wishes for your success.

R. Gajalakshmi

E-mail: talk2gjv@gmail.com

Acknowledgements

In compiling this book, I have extensively referred to a vast number of standard books, journals, proceedings of seminars and conferences. Primary acknowledgement must go to many dedicated scientists who have discovered the principles of food and nutrition. I express my deep sense of indebtedness to all these unnamed investigators.

In addition, I thank Mr YN Arjuna, Senior Director—Publishing, and Mr S Ramesh, General Manager, Chennai Branch, CBS Publishers & Distributors, for providing me this opportunity. I acknowledge the CBS staffs Mr Rajan, Mr Saravanan and Mr Prasath for their support in providing me the materials on time.

Our coworkers, especially Anusha Priyadharshini, Sowmya Balaji, Karthika, Jayaprakash, Hemamalini, Ramakrishnan, Venkatesh Kumar and Rudra Sri, deserve grateful recognition for their indispensable help.

R. Gajalakshmi

E-mail: talk2gjv@gmail.com

Contents

UNIT I

INTRODUCTION

Changing Concepts: Food Habits and Customs

1

Food habits, like other forms of human behaviour, do not develop in a vacuum. They result from many personal, cultural, social, and psychologic influences. For each of us these factors are interwoven to develop a whole, unique individual.

CULTURAL INFLUENCES

Food habits are among the oldest and most deeply rooted aspects of many cultures and exert deep influence on the behaviour of the people. The cultural and subcultural background determines what shall be eaten as well as when and how it shall be eaten. Food habits are primarily based on food availability, economics and personal food meanings and beliefs. Those food habits and customs, which have become meaningful to the group, are carefully held and not quickly changed. Regional culture communities are not the only subcultures of India. For each subculture, there are a number of religious and caste communities who have their own distinctive cultures.

The diets of Hindus in Gujarat and UP may have differences but there are similarities of ingredients or even taste. Often the diets of scheduled castes are decidedly non-vegetarian as opposed to that of Brahmins and Banyas. Not only are there differences between the higher and lower castes but also in the same caste with different social status.

Festivals and feasts can provide an opportunity of good nutritious food. Even the poor, who cannot afford, consume good foods on such occasions. Abstinence from some kinds of foods before or during a festival has been practiced throughout the recorded history across the globe. Many North Indians abstain from animal foods such as egg, meat and fish during Hindu festivals like "NAVRATRI". The examples presented above must have given you a good idea about the cultural influence on food behaviours.

SOCIAL INFLUENCES

The structure of a society is largely formed by grouping according to factors such as economic status, education, residence, occupation or family. Within a given society many of these groups exist, and their values and habits vary widely. Subgroups develop on the basis of region, religion, age, sex, social class, health concerns, occupation or political affiliation.

Food habits in any setting are highly socialized. First, within social relationships, food is a symbol of social acceptance, warmth and friendliness.

Food is often used to promote an individual or group's welfare, interpersonal sociability and feeling of belongingness. Often the place given to nutrition is considerably below than that given to prestigious items in expenditure.

Second, within family relationships, the primary social unit, strong food patterns develop. Food habits that are most closely associated with family sentiments are the most tenacious throughout life.

A pregnant mother among the North Indian family may be given plenty of sweet prepared of ghee during her pregnancy. Further, in the Indian population where sequential eating patterns are observed like the head of the family should eat first, then others and finally the wife and the mother. All the good items in the menu, which are limited, are given to men of the house and children. Such unequal distribution of meals affects the availability of food items and thereby nutrients.

Strong religious factors associated with food tend to have their origin and reinforcement within the family meal circle. Also, family income, community sources of food and market conditions influence food habits and ultimately food choices.

PSYCHOLOGIC INFLUENCES

Individual perceptions and senses have a fundamental role in human existence. Perception and sensation must be viewed as an integrated whole if the complex interactions that occur among human sensory processes, perceptions, cognitions and behaviour in everyday eating situations are to be understood. Investigators seek to understand both psychophysical and psychohedonic responses of foods.

Psychophysical measures are the relationship between sensory (affective) responses and physiology. Such differences may be particularly pertinent with the aging process, when atrophy of the sensory organs alters the perception of foods because of loss of sensitivity.

Psychohedonics is the pleasantness of a food and is influenced by cognitive (cultural, belief and attitudinal) factors expressed as subjective liking or disliking. Evidence suggests that psychohedonic responses play a major role in food choice. In this respect, investigators of food choice have claimed that the brain is the most important physical organ influencing human food choice. At an individual level, outcome measures of food choice can be taken as consumption, hedonic response (liking or disliking), preference, and acceptance.

RELATIONSHIP OF NUTRITION TO HEALTH

Nutrition is the science of foods, the nutrients and other substances therein, their action, interaction and balance in relationship to health and disease; the processes by which the organism ingests, digests, absorbs, transports and utilizes nutrients and disposes of their end products. In addition, nutrition is concerned with social, economic, cultural and psychological implications of food and eating. In short, nutrition science is the area of knowledge regarding the role of food in the maintenance of health. Health is defined by the World Health Organization as the "State of complete physical, mental and social well-being and not merely the absence of disease and infirmity".

The essential requisites (or dimensions) of "health" include the following:
- Achievement of optimal growth and development, reflecting the full expression of one's genetic potential.
- Maintenance of the structural integrity and functional efficiency of body tissues necessary for an active and productive life.
- Ability to withstand the inevitable process of ageing with minimal disability and functional impairment, and
- Ability to combat disease, such as
  a. Resisting infections (immunocompetence)
  b. Preventing the onset (and retarding the progress) of degenerative diseases and cancer, and
  c. Resisting the effect of environmental toxins and pollutants.
- Mental health
- Social well-being is the ability to live in harmony with others.

The word *nutrition* refers to nourishment that sustains life. The science and art of human nutrition both focus on nourishing human life. From the moment of conception until death, the body needs energy to carry out vital functions such as breathing. In addition, people need energy to support physical activity. They must constantly replenish these energy needs with food to sustain physical life.

Nutritional science comprises the body of scientific knowledge governing the nutritional requirements of humans for maintenance, growth, activity, and reproduction.

Good nutrition will always have a positive health results which include a well-developed body, ideal weight for body composition (ratio of muscle mass to fat) and height, and good muscle development and tone. The skin is smooth and clear, the hair glossy, the eyes clear and bright. Posture is good; facial expression is alert. Appetite, digestion and elimination are normal. Well-nourished persons are much more likely to be alert, both mentally and physically. They are meeting not only their day-to-day needs but also maintaining essential nutrient reserves for resisting infections diseases and generally extending their years of normal functioning. Clinical signs of nutritional status are shown in Table 1.1.

Table 1.1: Clinical signs of nutritional status

Features	Good	Poor
General appearance	Alert, responsive	Listless, apathetic, cachexic
Hair	Shiny, lustrous, healthy scalp	Stringy, dull, brittle, dry, depigmented
Neck glands	No enlargement	Thyroid enlarged
Skin, face, neck	Smooth, slightly moist, good colour, reddish pink mucous membranes	Greasy, discoloured scaly
Eyes	Bright, clear, no fatigue circles	Dryness, signs of infection, increased vascularity, glassiness, thickened conjunctivae
Lips	Good colour, moist	Dry, scaly, swollen, angular lesions (stomatitis)
Tongue	Good pink colour, surface papillae present, no lesions	Papillary atrophy, smooth appearance, swollen, red, beefy (glossitis)
Gums	Good pink colour, no swelling or bleeding, firm	Marginal redness or swelling, receding, spongy
Teeth	Straight, no crowding, well-shaped jaw, clean, no discolouration	Unfilled cavities, absent teeth, worn surfaces, mottled, malpositioned
Skin, general	Smooth, slightly moist, good colour	Rough, dry, scaly pale, pigmented, irritated; petechiae, bruises
Abdomen	Flat	Swollen
Legs, feet	No tenderness, weakness, swelling, good colour	Edema, tender, calf, tingling, weakness
Skeleton	No malformations	Bowlegs, knock-knees, chest deformity at diaphragm, beaded ribs, prominment scapulas
Weight	Normal for height, age, body build	Overweight or underweight
Posture	Erect, arms and legs straight, abdomen in, chest out	Sagging shoulder, sunken chest, humped back
Muscles	Well-developed, firm	Flaccid, poor tone, undeveloped, tender
Nervous control	Good attention span for age, does not cry easily, not irritable or restless	Inattentive, irritable
Gastrointestinal function	Good appetite and digestion, normal, regular elimination	Anorexia, indigestion, constipation or diarrhoea
General vitality	Endurance, energetic, sleeps well at night, vigorous	Easily fatigued, no energy, falls asleep in school, looks tired, apathetic

UNIT II

CLASSIFICATION OF FOOD

A. Classification by origin, chemical composition and sources

2   Carbohydrates

INTRODUCTION

"Carbohydrates", when people hear this word, the one thing comes to their mind is "Weight-Gain". Many weight-loss plans which captured the attention of public are designed with less carbs. As a result, more groups of people believe that carbohydrates are inherently bad. But the fact is not entirely true.

Carbohydrates are the chief sources:

i. Providing 40 and 85% of food energy in different population
ii. Used for oxidation of fat and
iii. Also for the synthesis of certain non-essential amino acids.

Carbohydrates are grouped into two categories. First, enzymatically digestible carbohydrates, starches and sugar that give glucose, which is a chief fuel for all tissues. Especially, brain cells and RBCs are almost wholly dependent on this for energy source. Almost all the starches and sugars that humans burn for energy come from plants; the only major exception is lactose, the sugar in milk. Second, non-digestible carbohydrates, fibre, which have important physiologic functions in gastrointestinal tract.

Occurrence

Carbohydrates get synthesized in plants through the process of photosynthesis.

Each plant is a complex food factory that takes water from soil, carbon dioxide from air, and energy from the sun to make glucose, a simple sugar that is later converted into starch. In animals it is stored as glycogen in the liver and muscles.

Starch and glycogen are stored in the form of polysaccharides. Carbohydrates also have a structural role, particularly in cell membranes, as a component of glycoproteins and glycolipids.

Classification

Carbohydrate components can be classified in a number of ways. *Chemically*, carbohydrates are classified according to the number of basic sugar, or saccharide units in their structure. There are four major groups of saccharides (Table 2.1).

9

Table 2.1: Classification of dietary saccharides

Class of saccharide	Type of saccharide	Digestibility	Dietary sources
Monosaccharides	Glucose	Readily absorbed and utilized.	Small amount of free glucose is present in fruits and vegetables and large amount is present in honey. Manufactured foods containing commercial glucose syrups are a major source. Most of the body's glucose is derived from the digestion and conversion of other saccharides.
	Fructose	Well absorbed at normal levels of intake (~10 g/day), but may cause osmotic diarrhoea in larger quantities, particularly in children. Can be directly oxidized without being converted to glucose.	Principal sugar in fruits, vegetables and honey. Component of sucrose. Commercial fructose syrups are used in the manufacture of some products (e.g. jams).
	Galactose	Absorbed by an active transport mechanism and rapidly converted to glucose.	Not found in its free state, but as a component of lactose, the principal sugar in milk and milk products.
Disaccharides	Sucrose	Broken down by the enzyme sucrase to *glucose and fructose*, which are rapidly absorbed.	Table sugar. Manufactured foods sweetened by the addition of sugar. Foods which are naturally sweet (e.g. fruits and young vegetables).
	Lactose	Broken down by the enzyme lactase to *glucose and galactose*. Some ethnic groups lose the ability to produce lactase beyond childhood, resultig in lactose intolerance.	Milk and milk products.

Contd.

Table 2.1: Classification of dietary saccharides (*Contd.*)

Class of saccharide	Type of saccharide	Digestibility	Dietary sources
	Maltose	Converted by the enzyme maltase to *glucose*.	Malted wheat and barley, germinating cereals, malt extracts, beers.
	Trehalose	Converted by the enzyme trehalase to glucose.	Mushrooms and edible fungi.
Oligosaccharides	Raffinose Stachyose Verbascose Inulin Fructo-Oligosaccharides (FOS) Galacto-Oligosaccharides (GOS)	Comprised of galactose, glucose and fructose units, but humans do not possess the enzymes to digest them. They can, however, be fermented in the colon.	Natural sources of oligosaccharides include legumes, onions, fennel, jerusalem artichoke, asparagus and chicory. FOS and GOS are added to certain "functional foods" as prebiotics and FOS is added to some commercial enteral feeds.
Polysaccharides	Starch	Comprised of amylose (linear molecules of 200–2000 glucose units) and amylopectin (branched-chain molecules of 10^4–10^6 glucose units). Broken down by pancreatic amylase to glucose once the starch has been released from its storage granules by heat and moisture. Raw uncooked starch is poorly absorbed. After heating, some types of starch also undergo retrograde conversion to a form which is resistant to amylase digestion. This "resistant starch" can be fermented in the large intestine.	The principal sources are cereal foods and potatoes. Smaller amount is present in root vegetables and unripened fruit. Dextrins are degradation products of starch where the polymers have been broken down to smaller units by partial hydrolysis. They may be used dietetically as a means of administering carbohydrate in an easily assimilable form.

Contd.

Table 2.1: Classification of dietary saccharides (*Contd.*).

Class of saccharide	Type of saccharide	Digestibility	Dietary sources
	Glycogen	Similar in composition to amylopectin, this is a storage form of glucose in living animals but is not present in foods derived from them.	
	Non-starch polysaccharides	A heterogeneous mixture of cellulose (a polymer of glucose), and non-cellulosic polysaccharides containing a variety of hexoses, pentoses, uronic acids and other components in their structure. Human digestive enzymes are unable to break these down into their constituent saccharide units. However, NSP can be partially or totally fermented by colonic bacteria to SCFA, which can be used as an energy source.	Vegetables, fruits, wholegrain cereals and cereal bran, pulses.
Sugar alcohols (polyols)	Sorbitol xylitol, mannitol lactitol	These are only partially absorbed and hence provide less energy per gram than other available carbohydrates. Large amounts of polyols can cause osmotic diarrhoea.	Small amount is naturally present in a few foods (such as certain fruits) but are usually only obtained in significant quantities from manufactured foods where they have been used as a substitute for sucrose.

Monosaccharides

Single (mono) molecule of sugar (saccharide), often called simple sugar. *Glucose, fructose, and galactose* are the simplest of all sugar. As basic units, these sugar molecules are absorbed "as is" without undergoing digestion.

Disaccharides

"Double sugar" composed of two (di) linked monosaccharides units, at least one of which is glucose. They are sucrose (glucose + fructose), lactose (glucose + galactose), and maltose (glucose + glucose). Disaccharides get split and becomes monosaccharides before being absorbed.

Oligosaccharides

It is a short-chain carbohydrates which are not enzymatically digestible but can be fermented by colonic bacteria. Stachyose, raffinose, inulin or fructo-oligo saccharides are few examples.

Polysaccharides

Carbohydrates consisting of many (poly) sugar molecules and can be broadly divided into starch (a glucose polymer linked by α-glucosidic linkages which can be broken down by pancreatic amylase) and non-starch polysaccharides (which are not enzymatically digestible by humans although many can be fermented by colonic bacteria).

Physiologically, carbohydrates are classified depending upon its availability after enzymatical digestion in the small intestine.

• Carbohydrates like starches and sugars are digested and absorbed as monosaccharides; therefore they are available to the body. And, this leads to a rise in blood glucose.

• Non-digestible carbohydrate, dietary fibre are not digested in the small intestine, they move and get fermented in the large intestine by colonic bacteria. Fermented carbohydrates have no effect on blood glucose levels, this has been termed "glycemic" and "non-glycemic" carbohydrates more appropriately reflect their physiological effects. (FAO/WHO–1998)

Intrinsic and Non-milk Extrinsic Sugars

As we seen before, any glycemic carbohydrates which are enzymatically digested are ultimately converted to glucose and are oxidized to provide the same amount of energy, i.e. 4 kcal per gram. However, there are different health implications depending upon their dietary origin. For example, starches are found with other important dietary components such as B vitamins, minerals, protein and fibre. Sugars are naturally found in micronutrient rich foods such as fruits, vegetables and milk. Sucrose is commercially extracted from these foods, and uses it as a sweetener, and also to prepare cakes, biscuits, soft drinks or confectionery. This extracted sucrose is high in sugars and energy but low in micronutrients and fibre. Therefore, dietary sugars should be divided into two distinct groups. They are as follows.

Intrinsic Sugars

Sugars present within intact cells (e.g. sugars in whole fruit). The sugars present in milk (lactose and galactose) are also regarded as intrinsic sugars (despite being present in a free state) because their metabolic effects are similar to those of intrinsic sugars.

Non-milk Extrinsic Sugars (NMES)

Sugars present in free and hence readily absorbable state, as a result of being added to foods (usually in the form of sucrose) or released from disrupted cells (e.g. the sugars present in fruit puree or fruit juice).

This is a classification of convenience rather than chemistry. The sucrose present in a bar of chocolate (extrinsic) is no different from that found in an apple (intrinsic), but the distinction is a useful one as an indicator of dietary quality. When diets contain high NMES foods, it is relatively high in sugar and energy but very low in other micronutrients and macronutrients. This diet is said to be imbalance diet and may lead to risk of obesity and others conditions.

GLYCEMIC INDEX

Glycemic index (GI) is the ratio of the area under the blood glucose curve resulting from ingestion of 50 g of digestible carbohydrates and the area under the curve after the ingestion of 50 g of a standard food, either glucose or white bread. It is a numeric measure of the glycemic response of 50 g of a food sample, the higher the number, the higher the glycemic response.

GI is calculated as

$$\frac{\text{Area under the 2h blood glucose response curve for test food containing } 50\,\text{g CHO}}{\text{Area under the 2h blood glucose response curve after } 50\,\text{g CHO as glucose or white bread}} \times 100$$

Glycemic response is the effect of a food on the blood glucose concentration: How quickly the glucose level rises, how high it goes, and how long it takes to return to normal.

Carbohydrates are often broadly classified into either "simple sugars" or "complex CHO's". Traditionally it was believed that simple sugars produce a greater glycemic response than complex carbohydrates because they are all rapidly and completely absorbed. However, glycemic response is influenced by many variables including its degree of ripeness, the amount of fat and fibre in the food, the method of preparation, and the amount eaten.

The types of carbohydrates eaten before, during and after prolonged exercise influences an athlete's endurance. Generally, athletes are advised to eat

- Low glycemic index carbohydrates before prolonged exercise.
- Moderate to high glycemic index carbohydrates during long distance events to ensure adequate glucose availability.
- High glycemic index carbohydrates after exercise appear to enhance glycogen (Table 2.2).

The glycemic response to a single food will also change when it is eaten in conjunction with other foods; for example, fat content and meal size

Table 2.2: Glycemic index (GI) of carbohydrate foods

	Lower GI foods (< 40)	Moderate GI foods (40–60)	Higher GI foods (> 60)
Breads	Wholegrain or mixed grain breads (e.g. granary, rye bread, linseed bread), fruit loaf	Pitta bread, bran muffin, crumpet, croissant	White, brown, wholemeal bread Baguette, bagel
Breakfast cereals	Oat-based cereals (e.g. porridge, muesli), bran-rich cereals	Cereal bars, popcorn, corn	Maize or wheat-based breakfast cereals (e.g. cornflakes, weetabix), rice cakes (Idli)
Pasta	Pasta and noodles	Cous cous	
Rice	Basmati rice	White rice, brown rice	
Beans and pulses	Green beans, peas, baked beans, kidney beans, lentils nuts		Broad beans
Potatoes	New potatoes in their skins	Boiled old potatoes french fries	Instant potato, jacket/ baked potato, mashed potato
Fruits	Most fresh fruits if not over-ripe, especially apple, pear, citrus fruits, plums, grapes.	Dried fruit, apricots, peaches, banana ripped, pineapple, orange.	Fruit juice, watermelon, lychees, raisins.
Vege-tables	All green and salad vegetables, carrots plantain, yam	Beetroot, sweet corn, sweet potato	Parsnips, pumpkin
Dairy foods	Milk, plain yogurt		Flavoured yogurt, ice cream
Sugars	Fructose	Sucrose, cola	Glucose, lucozade, honey, soft drinks

affect the rate of gastric emptying, amino acids from protein augment insulin release and soluble fibre present in one carbohydrate food may impact on the absorption of another.

An additional problem is that glycemic index compares the glycemic effect of foods containing 50 g of carbohydrate, but in practice foods are consumed in combinations. For this reasons, the glycemic load (GL) of a food or meal, defined as GI × g carbohydrate, is a more useful reflection of its glycemic potential.

GLYCEMIC LOAD

The estimated GL of the food, meals and dietary patterns is calculated by multiplying the glycemic index by the amount of carbohydrate in each food and then totalling the value for all foods in a meal or dietary pattern.

For diabetics, the glycemic index can help to fine-tune optimal meal planning. Athletes can use the glycemic index to choose optimal fuels before, during and after exercise.

GI and GL of a diet may have general implications for health. High glycemic index diets are associated with an increased risk of type 2 diabetes and cardiovascular disease.

Low-GI diets have a great role to play in management of obesity, diabetes and hyperlipidemia.

As general guidance, foods can broadly be divided into the categories of glycemic index shown. However, it should be borne in mind that factors such as the way in which a food is prepared or cooked, its degree of ripeness and other foods with which it is consumed may alter its glycemic effect (Table 2.3).

Table 2.3: Glycemic index (GI) and glycemic load (GL) of selected foods

	GI	GL
Breakfast cereals		
Kellogg's corn flakes	92	24
Kellogg's nutrigrain	66	10
Kellogg's special K	69	14
Grains/pastas		
Buckwheat	54	16
Bulgur	48	12
Rice		
Basmati	58	22
Brown	50	16
Instant	87	36
Noodles-instant	7	19
Pasta		
Egg fettuccine (avg)	40	18

Contd.

Table 2.3: Glycemic index (GI) and glycemic load (GL) of selected foods (*Contd.*)

	GI	GL
Spaghettic (avg)	38	18
Vermicelli	35	16
Tortellni, stouffer's	50	1
Bread		
Bagel	72	25
Croissant	67	17
Crumpet	69	13
"Grainy breads (avg)	49	6
Pita bread	57	10
Pumpernickel (avg)	50	6
Rye bread (avg)	58	8
White bread (avg)	70	10
Whole-wheat bread (avg)	77	9
Crackers/crisp bread		
Puffed crisp bread	81	15
Ryvita	69	11
Water cracker	78	14
Cookies		
Oatmeal	55	12
Milk arrowroot	69	12
Cake		
Chocolate, frosted	38	20
Oat bran muffin	69	24
Sponge cake	46	17
Waffles	76	10
Vegetables		
Beets	64	5
Carrots (avg)	47	3
Parsnip	97	12
Peas (Green, Avg	48	3
Potato		
Baked (avg)	85	26
Boile	88	16
French fries	75	22
Microwaved	82	27
Pumpkin	75	3
Sweet corn	60	11
Sweet potat (avg)	61	17
Yam (avg)	37	13
Legumes		
Baked beans (avg)	48	7

Contd.

Table 2.3: Glycemic index (GI) and glycemic load (GL) of selected foods (*Contd.*)

	GI	GL
Broad beans	79	9
Butter beans	31	6
Chickpeas (avg)	28	8
Cannelloni beans	38	12
Kidney beans (avg)	28	7
Lentils (avg)	29	5
Soya beans (avg)	18	1
Fruits		
Apple (avg)	38	6
Apricot (dried)	31	9
Banana (avg)	51	13
Cherries	22	3
Grpefruit	25	3
Grapes (avg)	46	8
Kiwi fruit (avg)	53	6
Mango	51	8
Orange (avg)	48	5
Papaya	59	10
Canned (natural juice)	38	4
Fresh (avg)	42	5
Pear (avg)	38	4
Pineapple	59	7
Plum	39	5
Raisins	64	28
Cantaloupe	65	4
Watermelon	72	4
Dairy foods		
Milk		
Full-fat	27	3
Skim	32	4
Chocolate-flavoured	42	13
Condensed	61	33
Custard	43	7
Ice cream		
Regular (avg)	61	8
Low-fat	50	3
Yogurt low-fat	33	10
Beverages		
Apple juice	40	12
Coca cola	63	16
Lemonade	66	13
Fanta	68	23
Orange juice (avg)	52	12

Contd.

Table 2.3: Glycemic index (GI) and glycemic load (GL) of selected foods (*Contd.*)

	GI	GL
Snack foods		
Tortilla chipst (avg)	63	17
Fish sticks	38	7
Peanut (avg)	14	1
Popcorn	72	8
Potato chips	57	10
Convenience foods		
Macaroni and cheese	64	32
Soup		
Lentil	44	9
Split-pea	60	16
Tomato	38	6
Sushi (avg)	52	19
Pizza, cheese	60	16
Sweets		
Chocolate	44	13
Jelly beans (avg)	78	22
Mars bar	68	27
Sugars		
Honey (avg)	55	10
Fructose (avg)	19	2
Glucose	100	10
Lactose (avg)	46	5
Sucrose (avg)	68	7

DIETARY FIBRE

- Dietary fibre can be described as intact and intrinsic plant material that is not digestible by endogenous enzymes and reach the large intestine, where they undergo fermentation. It is largely chemical in basis, encompasses a range of compounds including non-starch polysaccharides (NSP) and resistant starches.

- In relation to human nutrition, the principle NSP are those that comprise approximately 90% of plant cell walls. They are very heterogeneous group whose main constituents sugars are celluloses, hemi-celluloses, gums and pectins.

- Resistant starch that escapes digestion in the small intestine because of its highly intrinsical resistant to hydrolysis by pancreatic amylase. This starch remains intact throughout the cooking process or recrystalizes after cooling and resists enzyme breakdown. This yields limited amount of glucose for absorption (Table 2.4).

Table 2.4: Fibre fractions—definitions in use

Fraction	Examples	Physiological role	Food sources	Comments
Insoluble dietary fibre	Celluloses, some hemicelluloses, lignin	Laxation- increased stool weight and reduced transit time	Wheat bran, edible skins and seeds of fruit and vegetables	Division on the basis of solubility in aqueous solution (not necessarily physiological conditions) does not account for other variables, such as extent of colonic fermentation and binding capacity which may affect physiological response to "fibre".
Soluble dietary fibre	β glucans, pectins, gums, mucilages and some hemi-celluloses.	Blunt lipid and glucose absorption. Tend to be more fermen-table than insoluble fibre.	Fruits, oats, barley, beans	
Resistant starch (RS)	(RS1) Protected or physically enclosed starch. (RS2) Unswollen/ raw starch granules. (RS3) Retrograded starch. (RS4) Chemically modi-fied starches (ethers or esters)	Fermentable – produce SCFA	(RS1) Whole or partly milled grains or seeds. (RS2) Raw potato and green banana. (RS3) Cooked and cooled potato, bread, and rice. (RS4) Modified starches in processed foods	Difficult to assess intake. Levels of RS measured in the raw food may not accurately reflect in vivo amounts due to extrinsic factors such as extent of processing, cooking and chewing, transit time, concentration of digestive enzymes, pH, amount of starch and presence of other food components. RS4 not well studied in terms of intake or effect.
Prebiotics/ fructo-oligo-saccharide	Inulin, oligofructose, lactulose, oligo-	Selectively stimulate the growth and/or activity of one	Natural sources: Onion, leek, garlic, banana	"Colonic Nutrients".

Contd.

Table 2.4: Fibre fractions—definitions in use (*Contd.*)

Fraction	Examples	Physiological role	Food sources	Comments
(FOS)/ fructopoly saccharideh fructans	saccharides	or a limited number of bacterial species already resident in the colon—(re) equilibrate co- lon microflora. Fermentable— produce SCFA. Laxation	Functional foods, e.g. breakfast cereals with added inulin.	
Indigestible animal derived compounds	Chitin and chitosan	Chitin— cholesterol lowering	Derived from the shells of shrimps and crabs.	Would be included in gravimetric analysis. "Physiological Fibre".
Indigestible oligo- saccharides and glucose polymers.	Polydextrose	Fermentable and may have a role in (re) equilibration of microflora.	Added to "diet" or low energy manu- factured pro- ducts as a sugar/starch replacer.	Would be classified as a "Functional or Physiological Fibre". Inclusion in fibre definition varies between countries. Added to foods which are not traditionally good sources of "Dietary Fibre".

Functions

Physiologic Effects

The properties of fibre compounds, specifically their particle size, bulk volume, hydration, fluid flow, fermentation and surface area properties, and their effect on adsorption and entrapment of molecules explain the distinctive physiological effects.

Nutrient Absorption

Beneficial Effects

• Even after adequate processing, cooking, mastication a part of nutrients remain packed in it.
• Soluble, viscous polysaccharides can slow the digestion and absorption of nutrients from the gut; this may lead to eventual excretion of nutrients.
• By increasing the viscosity of the gastric contents, foods or meals with high soluble fibre content have been shown to blunt the postprandial lipid and glucose responses.

Table 2.5: Summary of food sources of various classes of dietary fibre

Dietary fibre class	Major chemical compound	Plant parts	Sources Grains	Fruits	Vegetables	Functions
Cellulose	Glucose (β-1-4 linkages)	Main cell wall constituent	Bran, whole wheat, whole rye	Apples pears	Beans, peas. Cabbage family. Root vegetable. Fresh tomatoes	*Insoluble;* binds minerals, increase water-holding capacity, thus increasing faecal volume and decreasing gut transit time.
Noncellulose polysaccharides hemicellulose	Xylose, mannose, galactose	Secretions, cell wall material	Bran, cereals, whole grains			*Mostly insoluble;* holds water, increases stool bulk, reduces colonic pressure; binds bile acids.
Pectins	Polygalacturonic acid	Intracellular cement material		Apples, citrus fruits, berries, especially strawberries	Green beans carrots	*Soluble;* binds cholesterol, bile acids and minerals thus decreasing serum cholesterol.
Gums	Galactose and glucuronic acid	Special cell secretions	Oatmeal, legumes, guar, barley	Food product thickener, stabilizer	Dried beans, other legumes, vegetable gums used in food processing	*Soluble;* binds cholesterol, bile acids; provides fermentable material for colonic bacteria with production of volatile fatty acids and gas. Cause gel formation, thus decrease gastric emptying, slow digestion, gut transit time, and glucose absorption.

Contd.

Table 2.5: Summary of food sources of various classes of dietary fibre (Contd.)

Dietary fibre class	Major chemical compound	Sources				Functions
		Plant parts	Grains	Fruits	Vegetables	
Mucilages		Cell secretions		Food product thickener, stabilizer		*Soluble;* slows gastric emptying time; fermentable substrate for colonic bacteria: binds bile acids
Algal substances		Algae, seaweeds		Food product thickener, stabilizer		*Soluble;* slows gastric emptying time; fermentable substrate; binds bile acids
Noncarbohydrate phenols Lignins		Woody part of plants	Whole wheat, whole rye	Strawberries, peaches, pears, plums	Mature vegetables	*Insoluble;* antioxidant; binds bile acids and metals, fermentation produces short-chain fatty acids associated with decreased risk of tumor formations.

- It provides a physical barrier to the digestion of sugars in plant foods by maintaining the integrity of cell walls, and the ion-exchange capacity of viscous fibres has been shown to interfere with the enterohepatic circulation of bile acids, which helps in LDL cholesterol reduction.
- Dietary fibre resisting digestion in the small intestine becomes substrates for bacterial fermentation. This increase in bacterial mass along with the production of gases and short chain-fatty acid (SCFA), which have been shown to exert a number of physiological effects.
- Resistant starch appears to be particularly effective in increasing SCFA and also butyrate production.
- Only 5% of SCFA produced are excreted in the faeces with the remaining 95% absorbed in the large bowel, from where they exert both local and distal effects as follows:
  - SCFAs are oxidized to provide 60–70% of the colonocyte's energy needs.
  - SCFAs are relatively week acids, lowering the pH of digesta. This may prevent the overgrowth of pH-sensitive pathogenic bacteria.
  - SCFAs have been shown to promote colonocyte health independently of their role as an energy source.
  - SCFA butyrate may promote apoptosis (cell death) in tumour cells.
  - It increases colonic blood flow (enhancing delivery of oxygen and nutrients to tissues) and reduces gastric tone and increase volume higher up in the gut (slowing passage of gastric contents to improve nutrient digestion).
  - SCFA stimulates electrolyte and fluid uptake, as shown by their ability to alleviate colonic based diarrhoea (antibiotic and infection-related).
  - It helps in release of regulatory hormones which stimulate growth of mucosal cells.
  - Prebiotic fibre exerts their effect by being selective substrates for beneficial bacteria in the gut, e.g. bifidobacteria and lactic acid bacteria.
  - A possible mechanism for prebiotic modulation of metabolic pathways by fibre is by their fermentation into SCFAs.
  - A low-fibre diet based primarily on meat, fat, and highly digestible carbohydrates is said to result in a higher ratio of "putrefactive" or potentially harmful bacteria such as *pseudomonas, clostridia, E. Coli,* and *proteus organisms.*

Adverse Effects

Some fibre fractions like phytates, bind with minerals such as magnesium, calcium, zinc and iron; this may therefore result in micronutrient deficiencies. In practice, this point has to be overlooked to avoid complications.

Effect of Faecal

Coarse bran is more effective than fine bran. Stools become soft, bulky, and readily eliminated due to water holding character of dietary fibre. It relieves us from constipation.

Diet rich in insoluble fibre primarily facilitated by its direct effect in diluting or binding toxins in the intestinal contents. Two main mechanisms which have direct impacts are, insoluble fibre like wheat bran contributes directly on increasing bulk. Fermentable fibres like oat bran provide bulk indirectly through an increase in bacterial mass.

SOLUBLE FIBRES

Soluble fibres can form gels, resulting in slow GI transit time and slow or decreased nutrient absorption. It also binds other nutrients such as cholesterol and minerals and increase excretion of these.

INSOLUBLE FIBRES

Increase the water-holding capacity of undigested material and lead to increased faecal volume (bulk) and decreased GI transit time (increases the frequencies of defecation).

The "prebiotic effect" may be influenced by the dose and duration of oligosaccharide intake, site of fermentation (proximal or distal colon) and baseline faecal flora composition (Table 2.6).

Fibre in diet (a practical view):

1. Increase cereal foods, specifically whole meal/whole grain products rather than "refined" forms.
2. Include dried fruits, nuts and legumes to your breakfast cereals.
3. Consume fruits and vegetables unpeeled whenever possible, e.g. apple, potatoes, chikku. Edible seeds, such as those found in strawberries, kiwifruit, tomatoes and cucumber can be consumed.
4. Add pulses and extra vegetables to soups, stews and sauces.
5. Half of the white flour can be substituted with whole meal flour when acceptable in baking.
6. Increase in dietary fibre should always be done gradually. Sudden hike or excess of dietary fibre may lead to distention, cramping, diarrhoea, intestinal obstruction and interference with absorption of mineral elements.
7. There should be increased fluid intake with fibre intake at the same time, as the effects of fibre on stool formation and passage rely on an adequate fluid intake (Table 2.7).

Fibre Requirement

Recommended dietary allowances (RDA) for fibre is 30 g/day for a normal healthy adult. Meeting the recommended levels of fibre is sufficient to achieve its benefit. Higher amount may lead to abdominal distention and excessive flatulence.

Table 2.6: Relationship between fibre and various health problems

Problem	Effect of fibre	Possible mode of action
Diabetes mellitus	Reduces fasting blood sugar levels, reduces glycosuria, reduces insulin requirements, increases insulin sensitivity	Slows carbohydrate absorption by: Delaying gastric emptying time, Forming gels with pectin or guar gum in the intestine, thus impeding carbohydrate absorption. "Protecting" carbohydrates from enzymatic activity with a fibrous coat. Allowing "protected" carbohydrates to escape into large colon where they are digested by bacteria.
	Inhibits postprandial (after meals) hyperglycemia	Alters gut hormones (for example, glucagon) to enhance glucose metabolism in the liver.
Obesity	Increases satiety rate	Prolongs chewing and swallowing movements.
	Reduces nutrient bioavailability	Increases faecal fat content.
	Reduces energy density	Inhibits absorption of carbohydrates in high-fibre foods. Decreases transit time.
	Alters hormonal response	Alters action of insulin, gut glucagon, and other intestinal hormones.
	Alters thermogenesis	
Coronary heart disease	Inhibits recirculation of bile acids	Alters bacterial metabolism of bile acids. Alters bacterial flora, resulting in a change in metabolic activity forms gels that bind bile acids. Alters the function of pancreatic and intestinal enzymes.
	Reduces triglyceride and cholesterol levels*	Reduces insulin level[+]. Binds cholesterol, preventing absorption. Slows fat absorption by forming gel matrices in the intestine.
Colon cancer	Reduces incidence of disease[++]	Bile acids or their bacterial metabolites may affect the structure of the colon, its cell turnover rate, and function.
Other gastrointestinal disorders:	Reduces pressure from within the intestinal lumen.	Decreases transit time.

Contd.

Table 2.6: Relationship between fibre and various health problems (*Contd.*)

Problem	Effect of fibre	Possible mode of action
Diverticular disease constipation hiatal hernia haemorrhoids	Increases diameter of the intestinal lumen, thus allowing intestinal tract to contract more, propelling contents more rapidly and inhibiting segmentations.**	Increases water absorption resulting in a larger, softer stool.

* This effect is based on epidemiologic studies, usually observed in combination with reduced fat intake.
+ Insulin is required for fat synthesis.
++ Preventive effect of fibre is assumed from epidemiologic studies that associate low fibre, high-fat diets with an increased incidence of disease.
** Segmentation increase pressure and weakness along the walls of the intestinal tract.

Table 2.7: Limitations of excess consumption of fibres

Disease	Type of fibre	Physiological mechanism
Increased risk of colonic cancer	Soluble fibres such as gum arabic, carrageenan, which are used as stabilizers and emulsifiers in food industry.	1. Reduce the ability of insoluble fibres to absorb and excrete carcinogen. 2. Soluble fibres are digested by colonic bacteria. The carcinogen formed can be deposited on the mucosal cells. 3. Soluble fibre may cross the intestinal epithelium and carry with it carcinogens in solution.
Decreased absorption of minerals such as calcium, iron, magnesium, zinc.	Insoluble fibres, seed coats	Phytates found in seed coat of legumes has the ability to bind metal ions like calcium, copper, iron and zinc and make them insoluble.

The proposition of soluble to insoluble fibre should be in the ratio of 1 : 2. In quality diet fibre should be in the form of foods such as fruits, vegetables, wholegrain breads and cereals, legumes, nuts and seeds, because they are not only rich in fibre but also excellent sources of vitamins, minerals, trace elements, antioxidants, and numerous protective phytochemicals.

Increasing the intake of fluid up to 2 L/day will facilitate the effectiveness of recommended fibre intake (Table 2.8).

Table 2.8: Dietary fibre content of foods g/100 g

Name of the foodstuff	Total dietary fibre g	Insoluble dietary fibre g	Soluble dietary fibre g
Cereals, grains and products			
Bajra	11.3	9.1	2.2
Jowar	9.7	8.0	1.7
Maize, dry	11.9	11.0	0.9
Ragi	11.5	9.9	1.6
Rice	4.1	3.2	0.9
Wheat	12.5	9.6	2.9
Pulses and legumes			
Bengal gram, whole	28.3	25.2	3.1
Bengal gram, dhal	15.3	12.7	2.6
Black gram, dhal	11.7	7.6	4.1
Black gram, whole	20.3	15.4	4.9
Green gram, whole	16.7	14.7	2.0
Green gram, dhal	8.2	6.5	1.7
Lentil, whole	15.8	13.5	2.3
Lentil, dhal	10.3	8.3	2.0
Red gram, dhal	9.1	6.8	2.3
Red gram, whole	22.6	19.8	2.8
Leafy vegetables			
Agathi	8.4	6.3	2.1
Amaranth	4.0	3.1	0.9
Ambat chukka	3.2	2.4	0.8
Cabbage	2.8	2.0	0.8
Colocasia, green	6.6	5.1	1.5
Coriander	4.3	3.0	1.3
Curry leaves	16.3	13.4	2.9
Drumstick	9.0	6.8	2.2
Fenugreek	4.7	3.2	1.5
Gogu	3.8	2.6	1.2
Mayalu	2.5	1.6	0.9
Mint	6.3	5.0	1.3
Paruppu keerai	3.9	2.9	1.0
Ponnaganni	7.9	6.9	1.0
Spinach	2.5	1.8	0.7
Tamarind leaves, tender	10.6	9.4	1.2
Roots and tubers			
Beetroot	3.5	2.6	0.9
Carrot	4.4	3.0	1.4
Potato	1.7	1.1	0.6
Radish	2.3	1.8	0.5
Sweet potato	3.9	2.6	1.3
Yam	4.2	3.2	1.0

Contd.

Table 2.8: Dietary fibre content of foods g/100 g (*Contd.*)

Name of the foodstuff	Total dietary fibre g	Insoluble dietary fibre g	Soluble dietary fibre g
Colocasia	3.0	2.3	0.7
Other vegetables			
Bananapith	2.2	2.0	0.2
Bitter gourd	4.3	3.2	1.1
Bottle gourd	2.0	1.7	0.3
Brinjal	6.3	4.6	1.7
Broad bean	8.9	6.7	2.1
Cauliflower	3.7	2.6	1.1
Chochomarrow	1.3	0.9	0.4
Cluster bean	5.7	4.2	1.5
Cucumber	2.6	2.0	0.6
Keera, green	1.1	0.8	0.3
Drumstick	5.8	4.8	1.0
Giant chilies	2.2	2.0	0.2
Kovai	2.5	1.5	1.0
Ladies finger	3.6	2.6	1.0
Mango, raw	3.0	1.4	1.6
Onion stalks	5.1	3.7	1.4
Peas, green	8.6	7.2	1.4
Plantain, green	3.5	2.6	0.9
Ridge gourd	1.9	1.4	0.5
Snake gourd	2.1	1.6	0.5
Tomato	1.7	1.2	0.5
Nuts and oilseeds			
Soya bean	23.0	17.9	5.1
Coconut fresh	13.6	12.7	0.9
Gingerly seeds	16.8	13.6	3.2
Groundnut	11.0	8.5	2.5
Mustard	13.6	10.2	3.4
Fruits			
Papaya	2.6	1.3	1.3
Zizyphus	3.8	2.8	1.0
Amla	7.3	5.8	1.5
Apple	3.2	2.3	0.9
Banana	1.8	1.1	0.7
Cherry	1.5	0.9	0.6
Dates, dry	8.3	6.9	1.4
Dates, fresh	7.7	6.9	0.8
Fig	5.0	2.6	2.4
Grapes, green	1.2	0.8	0.4
Guava	8.5	7.1	1.4
Jack fruit	3.5	2.1	1.4

Contd.

Table 2.8: Dietary fibre content of foods g/100 g (*Contd.*)

Name of the foodstuff	Total dietary fibre g	Insoluble dietary fibre g	Soluble dietary fibre g
Jambu	3.5	2.6	0.9
Sweet lime	2.7	1.3	1.4
Mango	2.0	1.0	1.0
Musk melon	0.8	0.5	0.3
Watermelon	0.6	0.3	0.3
Orange	1.1	0.6	0.5
Peach	1.6	1.1	0.5
Pear	4.3	4.0	0.3
Pineapple	2.8	2.3	0.5
Plum	2.8	1.7	1.1
Pomegranate	2.8	2.3	0.5
Sapota	10.9	9.1	1.8
Custard apple	5.5	4.0	1.5
Strawberry	2.3	1.6	0.7

Prebiotics, Probiotics and Synbiotics

Prebiotics

Non-digestible food, specifically oligosaccharides [fruto-oligosaccharides (FOS), inulin, lactulose and galacto-oligosaccharides (GOS)], from vegetables, grains and legumes, and also resistant starch, soluble dietary fibres and malabsorbed sugars, stimulate the growth of beneficial intestinal bacteria to improve the gastrointestinal health and immune function.

- Prebiotics may improve the gut microbionta of formula fed infants, reduce the toxicity of colonic contents and impact on lipid metabolism and mineral absorption.
- They boost beneficial bacteria in the gut and increasing SCFA butyrate production.
- During enteral feeding, use of prebiotics and probiotics may help to alleviate diarrhoea.
- Preterm infants fed formula supplemented with oligosaccharides had significantly increased levels of bifidobacteria.

Probiotics

Probiotics are not dietary fibres like prebiotics, for better clarification, probiotics may be described as "A preparation of or a product containing viable, defined micro-organism in sufficient numbers, which alter the microflora (by implantation or colonization) in a compartment of the host and by that exert beneficial health effects in this host" (Schrezenmeir and de Vrese 2001). Examples: Bifidobacteria and lactobacilli.

It is an orally consumed sources of bacteria used to reestablish the presence of beneficial intestinal flora and suppress potential harmful microbes.

Uses

- Probiotics in the form of cultured foods or supplements, has been modestly successful in antibiotic-related diarrhoea, travellers' diarrhoea, acute infections diarrhoea, bacterial overgrowth, and several types of pediatric diarrhoea (Teitelbaum, 2005). Post-operative pouchitis, inflammatory bowel disease, cancer may have a role in immune function.
- Probiotic supplement (*Lactobacillus GG*), has been found to improve gastrointestinal microflora, thus reducing the incidence of atopic march (process of developing any atopic disease) from atopic dermatitis to food allergy and asthma (Giudice et al. 2006).
- It inhibits pathogenic bacteria by production of inhibitory compounds, reduction of pH, competition for nutrients and adhesion sites on the gut wall, modulation of the immune response and the regulation of colonocyte gene expression (Tuohy et al. 2003). By this they provide nutrition for mucosa in the form of short-chain fatty acids and protect the intestinal tight junctions (which link intestinal epithelial cells together).
- Probiotics may play a role in the treatment of allergic disease as they appear to reduce the cytokines involved in IgE production (Kalliomaki et al. 2001).

There are investigation going on to find the evidence for probiotics effect on allergic disease, autism, inflammatory bowel disease, irritable bowel syndrome, pouchitis, on pre-term infants and many more.

Synbiotics

Synbiotics is a combined mixture of probiotic and prebiotic agents that is being tested in clinical settings. At present there are very less research about the character. But their benefits are similar to that of the individual pre-and probiotics like,

- Beneficial role in the pathogenesis of colorectal cancer.
- Modification of blood lipids.
- Facilitate the survival and implantation of live microbial supplements in the gut.
- Selectively stimulate the growth of beneficial bacteria.
- Activate the metabolism of bacteria.

FUNCTIONS OF CARBOHYDRATES

Glucose is the absorbed state of carbohydrates. The metabolism is a dynamic state of balance between burning glucose for energy (catabolism) and using glucose to build other compounds (anabolism). This process is a continuous response to the supply of glucose from food and the demand for glucose for energy needs.

Energy

Glucose is the principal fuel. Substrate for any body tissue. Glucose is burned more efficiently and more completely than either protein or fat. Although muscles use a mixture of fat and glucose for energy, the brain is totally dependent on glucose for energy. When oxidized 1 g of carbohydrates provides 4 kcal.

Protein Sparing

Carbohydrates need to be consumed adequately not only to meet energy but also to spare protein to do its special function. If not, body will oxidise, protein as a source of energy without using it for tissue building.

The function of carbohydrates by giving energy and sparing dietary . protein from being oxidized is called protein sparing action.

Preventing Ketosis

Carbohydrates are also needed to for energy from efficiently and completely oxidize fat. Ketone bodies are the intermediate, acidic compounds formed from the incomplete breakdown of fat when adequate glucose is not available. Ketone bodies are normally produced at a low level during fat oxidation, muscle and other tissues can use this little amount for energy. But, in extreme conditions such as starvation, uncontrolled diabetes, and practising very low-carbohydrate diets, makes fat to metabolize faster than the body can take care of the intermediate products and it starts to accumulate in body. An increased accumulation in the blood stream causes nausea, fatigue, loss of appetite, ketoacidosis. Dehydration and sodium depletion may follow as the body tries to excrete ketones in the urine. Sufficient amount of carbohydrates prevents ketosis under normal conditions.

Central Nervous System (CNS) Function

In CNS regulatory centre, the brain, glucose cannot be stored and supplied. So there should be a constant supply from the blood for proper functioning of the CNS. Sustained hypoglycemic shock may lead to irreversible brain damage.

Glycogen Reserves

After oxidizing for energy and other function excess of glucose is reserved as glycogen by liver and muscle cell, which can quickly release glucose in time of need.

In Muscle

Two-thirds of the body glycogen reserve is in muscle, which is available only for muscular contraction and relaxation. The stored glycogen is broken down to lactic acid while contracting. On recovery, this lactic acid is first oxidized to pyruvic acid and then to acetyl CoA which is then oxidized to CO_2 and H_2O, thus producing energy for muscular work.

In Liver

Typically one-third of the body's glycogen reserve is in the liver and can be released into circulation for all body cells to use.

The rate of oxidation of amino acids in liver is controlled if adequate supplies of carbohydrates are available.

In Gastrointestinal

Lactose (milk sugar) has several functions in the gastrointestinal tract. They are:
- Promoting the growth of desirable bacteria, some of which are useful in the synthesis of B-complex vitamins, enhancing the absorption of calcium.
- Dietary fibre stimulates peristaltic movements of GI track, gives bulk in intestinal contents. Dietary fibre helps in preventing many degenerative diseases.

In Heart Action

Glycogen reserve in cardiac muscle is an important emergency source of energy. Poor glycogen store or low carb intake may cause cardiac symptoms.

In Adipose Tissue

When body is in need of excess energy or when diet lacks in energy, it can be released from the adipose tissue.

Glucose remaining after energy needs are met, glycogen stores are saturated, and other specified compounds are made— is converted by liver cells to triglycerides and stored in adipose tissue. But body always prefers to make body fat from dietary fat, not from carbohydrates.

SYNTHESIS BY CARBOHYDRATES
- Galactose which is not found free in foods, produced by human digestion from lactose.
- The body converts glucose to other essential carbohydrates such as ribose, a component of ribonucleic acid (RNA) and deoxyribonucleic acid (DNA), keratin sulfate (in finger nails), and hyaluronic acid (found in the fluid that lubricates the joints and vitreous humor of the eye ball).
- If an adequate supply of essential amino acids is available, the body can use them and glucose to make nonessential amino acids.

DIGESTION, ABSORPTION AND METABOLISM
Digestion
The process of making the food available to the body is digestion. The digestion of carbohydrate foods are accomplished by two types of actions, mechanically breaking down into smaller particles and chemical breakdown of food nutrients into usable metabolic products (Fig. 2.1).

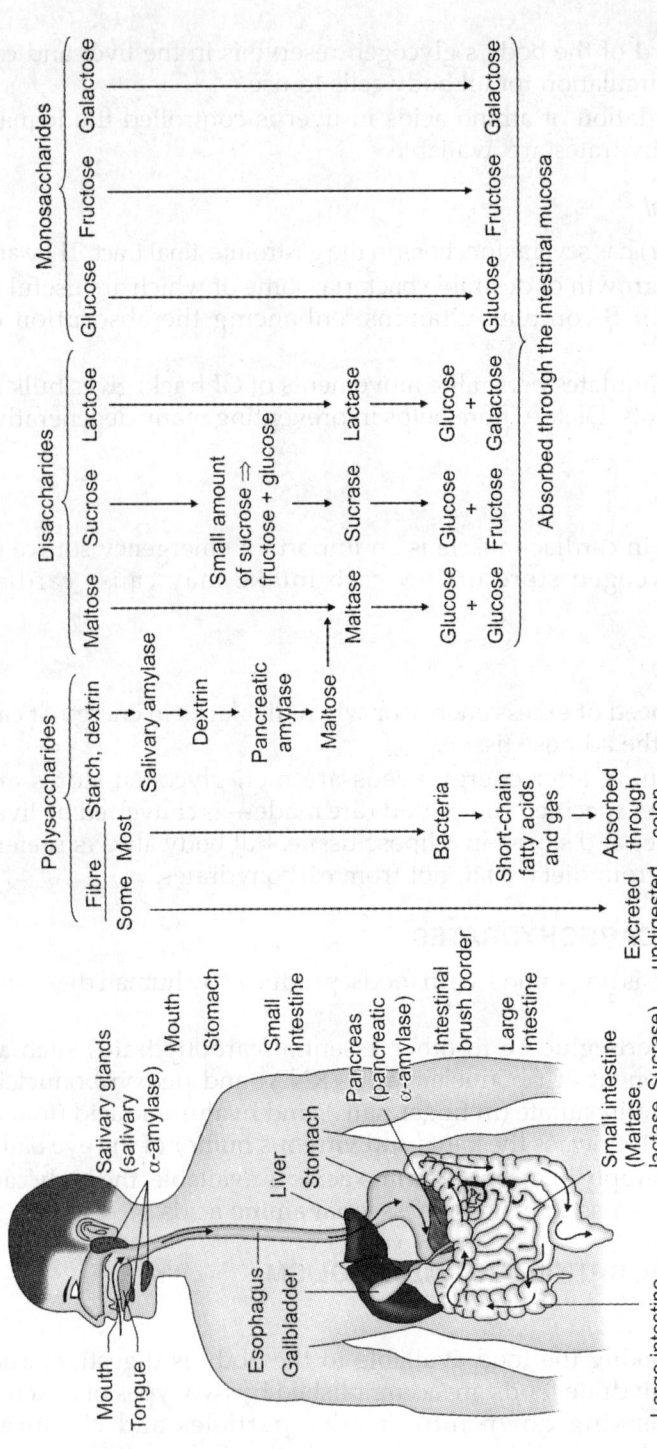

Fig. 2.1: Carbohydrate digestions. Dietary carbohydrates include the polysaccharides complex carbohydrates (fibre, starch, dextrin), the disaccharides (maltose, sucrose, lactose), and the monosaccharides (glucose, fructose, and galactose). Digestion begins in the mouth, where food is chewed into pieces and salivary amylase begins the process of chemical digestion. The stomach churns and mixes the carbohydrate, but stomach acids halt residual action of the salivary amylase. The small intestine is the site of most carbohydrate digestion, and pancreatic amylase reduces complex carbohydrates into disaccharides. Disaccharide enzymes (maltase, sucrase, and lactase) on the surface of the small intestine cells split maltose, sucrose, and lactose into monosaccharides, thus completing the process in the large intestine to yield gas, water, and short-chain fatty acids

In mouth, food particles break into fine parts and mixed with salivary secretion. Starch can be hydrolyzed by salivary amylase (ptyalin) secreted by parotid gland, if starch remains in mouth long enough. Starch, when hydrolyzed, breakdown into dextrins and maltose.

In stomach, there is no specific enzyme present to breakdown the carbohydrate. The hydrochloric acid in the stomach stops the action of salivary amylase. Muscle fibres of the stomach wall continue the mechanical digestestive process, and bring the food mass down to the lower part of the stomach.

In small intestine, chemical digestion of carbohydrate is completed by pancreatic and intestinal enzymes. Pancreatic enzyme (pancreatic amylase) breaks down the starch to dextrins and maltose. With intestinal enzymes, sucrase, lactase and maltase act on their respective disaccharides. Glycosidases break down dextrins, and the enzyme maltase, lactase and sucrase convert the disaccharides into their constituent monosaccharides (glucose, galactose and fructose).

The rate of digestion of starch varies with its physical structure and process (Fig. 2.2).

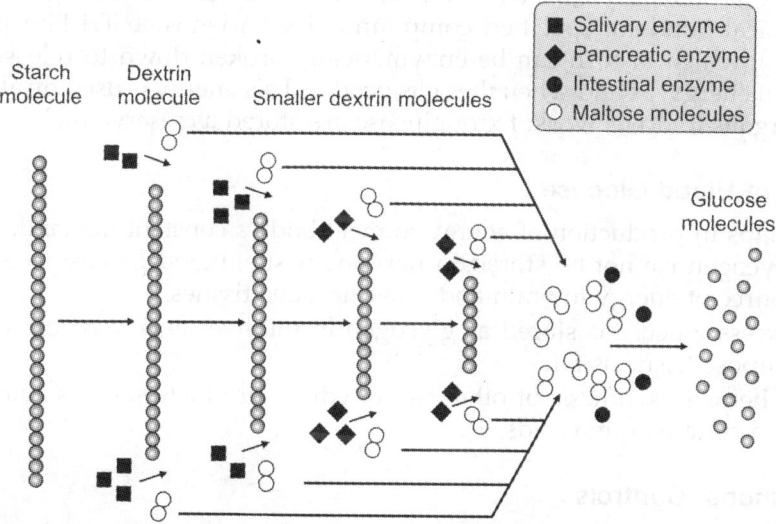

Fig. 2.2: The gradual breakdown of large starch molecules into glucose by digestion enzymes

- Starch processed into small fine particles, cooked long time in presence of water leads to extensive gelatinization and dispersion of starch granules and result in rapid digestion, e.g. baking the flour into bread.
- In cases like, starch in discrete structures is digested relatively slow, giving a modest glycemic index and may be excreted in the faeces, e.g. raw starch from cereals, banana, potato, food cooked with less water.

Absorption

These monosaccharaides are transported via the portal vein to the liver, where the galactose and fructose are removed and converted to other metabolites. Most of the glucose is transported via the blood directly to the peripheral tissues for use as a fuel source.

Glucose moves along with the sodium (Na^+) and is released inside the cell. The absorption of glucose is affected by the amount of Na^+ ions in the intestinal lumen. A high Na^+ facilitates glucose influx, whereas a low Na^+ inhibits influx. This is because glucose and sodium share the same cotransporter carrier protein. Glucose transport mechanism also transports galactose. Fructose is independent of Na^+ in transport and absorption. The rate of absorption is almost equal for glucose and galactose, but fructose is absorbed about half as rapidly.

Metabolism

The process, making the absorbed nutrients made available for the energy. The final end product of carbohydrates is glucose. Glucose is burned to produce energy through chemical reactions involving cell enzymes. This yields carbon dioxide, water and heat, which is captured in the high energy chemical bonds of specified compounds like Adenosine Tri Phosphate (ATP), which in turn can be enzymatically broken down to release the useful energy, as and when the cells need it. This energy is used by almost all organs to do its work. Extra glucose are stored as reserve fuel.

Use of Blood Glucose

- Helps in production of energy to meet body's constant demand. Since glycogen cannot be stored in nervous tissue, blood glucose acts as a source of energy to brain and other nervous tissues.
- Excess glucose is stored as glycogen in the liver and muscles, and in adipose tissue as fat.
- It helps in synthesis of other carbohydrate products such as galactose and certain amino acids.

Hormonal Controls

When carbohydrate is consumed, the release of hormones such as gastric inhibitory peptide (GIP) from endocrine cells in the gastrointestinal tract prime the body to expect or rise in blood glucose concentration.

Blood Sugar-lowering Hormone

The fasting blood glucose level is between 80 and 100 mg/dl of blood. After eating a meal, containing carbohydrates, blood glucose level normally rises from 130 to 140 mg/dl at 1 hour, but returns to fasting level 2 hours after the meal.

Insulin is the hormone, produced by β-cells of the islets of langerhans in the pancreas, regulates blood sugar through several actions: *Glycogensis* stimulates the conversion of glucose to glycogen in liver for constant energy reserve; *lipoprotein* stimulates conversion of glucose to fat for storage in adipose tissue; and *cell permeability* to glucose is increased, allowing it to pass into the cells for oxidation to supply needed energy.

Blood Sugar-raising Hormones

If the blood glucose levels fall to 30–50 mg/dl, then body is said to be hypoglycemic condition. A number of hormones effectively raise blood sugar levels:

* *Glucagon:* It is produced by α-cells of the islets of langerhans. It increases the breakdown of liver glycogen to glucose and maintaining blood glucose during fasting.

* *Epinephrine:* It is secreted by the chromaffin cells of the adrenal medulla. The liver and muscle glycogen breakdown occur to yield blood glucose and decreases the release of insulin. This happens during anger, fear or stress.

* *Glucocorticoids* (Steroid hormones): It is produced by adrenal cortex which reduces glucose utilization and also increases the rate at which protein is converted into glucose and act as insulin antagonists.

* *Thyroxine:* Released from thyroid gland, it influences the rate of insulin breakdown, increases glucose absorption from the intestine and enhances the action of epinephrine.

* *Growth hormone:* Released from anterior pituitary gland, this raises blood glucose level by protein synthesis and increasing the fat mobilization.

Carbohydrate Requirement

The recommended dietary allowance (RDA) for carbohydrate is not known, but 50–70 g/day may help to prevent ketosis. The acceptable distribution range for carbohydrates is that total carbohydrate should comprise about 50% energy intake (excluding any contribution from alcohol) and non-milk extrinsic sugars should not exceed 11% energy intake.

More than the percentages, it is all about the quality of carbohydrates. It is always recommended to eat a diet bas]ed on whole grains, cereals, with plenty of fruits, vegetables, and dried peas and beans, mainly unprocessed foods to avoid complications such as cardiovascular disease, obesity, dental caries, constipation, diverticular disease, type 2 diabetes, and breast and colon cancers.

Sources

The sources of different carbohydrates are given in Table 2.9.

Table 2.9: Sources of carbohydrates

Carbohydrate	Sources
Free Sugars	
Monosaccharides	
Glucose	Fruits, honey
Fructose	Fruits, honey
Galactose	Milk
Xylose	Fruits, vegetables, cereals
Disaccharides	
Sucrose	Cane and beet sugars, molasses
Lactose	Milk and milk products
Maltose	Malt products
Trehalose	Mushrooms
Sugar alcohols	
Sorbitol	Cherries
Xylitol	Fruits and vegetables
Sugar acids	
D-galacturonic acid	Pectin
Short chain carbohydrates	
Raffinose	Sugar beets, kidney beans, lentils and navy beans
Stachyose	Beans
Polysaccharides	
Digestible	
Rapidly digestible starch	Processed foods
Slowly digestible starch	Legumes, pasta
Resistant Starch	
Physically inaccessible	Whole grains
Resistant granules	Unripe banana
Retrograded amylose	Cooked starches
Indigestible	
Cellulose	Bran, whole wheat flour
Hemicellulose	Stalks and leaves of vegetables, outer covering of seeds

3   Protein

INTRODUCTION

Protein, a class of energy-yielding nutrients, is composed of individual building blocks known as amino acids. Amino acids are organic compounds made of carbon, hydrogen and oxygen atoms plus a nitrogen component, which distinguishes them from the other energy nutrients.

Proteins are neezded for the building blocks of the body, managing metabolism and organ function. Amino acids are versatile nutrients acting as precursors for protein synthesis and forming a wide range of other important metabolites.

Structure

Proteins are comprised of building block called amino acids. Every amino acid contains a central carbon atom, to which amino attached a carboxyl group (COOH), nitrogen containing amino group (NH_2), hydrogen atom and another group or side chain R specific to the particular amino acid. The general formula for an amino acid is

$$COOH - \overset{\overset{\text{H}}{|}}{\underset{\underset{\text{R}}{|}}{C}} - NH_2$$

During protein synthesis, amino acids become linked together through the amino group of one reacting with the carboxylic acid group of another to form a peptide bond. This allows the formation of polypeptides, which are chains of 50 or many amino acids, and one or more of these polypeptides comprise individual proteins.

Another consideration in protein structure is the shape. Amino acids may form proteins that are straight, folded, or coiled along one dimension or they may take on a three-dimensional shape as spheres or globes, even larger proteins are assembled when two or more three-dimensional polypeptides combine. A protein's shape determines its function. The sequence of the amino acids determines the ultimate structure and function of the protein and is determined by the genetic code stored in the cell nucleus as deoxyribonucleic acid (DNA).

In a solution at pH 7, all amino acids are *zwitterions*; that is, the amino group and carboxyl groups are both ionized and exist as COO^- and NH_3^+, respectively. Therefore, amino acids are *amphoteric*, can behave as an acid or as a base in water depending on the pH. When acting as an acid or proton donor, the positively charged amino group donates a hydrogen ion, and when acting as a base, the negatively charged carboxyl group gains a hydrogen ion, as follows:

Acid:

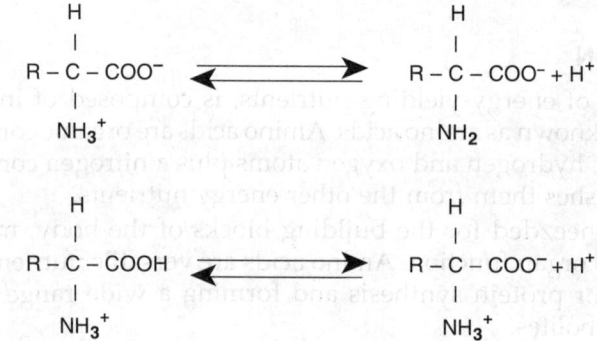

Base:

Occurrence in Body

- *Body structure and framework:* Almost 50% of protein in the body is found in skeletal muscle, 20% in bone, 10% in the skin and the blood.

- *Enzymes:* Enzymes are proteins that facilitate specific chemical reactions in the body without undergoing changes in themselves. Some enzymes break down larger molecules into smaller ones (e.g. digestive enzymes); others combine molecules to form larger compounds (e.g. enzymes involved in protein synthesis in which amino acids are combined).

- *Other body secretions and fluids:* Hormones (e.g. insulin, thyroxine, epinephrine), neurotransmitters (e.g. serotonin, acetylcholine) and antibodies are all made of amino acids.

- *Fluid and electrolyte balance:* Proteins help to regulate fluid balance because they attract water, thereby creating osmotic pressure. Circulating proteins, such as albumin, maintain the proper balance of fluid among the intravascular (within veins and arteries), intracellular (within the cells) and interstitial (in the fluid between the cells) compartments of the body.

- *Acid-base balance:* Amino acids are amphoteric in nature. This ability to buffer or neutralize excess acids and bases enables proteins to maintain normal blood pH, which protects body proteins from being denatured.

- *Transport molecules:* Globular proteins transport other substances through the blood. For instance, lipoproteins transport fats, cholesterol and fat-soluble vitamins; haemoglobin transports oxygen; and albumin transports free fatty acids and many drugs.

- *Other compounds*: Amino acids are components of numerous body compounds such as opsin, the light-sensitive visual pigment in the eye and thrombin, a protein necessary for normal blood clotting.
- *Fueling the body*. Like carbohydrates, protein provides 4 kcal/g. Although it is not the body's preferred fuel, protein is a source of energy when it is consumed in excess of need or when calorie intake from carbohydrates and fat is inadequate.

NUTRITIONAL CLASSIFICATIONS OF AMINO ACIDS

Protein comprises 21 unique amino acids. These include 10 nutritionally essential (indispensable) amino acids, 5 non-essential (dispensable) amino acids, 6 conditionally essential (indispensable) amino acids.

Essential Amino Acids

Amino acids which cannot be synthesized by the body and can be achieved only through diet are termed essential amino acids.

Synthesis of proteins requires the presence of all necessary amino acids during the process. Essential amino acids have carbon skeletons that human cannot make (or cannot make enough) and can obtain only from the diet. Many amino acids can be synthesized from carbon skeletons produced as intermediates in the major metabolic pathways by a process called transamination, which adds an amino group from amino acid without actually producing a free amino group.

Non-essential Amino Acids

These can be readily synthesized by the body from other carbon and nitrogen containing precursors. Transamination is the important process which allows essential amino acids to produce non-essential amino acids.

Conditionally Essential Amino Acids

Amino acids which are required in the diet under certain circumstances. In the conditions where the precursors are not available for synthesis of amino acids, e.g. a healthy new born baby may not have precursors to synthesise glycine and arginine. In conditions like intestinal metabolic dysfunction, arginine cannot be synthesized. Glutamine, arginine, proline, cysteine are examples where their need is conditionally essential in critically ill people (Table 3.1).

Functions of Protein

Protein is responsible for the structure, functions and metabolism within the body. There should be adequate availability of all types of amino acids to do its function. It includes building muscles, maintain and repair tissues, cell division, structural matrix within bones and teeth, enzymes for

Table 3.1: Classification of amino acid

Requirement	Amino acid	Chemical features
Essential (indispensable)	Isoleucine	Branched-chain amino acid.
	Leucine	Branched-chain amino acid.
	Valine	Branched-chain amino acid.
	Lysine	6-carbon chain, with basic properties.
	Methionine	4-carbon chain, containing sulphur.
	Phenylalanine	3-carbon chain with benzene ring.
	Threonine	4-carbon chain
	Tryptophan	Contains benzene ring.
	Histidine	Has an imidazole side-chain necessary for many catalytic reactions.
	Selenocysteine	A selenium-containing amino acid.
Conditionally essential (indispensable)	Arginine*	Similar in structure to lysine.
	cysteine	A sulphur-containing amino acid synthesised from the essential amino acid methionine.
	Glycine	The simplest amino acid in structure
	Proline	Contains an imino group.
	Tyrosine	Can be made from phenylalanine.
non-essential (dispensable)	Alanine	Non-polar, hydrophobic.
	Aspartic acid	Also exists in an amide form as asparagine+.
	Asparagine	Amide form of aspartate+.
	Glutamic acid	Also exists in an amide form as glutamine+.
	Glutamine	Amide form of glutamate.
	Serine	A hydroxyamino acid.

*An essential amino acid in infants.
+May be conditionally essential in critically ill people.

digestion, precursor for vitamin, regulate muscle contraction, transporting nutrients such as retinol, lipids, copper and zinc, regulating water balance, serve as buffer and maintain the pH.

- *Enzymatic function:* All enzymes are proteins. Enzymes which are all responsible for digestion are protein. These enzymes break down food into its constituent nutrients in the gastrointestinal tract; cellular enzymes catalyse and regulate metabolic processes.
- *Transport function:* Proteins act as carriers in blood and body fluids for many nutrients and other molecules, e.g. retinol is transported by retinol binding protein, metallothione transports copper and zinc, lipoproteins transport lipids and haemoglobin.

Proteins also act as carriers across cell membranes and help to regulate and channel the movement of nutrients and metabolites between the intracellular and extracellular compartments.

- *Hormonal function:* Hormones such as insulin, gastrin and growth hormone are proteins.
- *Immune function:* To fight against antigen the body produces antibodies. Antibodies are proteins synthesized by lymphocytes as part of the immune response.
- *Buffering function:* Protein such as albumin in blood helps to maintain acid-base by accepting and releasing hydrogen ions when necessary. Protein can also act as the source of energy at the rate of 4 kcal/g. when the diet is low in carbohydrate or an individual is starving, protein is the only good source of glucose obtained by gluconeogenesis process.

DIGESTION-ABSORPTION-METABOLISM

Digestion

Chemical digestion of proteins beings in the stomach. In stomach, pepsin transforms denatured protein into proteoses and then peptones, which are large polypeptide derivatives. Hydrochloric acid denatures protein to make the peptide bonds more available to the actions of enzymes. Rennin (present only in infancy and childhood) is important in the infant's digestion of milk. In the presence of Ca^{++}, rennin changes the casein of milk irreversibly to a paracasein which is then acted on by pepsin. By coagulating milk, rennin prevents the rapid passage of milk from the stomach.

In small intestine, majority of protein digestion occurs with the help of enzymes produced by pancreas. Trypsin acts on protein and large polypeptide fragments carried over from the stomach, producing smaller polypeptides and dipeptides. Chymotrypsin continues the same protein splitting action of trypsin. Carboxypeptidase makes smaller peptides and some free amino acids. Therefore, pancreatic proteases reduce polypeptides to shorter chains, tripeptides, dipeptides and amino acids.

Enzymes located on the surface of the cells that line the small intestine complete the digestion. They are amino peptidase which splits amino acids from the amino ends of short peptides and dipeptidase which reduces dipeptides to amino acids (Table 3.2) (Fig. 3.1).

Absorption

Amino acids, are absorbed through the mucosa of the small intestine by an energy-dependent active transport, using pyridoxine (vitamin B) as a carrier, into the blood circulation for transport to the liver via the portal vein.

Metabolism

The liver retains amino acids to make liver cells, non-essential amino acids and plasma proteins such as heparin, prothrombin and albumin. The liver regulates the release of amino acids into the blood stream and removes

Table 3.2: Summary of protein digestion

Organ	Inactive precursor	Activator	Active enzyme	Digestive action
Mouth			None	Mechanical only
Stomach (acid)	Pepsinogen	Hydrochloric acid	Pepsin	Protein→polypeptides
			Rennin (infants) (calcium necessary for activity)	Casein→coagulated curd
Intestine (alkaline)	Trypsinogen	Enterokinase	Trypsin	Protein, polypeptides →polypeptides, dipeptides
Pancreas	Chymotrypsinogen	Active trypsin	Czhymotrypsin	Protein, polypeptides →polypeptides, dipeptides
			Carboxypeptidase	Polypeptides →simpler peptides, dipeptides, amino acids
Intestine			Aminopeptidase	Polypeptides→peptides, dipeptides, amino acids
			Dipeptidase	Dipeptides→amino acids

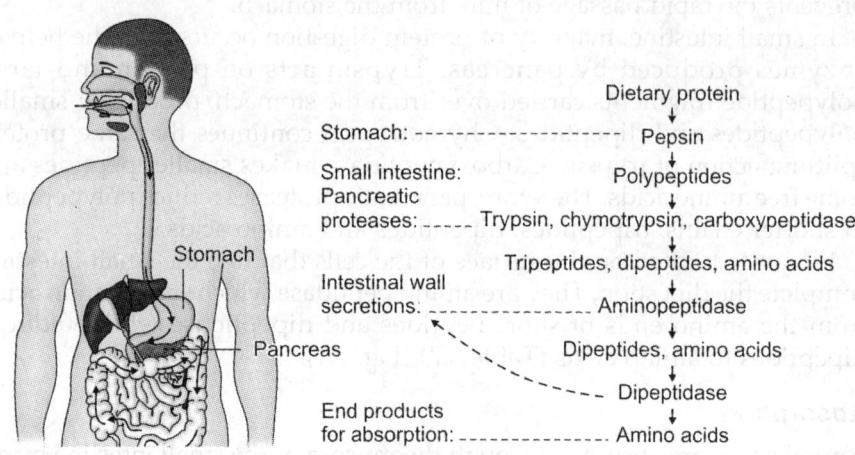

Dietary protein
↓
Stomach: -------------------- Pepsin
↓
Small intestine: Polypeptides
Pancreatic
proteases: _____ Trypsin, chymotrypsin, carboxypeptidase
↓
Tripeptides, dipeptides, amino acids
Intestinal wall
secretions: _____ Aminopeptidase
↓
Dipeptides, amino acids
↓
Dipeptidase
↓
End products
for absorption: _____ Amino acids

Fig. 3.1: Protein digestion

excess amino acids from the circulation. The liver removes the nitrogen from amino acids so that they can be burned for energy and it converts amino acids to glucose or fat as appropriate.

Protein Synthesis

Amino acids are used by all body cells to synthesise proteins that are either lost during normal wear and tear, needed to build new tissue during pregnancy or adolescent growth. Protein syntheses are related to metabolic pool, nitrogen balance, and protein turnover.

- *Metabolic pool*: Body will not store excess amino acids for later use. However, a limited supply of free amino acids exists within cells in a metabolic pool, which accepts and donates amino acids as needed. Amino acids derived from tissue breakdown and amino acids from dietary protein both contribute to a common collective metabolic "pool" of amino acids throughout the body available for use. A balance of amino acids is thus maintained to supply the body's constant needs. From this reserve pool, specific amino acids are supplied to synthesise specific body proteins.
- *Nitrogen balance*: Nitrogen balance is determined by comparing the rate of protein synthesis to protein breakdown. Positive nitrogen balance is when protein synthesis exceeds protein breakdown. Negative nitrogen balance is an undesirable state that occurs when protein breakdown exceeds protein synthesis, as occurs in conditions like long-term illness, a hypermetabolic wasting disease or starvation.
- *Protein turnover*: The constant breakdown and synthesis of endogenous protein is termed protein turnover. The rate of protein turnover varies in different tissues. It is the highest in the intestinal mucosa, liver, pancreas, kidney and plasma. It is lower in muscle, brain and skin. It is much slower in structural tissues, such as collagen and bone.

RECOMMENDED DIETARY ALLOWANCES

Table 3.3: ICMR recommended dietary allowances of proteins

Group	Protein g/day
Man	60
Woman	50
Pregnant woman	50 + 15
Lactation	
0–6 months	50 + 25
6–12 months	50 + 18
Infancy	
0–6 months	2.05/kg
6–12 months	1.65/kg
Children	
1–3 years	22
4–6 years	30
7–9 years	41

Contd.

Table 3.3: ICMR recommended dietary allowances of proteins (*Contd.*)

Group	Protein g/day
Boys	
10–12 years	54
13–15 years	70
16–18 years	78
Girls	
10–12 years	57
13–15 years	65
16–18 years	63

Estimation of Protein Requirement

Normally, nitrogen derived from amino acids, the catabolic product of proteins, is excreted in the urine and feces and lost from the skin. Unlike the energy that is retained and stored in triglyceride and glycogen, proteins and amino acids are not stored in the body. Therefore, protein or nitrogen requirements are often estimated by calculating nitrogen losses on a daily rather than a weekly basis. When excess protein is ingested, the amino acids not needed for new protein synthesis are transaminated so that the non-nitrogenous portion of the molecule can be used as a calorie source, for example, in pyruvate derived from alanine. The nitrogen that is not needed is converted to urea and excreted in the urine.

Urinary losses of nitrogen urea account for more than 80% of urinary nitrogen. Creatinine, porphyrins, and other nitrogen-containing compounds account for the remaining nitrogen.

Urinary nitrogen loss = [urea N_{urine}(mg/dL) × daily urine volume (dL)] ÷ 0.8

Urinary nitrogen excretion is related to the BMR. The larger the muscle mass in the body, the greater is the number of calories needed to maintain it. Also the rate of transamination is greater as amino acids and carbohydrates are interconverted to fulfill the energy needed in the muscle. Between 1 and 1.3 mg of urinary nitrogen is excreted for each kilocalorie required for basal metabolism. Nitrogen excretion also increases during exercise and heavy work.

Faecal and skin losses account for a relatively constant proportion of nitrogen loss from the body in normal conditions, but these may vary widely in disease states. Thus, measurement of urinary nitrogen loss alone may not provide a reliable prediction of the daily nitrogen requirement when it is most needed. Faecal losses are a consequence of the inefficient digestion and absorption of protein (93% efficiency). In addition, the intestinal tract secretes proteins into the lumen from saliva, gastric juice, bile, pancreatic enzymes, and enterocyte sloughing. These sources contribute, respectively, about 3, 5, 1, 8, and 50 g of protein daily to the total protein secreted into the intestinal lumen.

Total nitrogen (N) losses include those from urine, faeces, and skin. Faecal nitrogen averages 1 to 2 g per day in the absence of diarrhea. Skin losses average 0.3 g per day. The total faecal and skin losses can be estimated at about 2 g per day.

$$\text{Total N loss (g/day)} = N_{urine} + N_{stool} + N_{skin} \approx N_{urine} + 2$$

When faecal losses are measured, an estimated nitrogen loss of 1 g/day is used to cover losses in skin and other compartments.

Normal daily protein requirement is based on estimates of N loss and requirement (weight and extra requirement for growth and pregnancy). Obligatory losses of nitrogen are not altered by differences in age or sex, and urinary losses of nitrogen are proportional to body size and weight.

Women have a lower N requirement than men per kilogram of body weight, but they have a higher per cent of fat mass (28%) compared to men (15%). There is no difference in protein requirements by gender when corrected for lean body mass.

Protein requirement are the highest during infancy and adolescence. However, total body protein is the lowest in infancy, and obligatory losses are the greatest, so that protein deficiency is most common in infancy.

Calorie Requirement for Protein

Nitrogen ingested as amino acids without other sources of energy is not efficiently incorporated into protein because the energy consumed in heat loss during metabolism (thermal effect) is especially high for protein. Moreover, the incorporation of amino acids into peptides requires three high-energy phosphate bonds, so that 10 kcal is used for each molecule derived from the hydrolysis of ATP. Any excess of dietary energy over basic needs improves the efficiency of dietary nitrogen utilization. To achieve a positive nitrogen balance when protein intake is barely adequate, a positive energy balance of about 2 kcal/kg/day is required. In other words, when energy intake is limited, protein balance is negative, even when protein intake seems adequate but is not excessive. The exact amount of extra calories required to produce a positive nitrogen balance depends on a large number of factors, including body energy stores, body protein mass, and the ratio of energy to protein sources in the food. To ensure positive nitrogen balance in the depleted patient, it is advisable to provide an amount of calories near the estimated energy requirement. Excessive calories may not lead to improvement in meaningful lean body mass.

A safe ratio (protein energy to total energy) that avoid protein-calorie malnutrition in children seems to be 1 : 20, that is, for every kilocalorie provided by protein, 19 kcal of nonprotein energy is needed to prevent protein-calorie malnutrition in children. Each gram of protein produces 4 kcal of energy, so 4 × 19 or 76 kcal of non-protein energy is needed per gram of protein during the period of intense growth in children. When protein is present in excess of needs, even when non-protein calories are limited, some of the protein is converted to energy that can be metabolized, and the 1 : 20 ratio is not required.

Nitrogen Protein Requirement

Protein requirements are determined by measuring the amount of protein needed to maintain nitrogen equilibrium and to provide for any additional needs of growth, pregnancy and lactation. Protein is the only macronutrient that contains nitrogen. Approximately 16% of protein is nitrogen, so 1 g of nitrogen is equivalent to 6.25 g of protein.

Nutrition support should aim to keep the body in nitrogen balance, i.e. when nitrogen intake is equal to nitrogen loss from faeces, skin, urine and other losses (e.g. burns exudate, surgical drains). Where nitrogen balance is not achievable, nitrogen loss should be minimized.

Nitrogen/protein requirements can be assessed in a number of ways, estimating protein requirement by measuring nitrogen losses from the body.

A more precise estimate of nitrogen needs can be obtained by measuring daily nitrogen losses from the body via urine, faeces, fistulae, drains or burn exudates, although in practice this is difficult to achieve. Nitrogen losses from faeces and exudates are particularly difficult to measure. Fistulae content can be sent for analysis if volumes are significant enough to cause concern.

Urinary nitrogen excretion can be estimated by measuring urinary urea nitrogen (UUN) excretion from a 24-hour urine sample. Urea is a by-product of protein metabolism and measurement of urinary urea nitrogen can give an indication of nitrogen losses. Approximately 80% of total urinary nitrogen is urea nitrogen, the remaining 20% nitrogen comprising urinary creatinine, creatine, low molecular weight amino acids and other compounds.

Nitrogen excretion in grams is approximately equal to:

$$\text{g urinary urea excreted in 24 hours} \times \frac{28^{*}}{60} \times \frac{6^{\dagger}}{5}$$

*The molecular weight of urea is 60, of which 28 parts are nitrogen.
†Assume that 80% of the total urinary nitrogen is urea.

For practical purposes, this formula can be condensed to:

$$\text{nitrogen excretion (g)} = \frac{\text{mmol urinary urea per 24 hours}}{30}$$

or

$$\text{g protein lost per 24 hours} = \frac{\text{mmol urinary urea excreted in 24 hours}}{5}$$

Problems associated with urinary urea measurement

The following should be borne in mind:

- Urea production is influenced by liver failure, sepsis, starvation or stress, hence urinary urea is an insensitive and unreliable measure of nitrogen loss in clinically unstable patients.
- The ratio of total urea nitrogen to urinary urea nitrogen is not constant, varying with the degree of stress, course of an illness or different disease states (Konstantinides *et al.* 1991). In such circumstances, urinary urea nitrogen can represent between 10 and 90% of urinary nitrogen losses. Measurement of total urinary nitrogen is therefore a superior method but is technically difficult and beyond the resources of most hospital biochemistry departments.
- Nitrogen requiements are difficult to assess in renal failure, as urine production may be variable or absent. The following equation can be used for anuric patients and estimates the rate of urea nitrogen production form changes in serum urea concentrations:

$$\text{g urea nitrogen/day} = [(\text{urea } 2 - \text{urea } 1) \times (\text{wt} \times 0.6)$$

$$+ (\text{wt gain} \times \text{urea } 2)] \times 0.028$$

where urea 1 = serum urea at the start of period (mmol/l), urea 2 = serum urea at the end of period (mmol/l), 0.6 = factor to estimate total body water and wt = weight in kg.

Protein Quality

The nutritional value or quality of dietary proteins reflects both their ease of digestion (digestibility) and their amino acid content relative to that of the demand (biological value).

In animal source digestibility is generally high, whereas in plant protein, tough plant cell wall in some cereals or through anti-nutritional factors in legumes, limit the availability.

$$\text{Biological value} = \frac{\text{Nitrogen digested} - \text{Nitrogen lost in metabolism}}{\text{Nitrogen digested}} \times 100$$

$$= \frac{I - (F - F_m) - (U - U_e)}{I - (F - F_m)} \times 100$$

Where, I, F, U are dietary, faecal and urinary nitrogen on the test diet F_m and U_e are faecal and urinary nitrogen on a protein free diet respectively.

PROTEIN DEFICIENCY AND DEPLETION

Protein deficiency is defined as an inadequate protein intake, whereas protein depletion means insufficient body protein, i.e. thinness. Protein depletion (wasting) occurs, when the body demand for energy and to recover from disease is met by breaking down protein, removing the nitrogen from the amino acids and oxidizing the carbon skeleton in much the same way as those derived from glucose and fat. Inadequate intake of energy and several other nutrients such as zinc and vitamin B may also lead to protein depletion.

Protein deficiencies occur with diet in which only protein was inadequate. It leads to muscle-wasting and growth retardation and mental impairment in children. Protein-energy malnutrition (PEM) is the medical term for severe protein deficiency. Severe PEM is often associated with AIDS, tuberculosis, anorexia nervosa and cancer cachexia.

Protein depletion (wasting) is most likely to occur as a result of:

• If energy requirement is not met, resulting in use of dietary and tissue protein as an energy source.

• The catabolic response to trauma such as burns, surgery, injury or sepsis when breakdown of body protein exceeds the body's ability to replace it, resulting in the period of negative nitrogen balance.

• Failure to absorb or utilize dietary protein as a result of gastrointestinal disorders or liver disease.

• Excessive protein loss from body due to renal disease, haemorrhage or exudative losses.

Long-term depletion of protein can result in:

• Stunted growth in children.

• Increased susceptibility to infection.

• Poor wound healing.

• Anaemia.

Protein Surplus

Surplus protein cannot be stored or used by the body and it offers no benefits. Excess protein impairs renal function. The dietary protein content of many low-carbohydrate weight-management diets can be high. With such diets, the removal of most carbohydrate results in a high-protein, high-fat diet comparable to the traditional diets of carnivorous societies such as the Inuit. The long-term safety of such diets has not been evaluated, especially during weight maintenance. It is the case that high-protein, low-carbohydrate diets induce weight loss mainly through their satiating effect, so that the energy of the excluded carbohydrate is not completely replaced by increased protein or fat. This means that actual protein intakes may not be very different from normal diets. Nevertheless, if such diets are unbalanced, with insufficient alkali from fruits and vegetables to balance the acid derived from protein oxidation, there would be an increased risk for bone health. Clearly, there would also be other concerns associated with any exclusion of important food groups and increased intakes of saturated fat.

4

Lipids

Christie defines lipids (fat) as "a wide variety of natural products including fatty acids and their derivatives, steroids, terpenes, carotenoids and bile acids, which have in common a ready solubility in organic solvents such as diethyl ether, hexane, benzene, chloroform or methanol".

Fats and fatty acids have essential structural, storage and metabolic functions within the body. Lipids, a group of water insoluble, energy-yielding organic compounds composed of carbon, hydrogen and oxygen atoms.

LIPIDS CLASSIFICATION

Classification of lipids structures is possible based on physical properties at a room temperature (oils are liquid and fats are solid)—polarity (polar and neutral lipids), essentiality for humans (essential and non-essential fatty acids), or structure (simple or complex). A classification based on structure is preferable. Based on structure, lipids can be classified as derived, simple or complex.

The derived lipids include fatty acids and alcohols, which are the building blocks for the simple and complex lipids.

Simple lipids composed of fatty acids, and alcohol components, include acylglycerols, ether acylglycerols, sterols and their esters and wax (esters of fatty acid with high molecular weight alcohols). In general, simple lipids can be hydrolyzed to two different components, usually an alcohol and an acid.

Complex Lipids

Phospholipids

It is a compound of phosphoric acid, fatty acids, and a nitrogenous base. Glycerophospholipids (e.g. lecithins, cephalins, plasmologens), Glycosphingolipids (e.g. sphingomyelins).

Glycolipids

Compounds of fatty acids, monosaccharides, and a nitrogenous base (e.g. cerebrosides, gangliosides, ceramide).

Lipoproteins

Lipoproteins are globular, high molecular weight particles that are complex aggregates of lipid and protein molecules. A lipoprotein consists of a hydrophobic core, which mainly contains triacylglycerols and cholesterylesters and a polar, hydrophilic coat composed of phospholipids, unesterified cholesterol, and specific apolipoproteins. In this way, the hydrophobic core is protected from the watery surrounding, and transport of large amounts of cholesterol and triglycerols through the blood vessel is possible.

Lipoproteins are classified as five major classes. Chylomicrons, VLDL (very low density lipoproteins), IDLS (intermediate-density lipoproteins), LDL (low-density lipoproteins), HDL (high-density lipoproteins).

DIETARY FAT

Fatty Acids

Saturated Fatty Acids (SFA)

All carbon binding sites not liked to another carbon are linked to hydrogen and are therefore saturated. The saturated fatty acids begin with methanoic (formic) acid. Methanoic, ethanoic, and propanoic acids are uncommon in natural fats. However, they are found nonesterified in many food products, e.g. meat fat, lard, chocolate, milk, butter, cheese and cream. Foods of plant origin generally have a much lower content of SFA, although there are some exceptions, such as coconut and palm oil. Manufactured margarines and fat spread derived from plant oils also contain significant amount of SFA.

Saturated Fats

- Are solid at room temperature
- Are stable, less likely to become rancid than unsaturated fat.
- It raises the LDL-cholesterol, by regulating low-density lipoprotein (LDL) receptors and reduces the rate of LDL removal from the circulation. Hence, it enhances the risk of atherogenesis and cardiovascular disease.

Unsaturated Fatty Acid

Fatty acids that are not completely saturated with hydrogen atoms, so one or more double bonds form between the carbon atoms.

Unsaturated Fats

- Are soft or liquid at room temperature, e.g. oils and soft margarines
- Are susceptible to rancidity
- Include monounsaturated fatty acids (MUFA), which are the highest in canola, olive and peanut oils
- Include polyunsaturated fatty acids (PUFA), which are

- Omega-6 polyunsaturated oil, which are high percentage plant oil such as sunflower, safflower, corn, soya bean and cottonseed oils.
- Omega-3 polyunsaturated, found in fish oils and also in some plant oils such as canola oil, flaxseeds, walnut and hazelnuts.

Monounsaturated Fatty Acids (MUFA)

- It contains only one double bond.
- Liquid at room temperature.
- The most common MUFA is oleic acid (18 : 1 ω_9) which is the principal acid in olive oil.
- When substituted for SFA, MUFA are most beneficial fatty acid. It lowers low-density lipoprotein (LDL) cholesterol level and possesses less risk of lipid peroxidation.

Polyunsaturated Fatty Acids (PUFA)

- Contain two or more double bounds.
- Liquid at room temperature.
- Susceptible to oxidation.
- PUFA are divided into two types, omega-6 (ω_6) and omega-3 (ω_3) (Fig. 4.1).
- Linoleic acid (ω_6) and α-linolenic acid (ω_3), are termed essential fatty acids (EFA), since it cannot be synthesized in our body, therefore requires a dietary source.

ω_6 Polyunsaturated Fatty Acids

- Linoleic acid (ω_6) is the most common polyunsaturated fatty acid in food and is especially abundant in vegetable oil, nuts, seeds, leafy vegetables, whole grains and poultry fat.
- Derivatives of linoleic acid include arachidonic acid (20 : 4 ω_6) and γ-linolenic acid (18 : 3 ω_6) via omega-6 pathway (Fig. 4.1).

The most common of the omega 6 fatty acids in our diets is 18 : 2 ω_6. Often considered the parent of the ω_6 family, 18 : 2 ω_6 is first desaturated to 18 : 3 ω_6. The rate of this first desaturation is thought to be limiting in premature infants, in the elderly, and under certain disease states. Thus, a great deal of interest has been placed in the few oils that contain 18 : 3 ω_6, γ-linolenic acid (GLA). GLA is elongated to 20 : 3 ω_6, dihomo-γ-linolenic acid (DHGLA). DHGLA is the precursor molecule to the 1 series prostaglandins. DHGLA is further desaturated to 22 : 4 ω_6, precursor to the 2 series of prostaglandin. Sign of ω_6 fatty acid deficiency include decreased growth, increased epidermal water loss, impaired wound healing, and impaired reproduction.

- Arachidonic acid is the major component of cell structure and an important regulator of prostaglandin and leukotriene production.

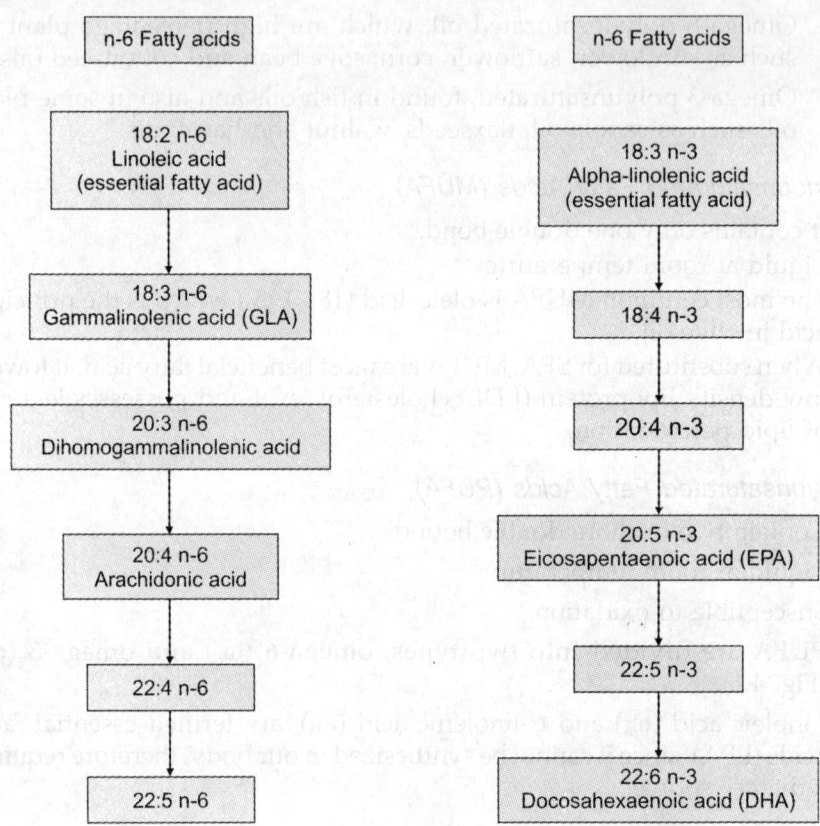

Fig. 4.1: Omega-6(n-6) and omega-3(n-6) fatty acid pathways

- γ-linoleic acid (GLA) also affects prostaglandin production and supplemental intakes of dietary GLA (usually as extracts from the seed oils of evening primrose, blackcurrant and borage) may have an anti-inflammatory effect, possibly by reducing the synthesis of inflammatory mediators derived from arachidonic acid, and by increasing production of anti-inflammatory eicosanoids.

ω₃ Polyunsaturated Fatty Acid

α-linolenic acid (ALA) (an 18 carbon ω₃ fatty acid) and its principal long-chain derivatives the 20 carbon eicosapentaenoic acid (EPA) and 22 carbon docosahexaenoic acid (DHA) comprise a much smaller proportion of dietary PUFA intake but have important physiological effects.

- ω₃ fatty acids are high in fish oil, salmon, tuna, mackerel, sardines and vegetables.
- ALA is present in certain nut and plant oil such as canola, walnut, soya bean and flaxseed oils.

- The main function of ω_3 fatty acids involves anti-thrombotic and anti-inflammatory effects, EPA and DHA being more potent in these respects than the parent compound ALA.
- Both ω_6 and ω_3 fatty acids are essential in the diet; excess ω_6 fatty acids in diet prevent the conversion of ALA into longer EPA and DHA forms. The optimal ω_6/ω_3 ratio has been estimated to be 2 : 1 to 3 : 1.

Trans Fatty Acid

Structure: Double bonds in unsaturated fatty acids may be in the cis- or trans-form. In the cis-form, the hydrogen atoms bonded to the carbon atoms at the end of the double bond or the same side; in the trans-form, these

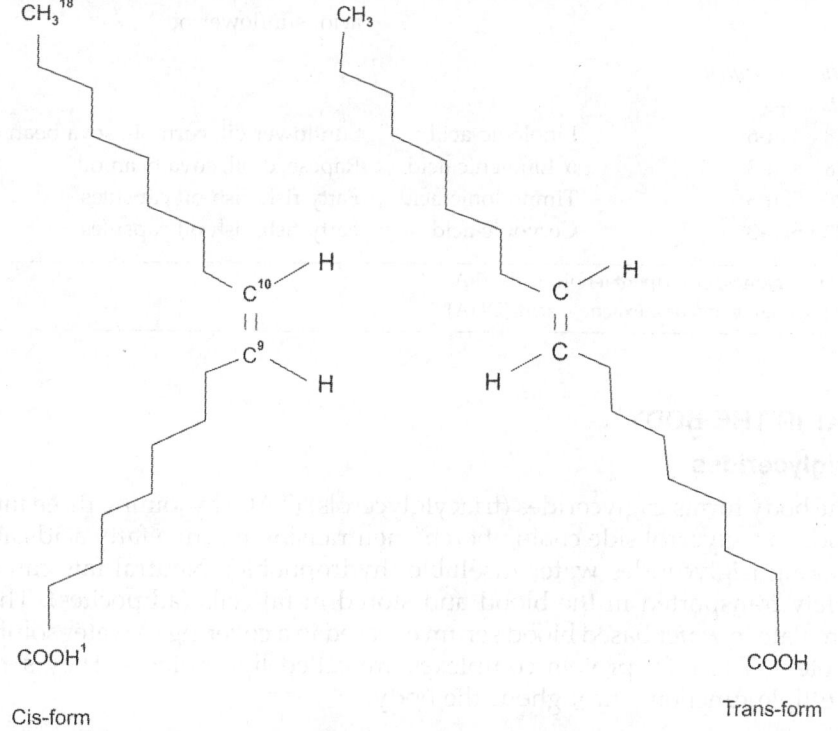

Cis-form   Trans-form

hydrogen atoms are on the opposite sides. Most dietary fatty acids contain cis double bonds, a characteristic which makes the fatty acids more rigid and bulky.

In our diet, the main origins of trans fatty acids are bacteria, deodorized oils and partially hydrogenated oils. The preponderance of trans fatty acids in our diets is derived from the hydrogenation process.

Trans fats raise serum LDL cholesterol levels and their intake should be kept as low as possible.

Table 4.1: Major fatty acids in some edible fats and oils

Formula	Fatty acid	source
Saturated fatty acids		
	Medium-chain fatty acids	Dairy fat, coconut oil, palm kernel oil
C12 : 0	Lauric acid	Dairy fat, coconut oil, palm kernel oil
C14 : 0	Myristic acid	Dairy fat, coconut oil, palm kernel oil
C16 : 0	Palmitic acid	Palm oil, meat
C18 : 0	Stearic acid	Meat, cocoa butter
Monounsaturated fatty acids		
C18 : 1, n-9	Oleic acid	Olive oil, rapeseed oil, high oleic acid, sunflower oil
Polyunsaturated fatty acids		
C18 : 2, n-6	Linolenic acid	Sunflower oil, corn oil, soya bean oil
C18 : 5, n-3	α-Linolenic acid	Rapeseed oil, soya bean oil
C20 : 5, n-3[a]	Timnodonic acid	Fatty fish, fish oil capsules
C22 : 5, n-3[b]	Cervonic acid	Fatty fish, fish oil capsules

[a] Trivial names, eicosapentaenoic acid (EPA).
[b] Trivial name, docosahexaenoic acid (DHA).

FAT IN THE BODY

Triglycerides

The body forms triglycerides (triacylglycerols) (TAG) by joining three fatty acids to a glycerol side chain, thereby neutralising reactive fatty acids and making triglycerides water insoluble (hydrophobic). Neutral fats can be safely transported in the blood and stored in fat cells (adipocites). They circulate in water based blood serum encased in a covering of water soluble protein. These fat protein complexes are called lipoproteins. They serve multiple functions throughout the body.

Phospholipids

Phospholipids are derivatives of phosphatidic acids, a triglyceride modified to contain a phosphate group. The formula of phosphatidic acid is a glycerolester with 2 fatty acids and one molecule of phosphoric acid. In phospholipids, one of the bases (choline, eithanolamine, serine) is attached to the phosphoric group.

Phospholipids make up most of the dietary lipids that is not triacylglycerol and they have important physiological functions as components of membranes and in the synthesis of a range of important regulatory molecules called the eicosanoids (e.g. prostaglandins). The phosphate group of phosphatidic acid can link with various other compound to produce a series of these phospholipids, e.g. phosphatidyl choline (lecithin), phosphatidyl inositol and phospatidyl serine.

Lecithin is a major phospholipid and it is the primary component of lipid in the membrane lipid bilayer. Lecithin is also a major component of lipoproteins used to transport fats and cholesterol. Lecithin is made by the body and is widely distributed in the food supply. Because all cells contain lecithin as a lipid bilayer component, animal products, especially liver and egg yolks are rich sources of lecithin. Plant products, such as soya beans, peanuts, legumes, spinach and wheatgerm.

Cholesterol

Cholesterol is a sterol, a waxy substance whose carbon, hydrogen and oxygen molecules are arranged in a ring. Cholesterol occurs in the tissues of all animals. It is found in all cell membranes and in myelin; brain and nerve cells are especially rich in cholesterol. The body synthesizes bile acids; steroids hormones, and vitamin D from cholesterol. If a person consumed no cholesterol at all, the body would still synthesize a needed supply. The body makes cholesterol from acetyl coenzyme A (acetyl CoA), which can originate from carbohydrates, protein, fat or alcohol.

Ketone Bodies

In normal human subjects, the degradation of fatty acids to acetyl CoA and the oxidation of acetyl CoA to CO_2 and water take place without appreciable accumulation of the intermediate products. Under some abnormal circumstances, e.g. starvation or diabetes mellitus, acetyl CoA accumulates leading to the formation of acetoacetic acid. This, in turn, is converted into β-hydroxy butyric acid and acetone. These products of fat metabolism are known as ketone bodies.

Ketone body formation takes place when large quantities of fats are oxidized to acetyl CoA in subjects who cannot oxidized carbohydrate adequately (diabetics) or who do not get a supply of carbohydrate due to lack of food intake (starvation). The tissues are not able to oxidise the large amounts of acetyl CoA formed through TCA cycle due to lack of oxalo acetate.

Ketosis is a condition in which large amounts of ketone bodies are produced in the liver and circulate in blood when the diet contains less than 100 g of carbohydrate. The level of ketone bodies in the blood of a normal person is about 3 mg/100 ml. This value can increase up to 70–80 mg/100 ml in ketosis.

FUNCTIONS OF LIPIDS IN BODY

Body Composition

All body cells contain some fat. In healthy non-obese women fat comprises about 18 to 25% of body weight and in healthy non-obese men about 15–20%, with aging the proportion of fat in the body generally increases as that of protoplasmic tissue decreases.

Adipose tissue consists of triglycerides is stored in the subcutaneous tissue and in the abdominal cavity. It is also surrounds the organs and is laced throughout muscle tissue.

Cell membrane contains lipids that facilitate the transfer of nutrients, cerebrosides, galactose containing lipids which are components of the myelin sheath of nerves and the white matter of the brain, gangliosides, glucose and galactose containing lipids which are constituents of brain tissue and of the synaptic membranes.

Energy Reserve

The primary function of fat is to provide energy as reserve—bank balance which can be drawn upon when necessary. Fat supply about 9 kcal (38 kJ) per gram. The short chain fatty acids like butyric acids from tributyrin of butter yield only 6.7 kcal (28 kJ) per gram. Excess reserves of fat cannot be excreted and can be reduced by the oxidation of the fat which occurs when there is insufficient intake of calories.

Tissues with high energy demands such as heart muscles, renal cortex and small bowel mucosa, show preferential oxidation of fatty acids. Skeletal muscle also utilizes fatty acids.

In the fasting state the major energy source is derived from mobilized fatty acids released from triglycerides of the fat deposit. Hormones that release fatty acids are epinephrine, non-epinephrine, ACTH and glucagon. These released fatty acids bound to albumin are transported to the liver, skeletal and heart muscle for energy. In the liver EFA are oxidized to CO_2 and ketones. The latter are utilized for energy by all the tissues except brain but with prolonged fasting even the brain utilize energy from ketones.

Essential Constituent of the Membrane of Every Cell

Fat is present not only in the outer membranes of all cells but also in the internal membranes of the nucleus, endoplasmic reticulum and the other membrane bound organelles.

Regulators of Body Function

As an essential component of all cell membranes fats indirectly help to regulate both the flow of materials into and out of the cells and change in cell size and shape such as those involved in growth.

Specific long chain ω_6 and ω_3 unsaturated fatty acids also act as the precursors of a range of hormone-like substances, the eicosaenoids, involves in the regulation of wide variety of processes in the body.

Eicosaenoids includes the classes of important physiological regulators known as prostaglandins, prostacyclins, thromboxanes and leukotrienes. Eicosaenoids perform many functions, including the regulation of blood pressure, the control of important aspects of the reproductive cycle. The stimulation of pain and fever and the induction of blood clotting.

Prostaglandins, is one of the eicosaenoids act within the brain, the wall of blood vessels, certain blood cells and blood platelets.

They are involved in promoting conception, including labour, effecting spontaneous abortions, regulating the transmission of nerve impulses and regulating blood pressure. Overproduction of some prostaglandins and other eicosaenoids from arachidonic acid may cause excessive clotting of the blood and narrowing of the arteries. The risk of these undesirable consequences can be reduced by eicosapentaenoic acid and docosahexaenoic acid which are both ω_3, fatty acids found in fish oil. These act to decrease the stickiness of the blood platelets involved in clotting, thus reducing possibility of a clot that could cause a heart attack.

Insulator

Deposits of fat beneath the skin known as the subcutaneous fat, serve as insulating material for the body and are effective at preventing heat loss. A certain minimal layer of fat is desirable, but too thick, a layer slows down heat loss considerably in hot weather causing discomfort.

Protector

Deposits of fat surround certain vital organs, such as kidneys and heart serving to hold them in position and protect them from physical shock. These protecting deposits are the last to be drawn on for energy supplies when energy in the diet is inadequate. These lipids have structural, storage and metabolic functions.

THE ROLE OF FAT IN THE DIET

Source of Energy

Fat is the most concentrated source of energy in the diet. Each gram of fat releases 9 kcals energy, when completely oxidized to CO_2 and water.

Satiety Value

Fat tends to leave the stomach relatively slow. It can still be released from the stomach up to 3.5 hours after a meal with the precise time depending on the size and composition of the meal. This prolonged stay in the stomach helps to delay the onset of hunger pangs and so contributes to a feeling of satiety after a meal. Due to this, moderate fat reducing diets are currently considered more successful in weight control than very low-fat diet.

Carrier of Fat-soluble Vitamins

Dietary fat serves as a carrier of vitamins A, D, E, and K. Also fat at a level of at least 10% of total energy intake appears to be required for the absorption of vitamin A precursors from non-fat sources such as carrots. Anything that interferes with absorption or use of fat such as abstruction of bile duct depresses the supply of fat-soluble vitamins to the body.

Palatability

The presence of fat in food or its addition to food is responsible for much of the texture and flavour of food. The marbling of fat throughout the lean muscle of a steak contributes greatly to its tenderness and flavour. Frying improves the taste of food. Many of the substances that are responsible for the flavours and aromas of foods are soluble in fat so that fat tends to carry these flavours and aromas mix them throughout the food as a whole.

DIGESTION, ABSORPTION AND METABOLISM

Digestion

The basic fat fuel various animals and plants fat (triglycerides) that naturally occur in foods is taken into the body with the diet. Then the task is to change these basic fuel fats into a refined fuel form of fat that the cells can burn for energy. This key refined fuel is the individual fatty acid. The body accomplishes this task through the process of fat digestion.

Mouth

No major chemical fat breakdown takes place in the mouth. In the first portion of the gastrointestinal tract, the main action is mechanical as fat is broken up into smaller particles through chewing and moistened for passage into the stomach with the general food mass.

Stomach

Little, if any, chemical fat digestion takes place in the stomach. General peristalsis continues the mechanical mixing of fat with stomach contents. No significant amount of enzymes specific for fats is present in the gastric secretion except a gastric lipase (tributyrinase), which acts on emulsified butter fat. As the main gastric enzymes act on other specific nutrients in the food mix, fat is separated from them and made readily accessible to its own specific chemical breakdown in the small intestine.

Small Intestine

Not until fat reaches the small intestine do the chemical changes necessary for fat digestion occur. Digestive agents from three major sources are present; the biliary tract consisting of the liver gallbladder which contributes a preparation agent, and the pancreas and small intestine itself which both release specific enzyme.

1. Bile from the Liver and Gallbladder

The presence of fats in the duodenum stimulates the secretion of cholecystokinin a local hormone from glands in the intestinal walls. In turn, cholecystokinin causes contraction of the gall bladder, relaxation of the sphincter muscle, and subsequent secretion of bile into the intestine via the common bile duct. The liver produces a large amount of dilute bile, and then the gall bladder concentrates and stores it ready for use with fat as needed.

Its function is that of an emulsifier. The process of emulsification is not a chemical digestive action itself, but it is an important and the first preparation step for the chemical digestion of fat through its specific enzymes. This preparation process accomplishes two important tasks.

a. It breaks the fat into small particles or globules which greatly enlarges the total surface area available for action of the enzyme and

b. It lowers the surface tension of the finely dispersed and suspended fat globules, which allow the enzymes to penetrate more easily. This process is similar to the wetting action of detergents. The bile also provides an alkaline medium for the action of the fat enzyme lipase.

2. Enzymes from the Pancreas

Pancreatic juice contains an enzyme for fat and one for cholesterol. First "pancreatic lipase" a powerful fat enzyme, break off one fatty acid at a time from the glycerol base of fats. One fatty acid plus a diglyceride, then another fatty acid plus monoglyceride, are produced in turn. Each successive step of this breakdown occurs with increasing difficulty. In fact, separation of the final fatty acid from the remaining monoglyceride is such a slow process that less than one-third of the total fat present actually breaks down completely.

The final products of fat digestion to be absorbed are fatty acids, diglycerides, monoglycerides and glycerol. Some remaining fat may pass into the large intestine for fecal elimination. Second, the enzyme "cholesterol enterase" acts on free cholesterol to form cholesterol esters by combining free cholesterol and fatty acids in preparation for absorption.

3. Enzyme from the Small Intestine

The small intestine secretes an enzyme in the intestinal juice called lecithinase. As its name indicates, it cuts on lecithin, a phospholipid, to break it down into its components for absorption (Fig. 4.2).

Absorption

The task of fat absorption is not easy. The problem is that fats are not soluble in water. Hence fat always requires some types of solvent carrier. To accomplish this task of transporting fat from the small intestine into the blood stream, the body has three basic stages of operation.

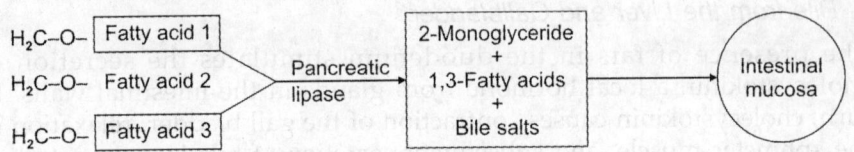

Fig. 4.2: Micellar complex of fats with bile salt for transport of fats into intestinal mucosa

Stage I

1. *Initial fat absorption:* In the small intestine bile combines with products of fat digestion in a micellar bile-fat complex. This unique carrier system, shown in Fig. 4.3, takes fat digestion products along its initial passage into the intestinal wall.

Stage II

Absorption within the intestinal wall: Once inside the wall of the small intestine, the bile separates from the fat complex and returns in the enterohepatic circulation to accomplises its task over and over again. Two important actions on the fat digestion products occur inside the intestine wall.

1. *Enteric lipase action:* An enteric lipase within the cells of the intestinal wall completes the digestion of the remaining glycerides.
2. *Triglyceride synthesis:* With the resulting fatty acids and glycerol, new human triglycerides are formed as body fats, now ready for final absorption and circulation.

Stage III

Final fat absorption and transport: This newly formed human fats triglycerides and other fat materials present are combined with a small amount of protein covering to form lipoproteins called chylomicrons. These packages of fat in a milk like liquid called chyle, cross the cell membrane intact into the lymphatic system and then into the portal blood. Here a final fat clearing enzyme, lipoprotein lipase helps clear the large meal loads of dietary fat from circulation. In the liver the fat is converted to other lipoproteins for transport to the body cells for energy and other structural functions (Fig. 4.3).

Metabolism

In the body cells, fatty acids are "burned" as concentrated fuel to produce energy. These derived units of fat have about twice the energy value of glucose products.

Essential Fatty Acids

The term essential and non-essential are applied to nutrients according to their relation necessary in the diet. The nutrient is essential if the body

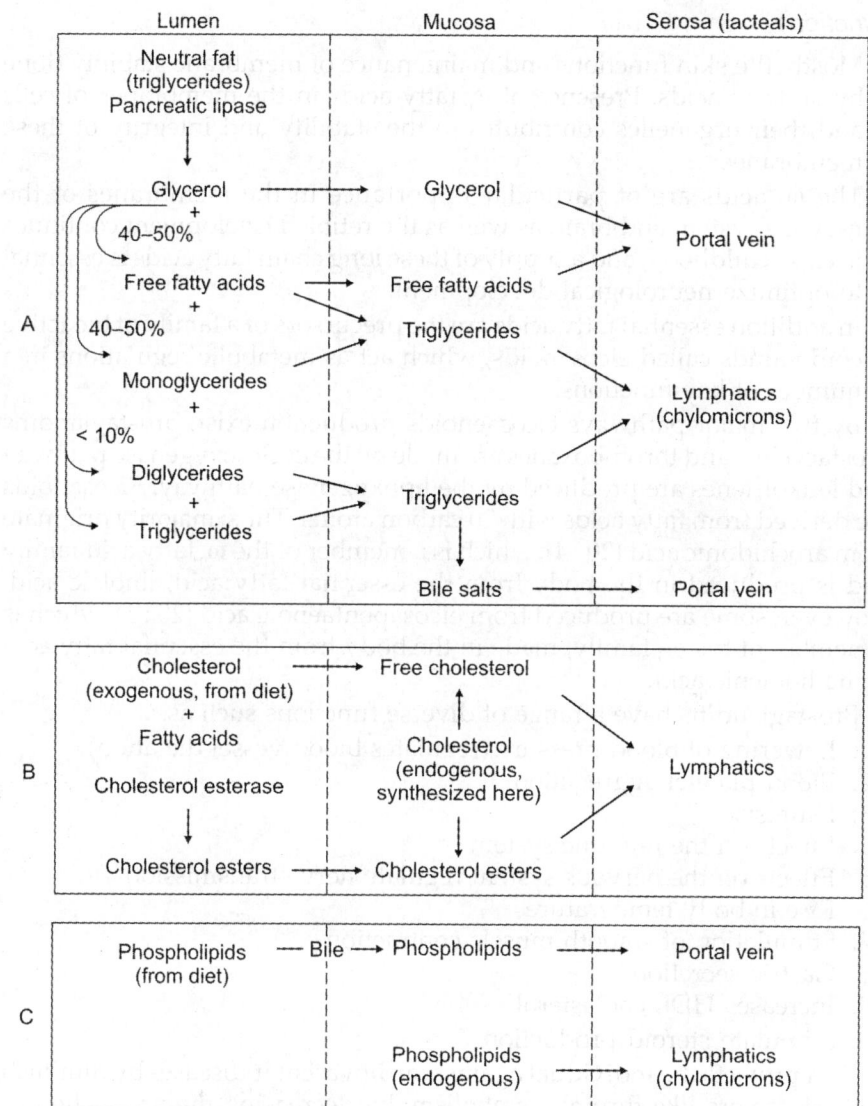

Fig. 4.3: Absorption of fat, cholesterol and phospholipids

cannot manufacture it and therefore must obtain it from the diet, because a failure to do so would result in a specific disease. If fat makes up only 10% or less of the diets daily kilocalories, the body cannot obtain adequate amounts of the essential fatty acids. Three fatty acids linoleic, linolenic acid, and arachidonic are the only ones known to be essential for the complete nutrition of humans. Actually only linoleic acid is a true essential fatty acid (EFA) because the other two may be naturally synthesized from it. These fatty acids—linoleic acid, along with linolenic and arachidonic acids serve important body functions.

Functions

1. Mostly, the skin functions and maintenance of membrane stability done by ω_6 fatty acids. Presence of ω_6 fatty acids in the membranes of cells and their organelles contributes to the stability and integrity of these membranes.
2. The ω_3 acids are of particular importance in the membranes of the nervous system and brain as well as the retina. Development continues in early childhood, and a supply of these long chain fatty acids is essential to optimize neurological development.
3. In addition essential fatty acids are the precursors of a family of bioactive compounds called eicosanoids, which act as metabolic regulations in a number of key functions.

By two major pathways eicosaenoids production exist, prostaglandins prostacyclins and thromboxanes are made by the cyclo-oxygenase pathway and leukotrienes are produced by the lipoxygenase pathway. Eicosanoids are derived from fatty acids with 20 carbon atoms. Thus, majority originate from arochidonic acid (20 : 4), which is a member of the ω_6 fatty acid family and is produced in the body from the essential fatty acid, linoleic acid. However, some are produced from eicosapentaenoic acid (20 : 5), which is a member of the ω_3 family, made in the body from the essential fatty acid alpha linolenic acid.

Prostaglandins have a range of diverse functions such as:

1. Lowering of blood pressure (regulates blood vessel dialation)
2. Blood platelet aggregation
3. Diuresis
4. Effects on the immune system
5. Effects on the nervous system regulate nerve transmission
6. Rise in body temperature
7. Stimulation of smooth muscle contraction
8. Gastric secretion
9. Increases HDL cholesterol
10. Stimulate steroid production.

EFA protects the individual against cardiovascular diseases by diminish the risk factors like thrombo embolism, by decreasing the production of LDL triglycerides and precursor of VLDL. It plays key role in transport of cholesterol.

Deficiency

Essential fatty acids deficiency is rare in humans. It may occur in infants who fed diets deficient in EFA. Babies fed a formula low in linoleic acid; such as a skim-milk formula, can develop EFA deficiency. EFA deficiency used to result from long-term TPN, if fat was not included.

Signs include scaly dermatitis, alopecia, thrombo cytopenia and in children growth retardation. Dietary replenishment of EFA reverses the deficiency.

Omega-6 deficiency may cause

a. *Eczema like skin Eruptions:* ω_6 fatty acids affect the capillary permeability. Increased swelling of mitochondria occurs and results in dermatitis of skin. Dry bumpy skin called "follicular hyperkeratosis", has also been known as toad skin or phrynoderma.

b. Behavioural changes

c. Water loss through skin

d. Susceptibility to infections

e. Male sterility

f. Arthritis-like condition

g. Growth retardation

h. Dry eyes

i. Hair loss

j. Kidney malfunction

k. Glands to dry up

l. Wounds fail to heal

m. Female miscarriages

n. heart beat abnormalities

o. Dry skin and hair

Omega-3 deficiency may cause

- Growth retardation
- Weakness
- Motor incoordination
- Behavioural change
- Vision and learning problems
- Tingling sensation in arms and legs.

Recommended Dietary Allowances

Studies relating fat intake to cardiovascular diseases suggests that an intake of fat energy at 30% or more of total calories is undesirable particularly in sedentary individuals. Daily visible fat intake should be kept below 50 g/day. WHO suggest that ratio of $\omega_6 : \omega_3$ should be 5 to 10 : 1 in the diet (Table 4.2).

Sources of Fat

The visible fats are ghee, butter and oil. Invisible fats are present in cereals, pulses, oilseed, milk and egg (Table 4.3).

Sources of EFA

1. Corn and cotton seed, safflower and soyabean oils are good sources of linoleic acid. Barley and oats contain appreciable amount of gamma linolenic acid which lowers cholesterol levels.

Table 4.2: Fat RDA of Indians suggested by ICMR

Group desirable	EFA requirement en%	Invisible fat* en%	Minimum visible fat** en%	g/day	Suggested visible fat intake g/day	en%
Adults**	3	10	5	12***	20***	9
Older children***	3	10	5	12	22	9
Young children	3	10	5	8	25	15
Pregnant women	4.5	10	12.5	30	30	12.5
Lactating women	5.7	10	17.5	45	45	17.5

*Contains 20% EFA about 6 per cent would be from cereals and pulses and rest from milk, nuts, spices, etc.
**EFA at least 20 per cent.
***Average of males and females

Table 4.3: Fat content of some foods

Name of foodstuff	Fat g/100 g
Ghee and oil	100
Butter	81
Coconut dry	62
Cashew nut	47
Groundnut	40
Cheese	25
Avocado	23
Soya bean	19
Egg hen	13

2. Cereals contain linoleic acid in small amounts. From cereals we get 15 g of invisible fat and this meets 50% of EFA requirements. It also presents in green leafy vegetable and algae.
3. Arachidonic acid is found in milk and butter (Table 4.4).

DIETARY FAT AND CORONARY HEART DISEASE

For more than 40 years epidemiologic studies, experimental studies, clinical trials have shown that numerous dietary risk factors effect serum lipids, atherogenesis, and CHD. Saturated fatty acids C_{12}, C_{14} and C_{16} promote hyper cholestriolemia while C_{14}, C_{16} and C_{18} potentiate thrombogenisis (Fig. 4.4).

Saturated Fatty Acids (SFA)

SFAs are restricted because they have the most potent effect, on LDL cholesterol, which rises in a dose response fashion when increasing levels of SFAs are consumed. The most hyper chlestrolemic promoting or atherogenic SFAs in order of potency are mysristic (C_{14} : O), palmitic

Table 4.4: Linoleic and linolenic acid content of edible oils g/100 g

Oil	Linoleic (ω_6)	Linolenic (ω_3)
Ghee	1.6	0.5
Coconut	2.2	–
Vanaspathi	3.4	–
Palmolein	12.0	0.3
Rape/Mustard	13.0	9.0
Groundnut	28.0	0.3
Rice bran	33.0	1.6
Sesame	40.0	0.5
Cotton seed	50.3	0.4
Corn oil	50.0	2.0
Sunflower	52.0	Trace
Soya bean	52.0	5.0
Safflower	74.0	0.5

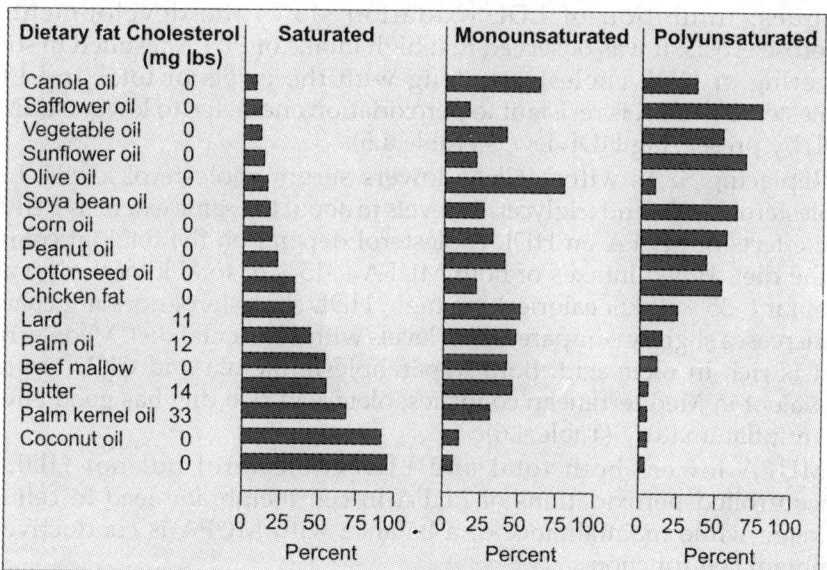

Source: Sienkiewicz Sizer Frances and Eleanor Noss Whitney, 2000, nutrition concepts and controversies, Wadsworth, Thomson Learning Belmont.

Fig. 4.4: Fatty acid composition of common food fats

($C_{16}:O$) and lauric ($C_{12}:O$) acids, palmitic acid is the most prevelant hyper cholestrolemic SFA. Most dietary plamitate comes from animal foods, mystiric acid (C_{14}) is found mostly in butterfat and coconut and palm kernel oils. Lauric acid, the only medium chain SFA, is also found in palm kernel and coconut oils.

SFAs raise serum LDL cholesterol by decreasing LDL receptor synthesis and activity. Regardless of form, all fatty acids lower fasting triglycerides if they replace carbohydrate in the diet.

Although milk fat and coconut oil contain short chain fatty acids (9 and 15%), the contents of most atherogenic C_{12}, C_{14}, C_{16} SFA are high (45 and 73%), particularly in the latter.

Lauric and mystiric acids raise HDL along with LDL cholesterol. Yet both have more atherogenic and thrombogenic than meat fat.

Plam oil contains α-tocopherol of α-tocotrienols and variety of carotenoids with potent antioxidant properties. Palmitic acid, the chief constituent of palm oil, raises serum cholesterol to a much lower extent than myristic acid of coconut oil and dairy fat.

Thus fatty acids affect disease progression through lipids and other mechanisms and possibly through inflammation and thrombosis.

Monounsaturated Fatty Acids

MUFA are a better replacement for saturated fatty acids than poly-unsaturated fatty acids because they are less susceptible for oxidation. Oxidized LDL is taken by macrophages and deposited in atherosclerotic plaques. Inhibition of LDL oxidation slows the development of atherosclerosis. It was observed that high intake of PUFA resulted in some lowering of HDL cholesterol along with the levels of total and LDL cholesterol. MUFA is resistant to peroxidation and helps to lower oxidized LDL by preserving HDL levels (Table 4.5).

Replacing SFAs with MUFAs lowers serum cholesterol levels, LDL cholesterol levels, and triglyceride levels to about the same extent as PUFAs. The effects of MUFA on HDL cholesterol depend on the total fat content of the diet. When intakes of both MUFA (>15% of total kilocalories) and total fat (>35% of kilocalories) are high, HDL cholesterol does not change or increases slightly compared with levels with a lower fat diet. Medetarrian diet is rich in oleic acid. Both hypercholesterolemia and CHD are less prevalent in Mediterranean countries, oleic acid rich diet has good effects of antinflammatory (Table 4.6).

MUFA lowers both total and LDL cholesterol but not HDL-C. Uncontrolled peroxidations of PUFA in cell membrane lead to cellular damage while maintainance of a balance with MUFA is conductive to maintain cell function.

Polyunsaturated Fatty Acids

Polyunsaturated fatty acids are divided into two types, omega-6 (ω_6) and omega-3 (ω_3), and these have distinctly different metabolic effects. The parent fatty acids in each of these groups, linoleic acid (ω_6) and α-linolenic acid (ω_3) are termed essential fatty acids. Long chain fatty acids derived from these essential fatty acids are precurrors of many metabolic intermediaries such as prostaglandins leukotrienes and thromboxanes and hence have variable influence on inflammatory processes, immune response and blood clotting. Other long-chain derivatives such as arachidonic acid, eicosapentaenoic acid (EPA) and docosahexaenoic acid

(DHA) play an important role in neural and optical development in foetal and early life

ω_6 Polyunsaturated Fatty Acids

Most dietary polyunsaturated fat is in the form of ω_6 fatty acids, principally linoleic acid derived from vegetable oils such as sunflower, safflower, corn, palm, groundnut, canola and soya oils.

ω_6 PUFA have a hypocholestrolaemic effect and their substitution for saturated fatty acids has in the past been actively encouraged in order to lower LDL and total cholesterol levels. This advice has now been moderated as a result of concerns over the possible adverse effects of excessive ω_6 PUFA intake. Although PUFA are effective at lowering blood LDL cholesterol, at intakes in excess of 8–10% dietary energy, they also lower HDL cholesterol concentration, necessary for atherogenic protection. PUFA are also susceptible to metabolic oxidation and high intake can enhance lipid peroxidation and free radical production with potentially adverse effects in terms of atherogenesis and carcinogenesis. Dietary intake of ω_6 PUFA therefore needs to be adequate but not excessive. Any beneficial effect of substitution of ω_6 PUFA for SFA is evident only when diet is rich in antioxidants.

ω_3 Polyunsaturated Fatty Acids

α-linolenic acid (ALA) and its principle long-chain derivatives the 20 carbon eicosapentaonic acids (EPA) and 22 carbon docosahexaenoic acid (DHA) comprise much smaller proportion of dietary PUFA intake but have important physiological effects. ω_3 can reduce fasting and postprandial triglyceride concentrations. The main interest in ω_3 PUFA is in their anti-thromboitic and anti-inflammatory effects, EPA and DHA being more potent in these respects than the parent compound ALA.

EPA and DHA have important anti-thrombogenic influences, increased consumption of fish, especially oily fish is now recognized as an important dietary protective measure against myocardial infarction.

Omega-3 fatty acids lower the triglyceride levels by inhibiting VLDL and apo B-100 synthesis and by decreasing postprandial lipemia. Therefore high intake prolong bleeding times, a condition that is common in eskimo populations with high omega-3 fat dietary intake and low incidence of CHD.

The ω_6 and ω_3 fatty acid pathways share common enzymes (e.g. ω_6 linoleic acid and ω_3 α-linolenic acid both compete for the enzyme delta 6-desaturase), it is likely that the balance between the two influences the type and amount of long chain fatty acids and eicosanoids formed as a result of their metabolism. Diets containing a high proportion of ω_6 relative to ω_3 fatty acids may increase production of the more proinflammatory eicosanoids derived from arachidonic acid rather than the more anti-inflammatory eicosanoids from DHA and EPA.

Amount of Dietary Fat

Total fat intakes are related to obesity which affects many of the major risk factors for atherosclerosis, also, high fat diets increases postprandial lipemia and chylomicron remnants, both of which are associated with increased risk of CHD. When fat is reduced in the diet and carbohydrate is the replacement source of calories, triglycerides and HDL levels affected. Low fat diets (< 25% of total kcal from fat) raise triglyceride levels and lower HDL levels. Although these changes appear to be negative, they are not associated with CHD risk because

1. LDL cholesterol levels are low in person consuming low-fat diets and
2. The VLDLs that are produced are large, triglyceride-rich VLDLs which are not associated with risk.

Table 4.5: Summary of fatty acids in atherosclerosis

	SFA	Oleic	n-6	n-3
Blood cholesterol	↓	↓	↓	↓
HDL cholesterol	↓	No change	↓	No change
Triglycerides	↓	No change	No change	↓
Platelet aggregation	↑	No change		↓↓↓

Source. Ghafoorunissa, nutrition aspects of fats in Indian diets, proceedings of the Nutrition Society of India, 35, 1989.

Table 4.6: Desirable percentage of calories from different fats

Recommended fat	% of kcal
Total fat	<30
Saturated	8–10
Polyunsaturated	5–8
Monounsaturated	Difference
Ratio ω_6 to ω_3	5–10 : 1

To prevent heart disease one needs to control total energy, total fat and saturated fat and cholesterol content of the diet and proper balance between ω_6/ω_3 fatty acids. Blended oils are the solution to prevent atherosclerosis as no single oil has absolutely desirable composition. Government of India has permitted admixture of any two vegetable oils. Consumption of blended oils could ensure optimum balance of fatty acids in Indian diets.

5 Minerals

The minerals are divided according to the requirement in our body. Minerals which are required and present in our body in a large amount are called macro minerals and which are present and required in a small amount are called micro minerals.

CALCIUM

Calcium is the most abundant mineral in the body. An adult has 1.5 to 2% of calcium in his body, 99% of which is in the skeleton and teeth. The remaining 1% is found within plasma, lymph and other body fluids, where it regulates many important metabolic functions. About 45% of plasma calcium exists as free ions (ionised calcium), the remainder 45% being bound to plasma proteins and 10% complexed with citrate, phosphate or bicarbonate.

Absorption

Most food calcium occurs in complexes with other dietary components. These complexes must be broken down and the calcium released in a soluble form before it can be absorbed.

Calcium is absorbed by two mechanisms:

i. Active transport, which operates predominantly at low luminal concentrations of calcium ions. Active calcium absorption depends on vitamin D intake and the presence of calbindin (calcium-binding protein) in duodenal enterocytes.

Calcium absorption is limited in duodenum and proximal jejunum because transit time through the duodenum is so short and also it is controlled through the action of 1, 25-dihydroxyvitamin D (1, 25 [OH]$_2$ D$_3$). This vitamin/hormone increases calcium uptake at the brush border of the intestinal mucosal cell by also stimulating the production of calbindins and other mechanisms. Calbindins store calcium ions temporarily after a meal and ferry them to the basolateral member for the finel step of absorption.

ii. Passive transport, paracellular transfer, which operates at high luminal concentrations of calcium ions.

In this mechanism, nonsaturable (with no limit), and independent of vitamin D, occurs along the entire length of the small intestine. When a large amount of calcium is consumed in a single meal like dairy food or a supplement, much of the calcium that is absorbed occurs by this passive route.

Until puberty, calcium absorption is increased up to two fold (60%) in comparison with absorption in adults. In pregnancy, absorption and retention of calcium are increased. At old age, calcium absorption decreases, and the ability of the intestine to respond to a low-calcium diet by increasing the rate of absorption is impaired.

FACTORS INCREASING CALCIUM ABSORPTION
Vitamin D Hormone

This hormone controls the synthesis of calcium-binding protein carries in the duodenum that transports the mineral into the mucosal cells and blood circulation. The presence of the active form of vitamin D can result in a 10–30% increase in calcium absorption.

Protein

Calcium absorption is increased when the diet is high in protein but it has no effect when the diet is high in protein and calcium intake is less. When calcium absorption is increased, it results in increased, renal excretion, with a negative calcium balance following.

Any protein-rich food also rich in phosphate. Phosphate in diet will reduce the calcium excretion. So, the net effect of increased protein intake on calcium losses via urine is considerably less than is expected from the effect of the protein alone. Protein supplements composed of purified protein practically devoid of phosphate, however, may have an adverse effect of calcium balance if consumed in a large amount.

Lactose

Lactose enhances calcium absorption through the action of the lactobacilli, which produce lactic acid and lower intestinal pH. The lactose in breast milk and formula improves calcium absorption in human infants. In infants, there is 15% additional raise in absorption of dietary calcium due to lactose. High ratio of lactose to calcium is required to promote calcium absorption. However, this effect is not consistent after infancy period.

Acidity

Lower pH (increased acidity) favours solubility of calcium and consequently its absorption. The normal decline in the efficiency of calcium absorption with age is partly caused by an associated decline in hydrochloric acid secretions into the stomach.

Body Need

Body calcium absorption increases with body demand, such as growth or depletion states. In pregnancy, lactation and adolescence when the need of calcium is too high, the absorption efficiency is as high as 50%. In old age and postmenopausal, the ability to absorb calcium is reduced.

FACTORS DEPRESSING CALCIUM ABSORPTION

Vitamin D Deficiency

Deficiency in vitamin D hormone along with parathyroid hormone will depress the absorption of calcium.

Steatorrhoea

Excess dietary fat or poor absorption of fats results in steatorrhoea (excess unabsorbed fat in faeces) in which calcium absorption is certainly reduced. Because malabsorbed fat combines with calcium to form insoluble soaps which results in reduction of calcium absorption.

Oxalic Acid

Oxalic acid combines with calcium to produce insoluble complex of calcium oxalate which cannot be absorbed. Green leafy vegetables are rich sources of oxalic acid, but the amount of oxalates in them varies, making some of them better sources of calcium than the others, e.g. spinach is the rich source of oxalic acid which can reduce absorption of calcium, whereas cocoa is insufficient to depress calcium absorption.

Phytic Acid

Phytic acid, a phosphorous-containing compound present in outer husks of cereals combines with calcium to form calcium phytate prevents calcium absorption. The effect of rachitogenic is high in whole wheat flour than in white flour and oatmeal worse than either. Fermentation reduces phytic acid because of phytase present in yeast.

Fibre

Increased dietary fibre binds calcium and other minerals within its structure and hinders the availability for absorption.

Fibre will increase the gastrointestinal motility, which in turn increase the rate of passage of food through the intestinal tract. This decrease the absorption since the time available for the absorption is reduced.

Ageing

Calcium absorption is decreased during old age. Associated with vitamin D deficiency and hyperparathyroidism may increase the risk of fractures.

Caffeine

A high intake of caffeine affects the bioavailability of calcium by increasing the loss of calcium in urine and stimulating the secretion of calcium into the gastrointestinal tract.

Drugs

Some medicines including anticoagulants, cortisone and thyroxine reduce calcium absorption as a side effect.

Metabolism

After the absorption calcium is transported in the blood and released into the fluids bathing the tissues of the body. From extracellular fluids the cells take up the amount of calcium needed for their normal functioning and growth. During the postprandial period bone also takes up calcium and other minerals from the blood when they are consumed. Bone is a dynamic tissue that returns calcium and other minerals to the extracellular fluids and blood on demand (Fig. 5.1).

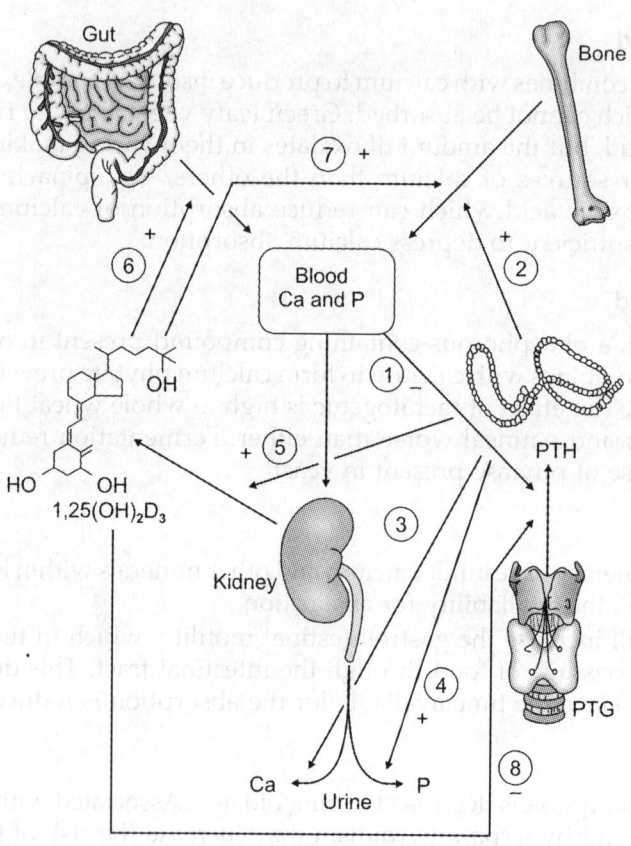

Fig. 5.1: Pathways of calcium metabolism. The regulation of calcium metabolism involves intestinal absorption (gut), blood calcium (Ca) and phosphate (P) concentrations, bone, the kidneys—which produce the hormonal form of vitamin D (1, 25[OH]$_2$D$_3$)—and the parathyroid glands (PTG), which secrete parathyroid hormone (PTH). Steps 1 through 8 are specific regulation points. A low serum calcium or high serum phosphate level stimulates PTH secretion (Step 1) through negative feedback

ROLE OF HORMONES

The external balance of calcium, i.e. the difference between intake and output is determined by exchange between the skeleton, the intestine and the kidney. These fluxes are controlled by the action of the calciotrophic hormones, parathyroid hormones, 1,25, dihydroxy cholecalciferol and calcitonin. They are also influenced by a variety of locally acting hormones. Physiological changes in calcium balance occur during growth, pregnancy, lactation and with increasing years. Calcium metabolism is regulated at three levels—absorption, renal reabsorption and bone resorption. Parathyroid hormone and calcitonin (from the thyroid gland) regulate deposition and release of calcium from bone and also the rate of excretion of calcium in the urine.

Parathyroid Hormone

Decreased plasma calcium or increased phosphate will trigger secretion of parathyroid hormone:

- Parathyroid hormone mobilises calcium from the bones in the fasting condition, to maintain the plasma calcium. The action of parathyroid hormone on bones is called "calcium mobilizing action".
- At the same time, it lowers the serum phosphate concentration. This is brought about by decreasing the reabsorption of phosphate and causing "phosphaturic action" (Fig. 5.2).

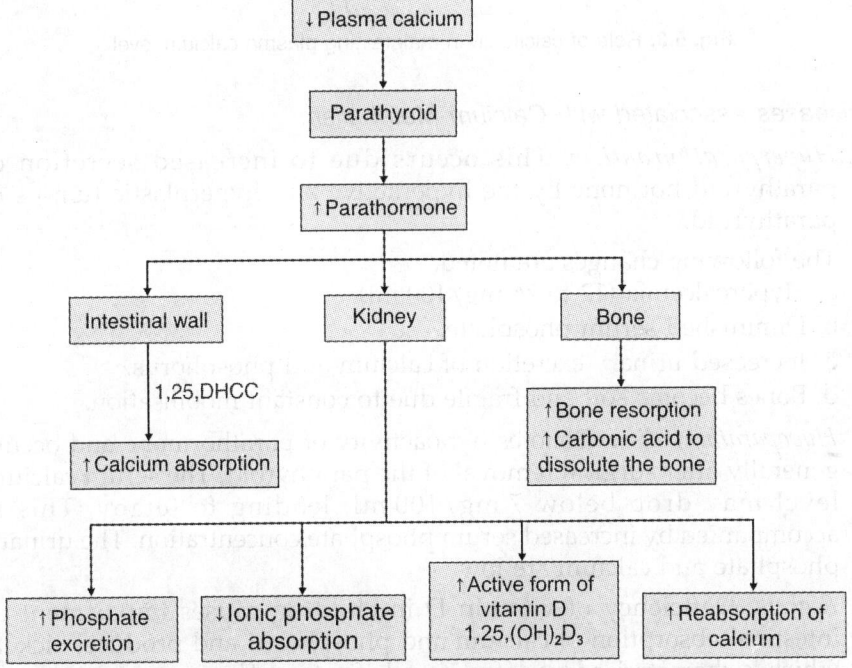

Fig. 5.2: Role of parathyroid hormone in maintaining calcium levels

Calcitonin

Calcitonin released when plasma calcium levels rise too high. calcitonin lowers plasma levels of both calcium and phosphorus by inhibiting the release of these minerals into the blood from bone (Fig. 5.3).

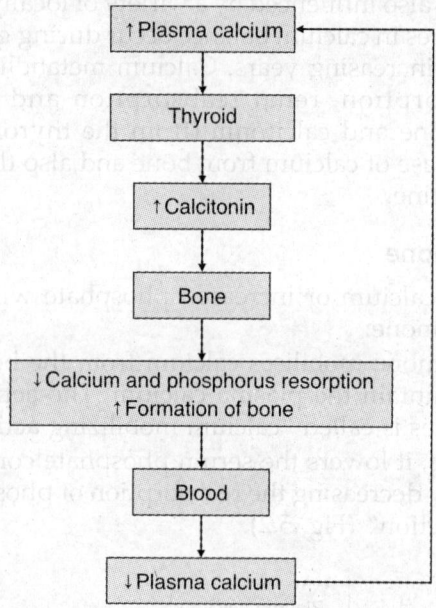

Fig. 5.3: Role of calcitonin in maintaining plasma calcium level

Diseases associated with Calcium Metabolism

1. *Hyperparathyroidism:* This occurs due to increased secretion of parathyroid hormone by the hyperactive and hyperplastic tumors of parathyroid.

   The following changes are noted.
   a. Hypercalcemia (12 to 24 mg/100 ml).
   b. Diminished serum phosphate.
   c. Increased urinary excretion of calcium and phosphorus.
   d. Bones become soft and fragile due to constant mobilisation.

2. *Hypoparathyroidism:* Denotes hypoactivity of parathormone and occurs generally after surgical removal of the parathyroid. The serum calcium level may drop below 7 mg/100 ml, leading to tetany. This is accompanied by increased serum phosphate concentration. The urinary phosphate and calcium are low.

3. *Rickets:* Deficiency of vitamin D in children causes impairment of intestinal absorption of calcium and phosphorus and produces rickets which is characterised by defective calcification. The serum calcium and

phosphorus remain normal or may be slightly lowered. But the faecal excretions of both are increased because of their poor absorption. The alkaline phosphatase activity is raised because of increased osteoblastic activity. Another type of rickets known as renal rickets is caused by an inherited defect in the renal tubules by which the reabsorption of phosphates is impaired. This disease in not relieved by vitamin D therapy.

Serum Calcium

Total serum calcium consists of three distinct fractions:

i. Free, or ionized, calcium (47.6%).

ii. Complexes between calcium and anions such as phosphate, citrate, or other organic anions (6.4%).

iii. Calcium that is protein bound, primarily with albumin (46%).

Ionized calcium is regulated and equilibrates rapidly with protein-bound calcium in blood. The serum ionized calcium concentration is controlled primarily by PTH, although hormones such as calcitonin, vitamin D, estrogen and others have minor role in its regulation. Several factors affect the relative distribution of calcium in blood serum or plasma. One of these is pH; the ionized calcium fraction is higher in acidosis and lower in alkalosis. Total calcium changes concurrently with changes in plasma protein level; however, the ionized fraction usually remains within normal limits. Serum levels of calcium are highest early in life, gradually decreasing throughout life and reaching the lowest levels during the older years.

The strict regulation in ionized calcium makes it a useful diagnosed tool in assessing parathyroid gland function, monitoring kidney diseases, and monitoring sick neonates for whom hypocalcemia could be life threatening.

REGULATION OF SERUM CALCIUM

Calcium in bones is in equilibrium with calcium in the blood. PTH plays the major role in maintaining serum calcium. When the blood calcium concentration falls below this level, PTH stimulates the transfer of exchangeable calcium from the bone into the blood. At the same time, PTH promotes renal tubular resorption of calcium, and it indirectly stimulates increased intestinal absorption of calcium by increasing kidney production of vitamin D (1, 25 $[OH]_2 D_3$). Other hormones such as glucocorticoids, thyroid hormones, and sex hormones also have important role in calcium homeostasis. In women normal bone balance requires serum estrogen concentrations to be within normal limits. The rapid decrease of serum estrogen concentration during menopause is a major factor contributing to bone resorption. Treating postmenopausal women with estrogen slow-down the rate of bone resorption. Bone resorption is also inhibited by testosterone.

Excretion

Urinary calcium excretion increases as protein intake increases, but the effect is not always proportional to the protein intake. In balance studies, when phosphorus intake was stable, 1 g of dietary protein increased urinary calcium excretion by 1 to 1.5 mg. Thus, diets high in protein but with limited calcium intake may increase urinary calcium loss and alter daily requirements.

Calcium and sodium share the same transport system in the proximal tubule. Every gram of sodium excreted carries about 8 to 25 mg of calcium with it. Sodium bicarbonate does not have the same effect on urinary calcium loss as sodium chloride. In addition, 1 mg of calcium is lost with each 1 g of protein metabolized in the body. This effect may be related to calcium binding to the sulphate derived from sulphur-containing amino acids.

Renal Excretion

The bowel and kidney excrete about 160 mg of calcium daily even when calcium intake is low.

Dermal Losses

In addition, about 40 mg is lost per day through the skin. Thus, an intake of 200 mg per day is needed to offset these obligatory losses. Net calcium absorption will not occur until these obligatory losses have been satisfied.

Functions

In Bone

Calcium provides part of the matrix structure of bone along with phosphate and magnesium. Bone tissue serves as a reservoir of calcium and other minerals that are used by other tissues of the body. Calcium homeostasis, or the process of maintenance of a constant serum calcium concentration, is almost totally reliant on this bone tissue source of calcium when the diet is inadequate. Bone tissue is also slowly dynamic, since it undergoes bone turnover via both modelling early in life and remodelling after skeletal growth ceases.

Bone Modelling

Bone modelling is the term applied to the growth of skeleton until mature height is achieved. Bone modelling is typically completed in girls by ages 16 to 18 and in boys by ages 18 to 20. After growth ceases, gains in bone tissue may continue by the process known as bone consolidation. The major event of the skeleton in early life is growth, whereas in later life it is loss of bone. During bone modelling long bones elongate and widen by undergoing great internal changes as well as external expansions in their structures.

Bone Remodelling

Bone remodelling is the process in which bone is continuously resorbed through the action of the osteoclasts and reformed through the action of the osteoblasts. After skeletal growth is completed, bone continuously undergoes remodelling in response to strains on the skeleton, adapts to changes in lifestyle factors and dietary intakes, maintains the set calcium concentration in extracellular fluids, and repairs microscopic fractures that occur over time.

In Tooth

Vitamin D is essential to the process by which calcium and phosphorus are deposited in crystals of hydroxyapatite, a naturally occurring form of calcium and phosphorus, that is the mineral component of dental enamel and dentin.

IN METABOLIC FUNCTIONS

Blood Clotting

At the time of injury by cuts, fibre polymers, in the presence of calcium and a serum factor (factor XIII), and fibrinase, form the more solidified and coarse physiological clot, the fibrin (Fig. 5.4).

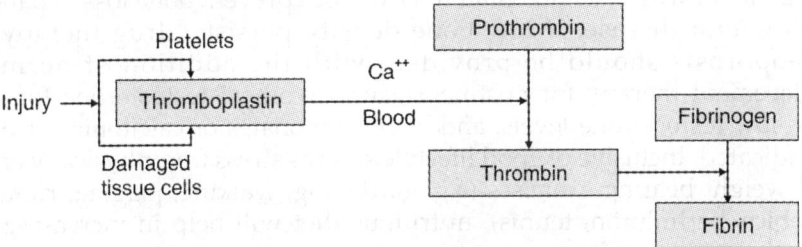

Fig. 5.4: Role of calcium in blood clotting

Muscle Contraction

Muscle contraction is impaired when there is a deficiency of calcium ions. Excess calcium increases the contractility of heart muscles and the heart stops during systole.

Nervous System

Normal transmission of nerve impulses along axons requires calcium. A current of calcium ions triggers the flow of signals from one nerve cell to another and on to waiting target muscles.

CELL MEMBRANE PERMEABILITY

Ionized calcium controls the passage of fluids and solutes through cell membranes by affecting membrane permeability. It influences the integrity of the intercellular cement substance.

Enzyme Activation

Calcium ions are important activators of specific cell enzymes, especially ones that release energy for muscles contraction. They play a similar role with other enzymes, including lipase, which digests fat, and with some membrane of the protein splitting enzyme system.

Deficiency

Osteoporosis

The term osteoporosis is of Greek origin and literally means "porous bone". In this condition the total amount (quantity) of bone is reduced, but the remaining bone is of normal composition and quality. The major symptom is an increased vulnerability to bone fractures.

Physical activity and adequate nutrition should be promoted. Cigarette smoking, alcohol, caffeine, high salt intake, sedentary lifestyle, emotional stress, inappropriate diet should be discouraged.

In certain intestinal diseases, fecal calcium loss is increased by diarrhea or malabsorption. Patients with celiac disease and inflammatory bowel disease should be given adequate dietary calcium and supplementation.

Treatment

Supplement with calcium, vitamin D, or both prevent bone loss in patients with Crohn disease. If low bone density persists, drug therapy for osteoporosis should be provided, with the addition of hormone replacement therapy for postmenopausal women, testosterone for men with low testosterone levels, and bisphosphonates or calcitonin for other as indicated. Inclusive of good lifestyle such as stress free, physically active and weight bearing exercises (e.g. gardening, walking, jogging, running, aerobics, badminton, tennis), nutritious diet will help in increasing the situation.

Hypertension

A small decrease in systolic, but not diastolic pressure was observed with calcium supplementation. However, the use of natural calcium-rich diet produced a greater fall in pressure. Thus, calcium supplements are not often indicated for the treatment of hypertension.

Colon Cancer

One large study measuring the effect of calcium on colonic proliferative showed a modest effect of calcium supplementation in preventing colorectal polyps.

PREMENSTRUAL SYNDROME

The use of 1,200 mg of calcium per day for three cycles led to fewer symptoms in women ages 18 to 45 years.

Hypercalcemia

A very high intake of calcium, especially in a person with a high level of vitamin D is a potential cause of hypercalcemia. High intake of calcium may also interfere with the absorption of other divalent cations such as iron, zinc and manganese.

Hypocalcemia

Inadequate intake of calcium leads to hypocalcemia. This may occur after operation on the thyroid gland, if too much parathyroid tissue is removed or due to impaired alimentary absorption. It may also occur in malabsorption syndrome condition.

Sources

Calcium is present in both animal and plant foods. The richest sources of calcium are milk and green leafy vegetables. Among the leafy vegetables, amaranth, fenugreek and drumstick leaves are particularly rich in calcium. Most cereals and millets contain some amount. Ragi is a particularly rich source of calcium. Some of the pseudocereals like grain amaranth (Rajkeera) is a good source of calcium (Table 5.1).

Table 5.1: Calcium content of foods

Name of the foodstuff	Calcium mg/100 g
Crab small	1606
Colacasia leaves	1546
Gingelly seeds	1450
Skimmed milk powder	1370
Agathi	1130
Whole milk powder	950
Cheese	790
Drumstick leaves	440
Milk, buffalo	210
Aavin milk	120

PHOSPHORUS

Next to calcium, phosphorus is present in abundance in human tissues. It is an essential elemant for many metabolic processes and for bone health. Around 85% of the body phosphorus is in bone in the form of hydroxyapatite. Phosphorus is essential for the release of oxygen and energy to the cell via high-energy compounds such as ATP and NADP. Phosphate excretion through the kidney is one of the mechanisms for regulating acid-base balance in the body.

Phosphorus shares similar homeostatic mechanisms with calcium. Parathyroid hormone (PTH) is the major regulator of the balance between phosphorus and calcium. PTH decreases high serum phosphate levels by reducing the renal reabsorption of phosphate and thus increasing its urinary excretion. The kidney is the major site for regulating the amount of phosphorus retained in the body.

Absorption, Transport, Storage and Excretion

Approximately 60% of dietary phosphorus is absorbed. Organically bound phosphate is hydrolyzed in the lumen of the intestine and released as inorganic phosphate, primarily through the action of pancreatic or intestinal phosphatases. Bioavailability depends on the form of the phosphate and the pH. The acidic milieu of the most proximal portion of the duodenum is important in maintaining phosphorus solubility and therefore bioavailability.

In vegetarian diet the major portion of the phosphorus exists as phytate, which is poorly digested by humans. Humans do not have the phytase enzyme to cleave the phosphorus from the phytate; however, intestinal becteria have the enzyme needed to hydrolyze phosphates. The yeast used in making bread contains a phytase, which releases phosphate.

The primary route of phosphorus excretion is renal, which also is the primary site of phosphate regulation. Major determinants of urinary phosphorus loss are increased intake of phosphate, an increase in phosphate absorption, and the plasma phosphorus concentration. Other factors contributing to increased urinary phosphate loss are hyperparathyroidism, acute respiratory or metabolic acidosis, the intake of diuretics, and the expansion of extracellular volume. If PTH levels are high, the urinary route excretes additional phosphate. Starvation or chronic under nutrition typically contributes to most of the alterations in metabolism that result in hypophosphatemia and renal losses of phosphate. Regulation of serum phosphate and hence urinary phosphate losses is not as precise as it is for calcium, but endogenous fecal phosphate excretion may be better regulated and provides a way to eliminate some of the excessive phosphate when PTH levels are elevated. The latter route of excretion may increase when the phosphate load in the blood and tissue is excessively high. Reduced phosphate excretion is associated with dietary phosphorus restriction; increases in plasma insulin, thyroid hormone, growth hormone, glucagon, or glucocorticoids; metabolic or respiratory alkalosis; and extracellular volume contraction.

Functions

Bone and Teeth Formation

Phosphate ions combine with calcium ions to form hydroxyapatite, the major inorganic molecule in teeth and bones. The bone mineral provides phosphate ions via homeostatic regulation of serum calcium by PTH.

ENERGY METABOLISM

Phosphorus contributes to the formation of high energy bond compounds such as ATP, ADP and creatine phosphate. These are required for phosphorylation of sugars in carbohydrate metabolism.

Absorption of Glucose and Glycerol

Phosphorus combines with glucose and glycerol to assist in their intestinal absorption. It also promotes renal tubular reabsorption of glucose to return this sugar to the blood.

Regulation of Acid-base Balance

Phosphate ions, hydrogen phosphate ions and dihydrogen phosphate ions are the major anions in blood plasma. These ions maintain acid base balance by combining with excess hydrogen ions when condition becomes too acidic and yet release hydrogen ions when a condition threatens to become too alkaline. The phosphate ions and phosphate containing compounds act as buffers against excessive variation in the pH level of fluids in body.

Deficiency

Phosphate deficiency is very rare, since there is widespread distribution of phosphorus in foods. But in conditions that occur in intestinal diseases such as sprue and celiac diseases, the phosphorus absorption is hindered which leads to low serum phosphorus level. In bone diseases such as rickets or osteomalacia, the calcium-phosphorus serum balance is disturbed. In primary hyperparathyroidism, in which the excess secretion of parathyroid hormone causes excess renal tubular excretion of phosphorus. Long-term administration of glucose or TPN without sufficient phosphate, excessive use of phosphate-binding antacids, hyperparathyroidism, or treatment of diabetic acidosis, those who have alcoholism with or without decompensated liver disease, develop hypophosphatemia. The consequences of severe phosphorus depletion reflect its ubiquitous role in body funcitons. Symptoms result primarily from decreased synthesis of ATP and other organic phosphate molecules. Neural, muscular, skeletal, hematologic, renal and other abnormalities occur (Table 5.2).

Table 5.2: ICMR recommended dietary allowance of calcium and phosphorus mg/day

Group	Calcium	Phosphorus
Men	400	400
Women	400	400
Pregnancy and lactation	1000	1000
Infants	500	750
Children 1–9 years	400	400
10–15 years	600	600
16–18 years	500	500

Sources

Practically all foods contain significant amount of phosphorus, although it is particularly abundant in protein-rich foods. Meat, fish, poultry, egg, dairy products and cereal products like rice are the primary sources of phosphorus in the average diet (Table 5.3).

Table 5.3: Causes of altered plasma phosphate levels

Condition	Mechanism
Hypophosphatemia	
Increased urinary excretion	Urinary loss, decreased replacement on IV therapy, acute alcoholism, vitamin D deficiency, hypophosphatemic rickets, kidney transplantation, volume expansion, renal tubular defects, metabolic or respiratory alkalosis, hyerpara-thyroidism, (decreased tubular reabsorption of phosphate)
Decreased intestinal absorption	Vitamin D deficiency, dietary phosphorus restriction (severe), antacid abuse (phosphate binding), chronic diarrhea
Phosphate Compartmentalization	Rapid shift of phosphate between body compartment, TPN Recovery from diabetic ketoacidosis, respiratory alkalosis, sepsis, refeeding syndrome, hormonal therapy (insulin, glucagon, corticosteroids), carbohydrate infusion (glucose, fructose, lactate)
Hyperphosphatemia	
Increased exogenous load	Feeding cow's milk to premature infants, IV infusion, oral supplements, vitamin D toxicity, phophate enemas
Increased endogenous load	Hemolysis, lactic acidosis, respiratory acidosis, rhabdomyolysis
Decreased urinary excretion	Renal failure, hypoparathyroidism, acromegaly, vitamin D toxicity, bisphosphonate therapy, magnesium deficiency
False (pseudo) hyperphosphatemia	Hemolysis in vitro, hypertriglyceridemia, multiple myeloma

IV, intravenous; TPN, total parenteral nutrition.

IODINE

Iodine is a nonmetallic halogen element required for the synthesis of thyroid hormone. The body contains 15 to 20 mg of iodine, 60% to 80% of which is in the thyroid gland. The concentration of inorganic iodine is low, and organic compounds are the usual circulating form (thyroxine, triiodothyronine, diiodotyrosine and monoiodotyrosine). Dietary iodine is needed for the synthesis of thyroid hormones.

Absorption, Transport, Storage and Excretion

Food contains mostly inorganic iodide, which is reduced in the gut lumen and nearly completely absorbed. Some iodinated compounds (e.g. thyroid hormones, amiodarone) are absorbed intact. Iodide passes easily across membranes, unlike other trace minerals. It is concentrated in the thyroid and salivary glands by the action of the sodium/iodide cotransporter. It is present in basolateral membranes of the thyroid, breast, colon and ovary. It is secreted as inorganic iodine in saliva and milk but only as the organic form from the thyroid.

The iodide pool is replenished from the diet, saliva, gastric juice, and the breakdown of organic thyroxine derivatives. The thyroid gland, kidneys and salivary and gastric glands all compete for free iodide. The thyroid must trap about 60 µg of iodide per day to maintain thyroxine levels.

If the hypothalamus detects a fall in the blood thyroxin level, it releases a substance known as thyroxine releasing factor (TRF) into the plasma. The TRF travels to the pituitary gland, where it stimulates, the release into plasma of a hormone called thyroid stimulating hormone (TSH) (Fig. 5.5).

The TSH is transported to the thyroid gland, where it stimulates the production of an enzyme that acts on thyroglobulin to release the iodine containing tyrosine residues from the protein. These residues are then

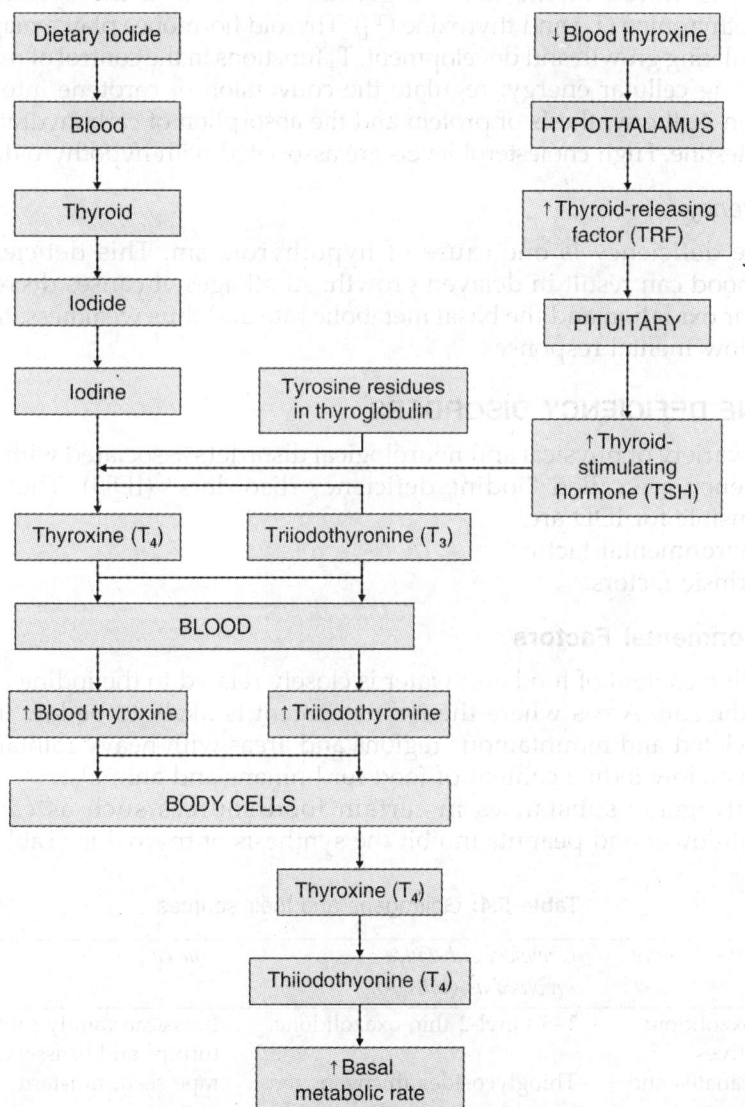

Fig. 5.5: Absorption and metabolism of iodine, including the synthesis of thyroxine and triiodothyronine.
Source: Guthric Helen A. and Mary Frances Picciano,1999, human nutrition, WCB

converted into the two thyroid hormones T_3 and T_4 which are released into blood plasma in a ratio of four T_4 molecules for each T_3 molecule.

Iodine is excreted as inorganic iodide. The major route of excretion is through kidneys. 40 to 80% is excreted in the urine. Some amount is also excreted by liver, skin, lungs, milk and saliva. Lesser amount is excreted in faeces.

Functions

Iodine is stored in the thyroid gland. It is used in the synthesis of triiodothyronine (T_3) and thyroxine (T_4). Thyroid hormones play a major role in regulating growth and development. T_4 functions in the control of reactions involving cellular energy: regulate the conversion of carotene into active vitamin A, the synthesis of protein and the absorption of carbohydrate from the intestine. High cholesterol levels are associated with hypothyroidism.

Deficiency

Iodine deficiency is one cause of hypothyroidism. This deficiency in childhood can result in delayed growth. At all ages, it causes decrease in cellular oxidation and the basal metabolic rate and thus weakness, fatigue, and slow mental responses.

IODINE DEFICIENCY DISORDERS

Wide variety of physical and neurological disorders associated with iodine deficiency are called "iodine deficiency disorders" (IDD). The factors responsible for IDD are
- Environmental factors
- Intrinsic factors.

Environmental Factors

- Iodine content of food and water is closely related to the iodine content of the soil. Areas where the iodine content is likely to be low include glaciated and mountainous regions and areas with heavy rainfall. This causes low iodine content of food for humans and animals.
- Goitrogenic substances in certain food sources such as cabbage, cauliflower and peanuts inhibit the synthesis of thyroxine (Table 5.4).

Table 5.4: Goitrogens and their sources

Name of substance	Chemical substance involved as goitrogen	Source
Thio-oxzolidone derivatives	1–5 vinyl-2 thio-oxazolidone.	Brassicae family-cabbages, turnips and Brussels sprouts
Thiocyanates and isothiocyanates	Thioglycosides thicoyanogens formed from cyanoglycosides.	rape seed, mustard.
Indolyl acetonitrile	1, 2, diethiacyclopentyl-4-ene-3-thione, phenolic glycoside.	Brassicae family, red skin of groundnut.

Intrinsic Factors

Rare congenital defects can occur in the hormone synthesis and secretion and peripheral resistance to thyroid hormones can also result in goitre.

Goitre

Very low iodine intakes are associated with the development of endemic or simple goitre, which is an enlargement of the thyroid gland. The direct stimulus of the enlargement is abnormally high level of thyroid stimulating hormones. The TSH causes an increase in both the number and size of the cells of the thyroid gland.

Lack of dietary iodine reduces negative feedback and leads to over-production of thyrotropin, which causes over-stimulation and swelling of the thyroid-goitre (Fig. 5.6).

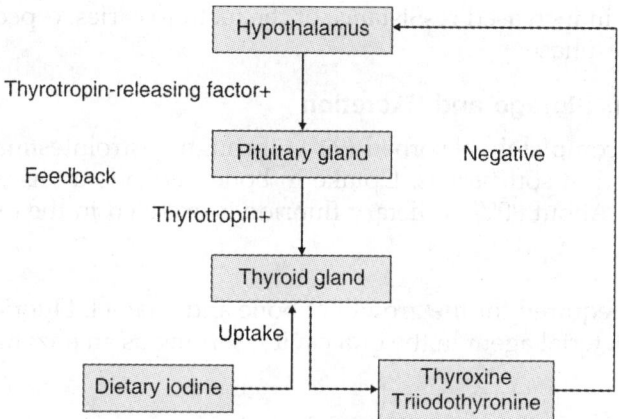

Fig. 5.6: The regulation of thyroid hormone output and the origins of goitre

The Goitre Grade

The new classification of goitre severity has recently been adopted by World Health Organization (Table 5.5).

Table 5.5: Proposed classification of goitre

Grade	Signs and symptoms
Grade 0	No palpable or visible goitre.
Grade 1	A mass in the neck that is consistent with an enlarged thyroid, that is palpable but not visible when the neck is in normal position. It moves upward in the neck as the subject swallows. Nodular alterations can occur even when the thyroid is not enlarged.
Grade 3	A swelling in the neck, that is visible when the neck is in a normal position and is consistent with an enlarged thyroid when the neck is palpated.

Source: Joint WHO/UNICEF/ICC/DD consultation (World Health Organization, 1994)

Cretinism

In children, iodine deficiency can lead to cretinism, a condition characterized by impaired mental and physical development.

Myxoedema

Myxoedema, a dry, waxy type of swelling (nonpitting edema) with abnormal deposits of mucin in the skin (mucinosis) and other tissues, associated with hypothyroidism.

FLUORIDE

Though fluoride is not an essential nutrient element, this anion is known to be important for the health of bones and teeth. The average skeleton contains 2.5 mg of fluoride. Fluoride is concentrated in bone and teeth, where it is incorporated into the crystalline structure of hydroxyapatite. This results in increased resSistance of the teeth to caries, especially in the pre-eruptive phase.

Absorption, Storage and Excretion

Fluoride is completely absorbed (90%) through gastrointestinal tract and is distributed in soft tissues. Uptake in bone depends on its growth and vascularity. About 80% of dietary fluoride is excreted in the urine.

Function

Fluoride is required for the growth of bone and enamel. Fluoride also acts as an antibacterial agent in the oral cavity, serving as an enzyme inhibitor.

Deficiency

Fluoride is present in almost all water supplies, plants, and animals, therefore deficiency do not occur. Moreover, no known metabolic function exists for fluoride.

Toxicity

Excessive intake of fluoride causes fluorosis.

Dental Fluorosis

The most common form of fluorosis is hypermineralization of tooth enamel from excessive systemic fluoride during the period of enamel development, but before tooth eruption. Dental fluorosis is characterized by mottling or pitting of the surface of the enamel which becomes bleached shouring chalky white patches in the initial stage. In later stages, the enamel becomes abnormally fragile and chips off.

Skeletal Fluorosis

When intake is too high for years, a syndrome including osteosclerosis, genuvalgum, kyphosis and spine stiffness can occur.

Food Source

The major dietary sources are drinking water. The water should contain >1 ppm of fluoride. The source of the food (where it is grown) is more important than the type, one exception is ocean fish. Tea is the other food naturally high in fluoride.

ZINC

The second most abundant "trace" mineral in the body, after iron is zinc. The body (adult) contains between 1.5 and 2.5 g of zinc.

Absorption, Transport and Excretion

About 20% to 30% of ingested zinc is absorbed, particularly in the proximal bowel. Both carrier-mediated and non-saturable diffusion components have been reported, but the former is more active when zinc intake is low. Zinc absorption is affected not only by the level of zinc in the diet but also by the presence of interfering substances, especially phytates. Protein-rich diet promotes zinc absorption. Zinc absorption is slightly higher during pregnancy and lactation. Copper and cadmium, high intake of iron, calcium, folic acid may also reduce the zinc absorption. On the other hand, high doses of zinc can impair absorption of iron from ferrous sulfate, the form usually found high in vitamin and mineral supplements.

Albumin is the major plasma carrier of zinc, and the amount of zinc transported in the blood depends not only on zinc but also on the availability of albumin, a transport protein for many mineral cations. Some zinc is transported by transferrin and by α_2-macroglobulin. The major route of excretion is in the faeces.

Deficiency

Acquired zinc deficiency may occur as a result of malabsorption, starvation or increased losses via urinary, pancreatic or other exocrine secretions.

- Overt zinc deficiency is rare and usually only seen in people with acrodermatitis enteropathica, a rare genetic disorder which causes impaired zinc absorption and results in severe skin lesions, hair loss and diarrhoea.
- Zinc deficiency causes a rapid decline in antibody and cell-mediated immune responses.
- *Zinc deficiency symptoms:* Growth retardation, delayed sexual maturation, hypoganadism and hypospermia, alopecia, delayed wound healing, skin lesions, impaired appetite, immune deficiencies, behavioural disturbances, eye lesions, including photophobia and night blindness, impaired taste (hypogeusia).

Toxicity

Very high doses have induced copper with sideroblastic anaemia. Large acute overdoses can produce nausea, vomiting, rash, dehydration and gastric ulceration.

A major form of zinc toxicity develops in patients receiving hemodialysis for renal failure. The toxic syndrome in these patients is characterized by anaemia, fever and central nervous system disturbances.

SODIUM

Sodium is one of the most plentiful minerals in the body. Sodium is the principal cation in extracellular fluid and plays a vital role in the regulation of fluid balance, blood pressure and transmembrane gradients. Sodium and chloride are mostly found together in foods, sodium chloride is the only mineral which takes in more or less pure form in addition to the amount present in natural foods.

About 120 mg (4 oz) is in the body of an adult, with one-third in the skeleton as inorganic bound material. The remaining two-third is free ionized sodium, the major electrolyte in body fluids outside the cells (extracellular fluids) (Table. 5.6).

Table 5.6: Sodium content of blood and muscle

Tissue	Sodium content	
	mg/100 ml	mEq[1]/litre
Whole blood	160	70
Plasma	330	143
Red blood cells	85	27
Muscle	60*	26*
	*per 100 g	*per kg

Intake

The daily intake of sodium in the form of (NaCl) sodium chloride in adults will vary from 5 to 20 g depending on climate. In temperate region, the NaCl intake may be from 5 to 8 g while in tropical countries, the intake ranges from 10 to 20 g. The intake of sodium from the foodstuff may range from 100 to 200 mg as the common foods are poor sources of sodium.

Absorption

Sodium intake is readily absorbed from the intestine. Normally only about 5% remains for elimination in the faeces, a large amount is lost in abnormal states such as diarrhoea.

Excretion

The total quantity of sodium excreted in urine, faeces and sweat is equal to the intake of sodium in normal individuals.

The minimum daily sodium need can be met by a daily intake of 250 mg of sodium (equivalent to 525 mg NaCl). Since the daily NaCl consumption is higher than the requirement, the excess NaCl consumed is excreted in urine.

The major route of excretion is through the kidney, under the powerful normal control of aldosterone, the sodium conserving form the adrenal glands.

FUNCTIONS OF SODIUM

Sodium ion exists in the body in association with Cl, BCO_3, phosphate, lactate and protein. Its functions are as follows:

Water Balance

The predominant cation of the ECF is Na^+, it makes up more than 90% of total base, and its concentration is 142 meq/l. The high concentration of Na^+ in the plasma and the relative impermeability of Na^+ ions across the cell wall membrane are important factors in controlling the distribution of water throughout the body. It is this function of Na^+ which makes it important in maintaining fluid balance. Drops of Na^+ in the serum will initiate loss of fluid from the body.

Cell Permeability

The sodium pump in all cell membranes helps exchange sodium and potassium and other cellular materials. A major substance carried into cells by this active transport system is glucose.

Muscle Action

Na^+ ions play a large part in transmitting electrochemical impulses along nerve and muscle membranes and help maintain normal muscle action. Potassium and sodium ions balance the response of nerves to stimulation. The travel of nerve impulses to muscle, and then result in contraction of the muscle fibre.

Sodium Requirement

The body can function on a rather wide range of dietary sodium by mechanisms designed to conserve or excrete the mineral. Thus there is no specific stated requirement. The body of a 70 kg man may contain between 3,600 and 4,200 mmol of sodium (83 and 97 g). About one-fourth of this, largely in skeleton, is not exchangeable. Exchangeable Na^+ averages 40 mmol per kg in males and 37 mmol per kg in females. This RDA standard estimates a minimum sodium requirement for healthy persons over age 18 to be about 500 mg/day to cover wide variations in individual patterns of physical activity and climate.

Food Sources

Cereals: Cereals are poor sources containing 4 to 18 mg/100 g. Some cereal products, e.g. bread, biscuits, and corn flakes are rich sources as NaCl is added to them during the processing.

Pulses: Pulses are moderate sources of sodium containing 29–95 mg/100 g.

Nuts and oilseeds: Nuts and oilseeds are poor to moderate sources (6 to 41 mg/100 g). Salted peanuts or cashew nut are rich sources of sodium.

Milk and milk products: Cow's milk is a good source of sodium containing about 50 mg/100 ml. One litre of milk will supply about 500 mg salted butter and processed cheese which are rich sources of sodium as NaCl is added to them during processing.

Egg, meat and fish: These foods are moderate sources of sodium. Cured pork and salted fish are very rich sources of sodium as salt is added to them during processing.

Vegetables: Vegetables are poor to fair sources of sodium (4 to 71 mg/100 g).

Fruits: Fruits are poor sources of sodium (1–3 mg/100 g).

Hyponatremia: When serum sodium level is below normal, the condition is called hyponatremia.

Severe hyponatremia will cause:
1. Severe dehydration.
2. Decrease in blood volume.
3. Decrease in blood pressure.
4. Circulatory failure.

Clinical conditions causing hyponatremia are:
1. Prolonged vomiting and diarrhoea resulting in excessive loss of digestive juice rich in sodium ion.
2. Chronic renal disease with acidosis due to poor reabsorption of sodium in the tubules.
3. Adrenocortical deficiency leading to Addison's disease.

Hypernatremia: When plasma sodium ion content is higher than the normal, then the condition is hypernatremia.

Hypernatremia occurs in:
1. Hyperactivity of adrenal cortex as in cushing's syndrome.
2. Prolonged treatment with cortisone, ACTH and sex hormones.

The symptoms of hypernatremia are:
1. Increased retention of water in the body.
2. Increased blood volume.
3. Increased blood pressure.

POTASSIUM

Potassium is about twice as plentiful as sodium in the body. It is present in small amount in the ECF (extra cellular fluids). An adult body contains about 270 mg (4000 mcg). About 90% of quantity is present in the cells of various tissues and RBC, remainder in the ECF (extra cellular fluids) (Table 5.7).

Table 5.7: Potassium content of blood and muscle

Tissue	Potassium content	
	mg/100 ml	mEq^1/litre
Whole blood	200	50
Plasma	20	5
Red blood cells	440	112
Muscle	250–400*	63–100*
	*per 100 g	*per kg
	1 mEq/litre K = mg/100 ml × 10/39	

Absorption

Dietary potassium is easily absorbed in the small intestine. Potassium also circulates in the gastrointestinal secretions, and is reabsorbed in the digestive process. However, disease such as prolonged diarrhoea causes dangerous losses.

Excretion

Urinary excretion is the principal route of potassium loss. There is excess loss with some diuretic drugs. Since maintainance of serum potassium within the narrow normal range is vital to heart muscle action and electrolyte balance, kidneys guard potassium carefully. However, they cannot guard potassium as effectively as sodium in the renal aldosterone mechanism for sodium conversion. Potassium is lost in exchange for sodium. The normal obligatory loss is about 160 mg/day. The normal kidney can adjust the amount of potassium excretion from 5 to 1000 meq/day.

PHYSIOLOGIC FUNCTION OF POTASSIUM

Water and Acid-base Balance

As the major guardian of cell water, potassium inside the cells balances with sodium outside the cells to maintain normal osmotic pressures and water and balance to protect cellular fluid potassium also works with sodium and hydrogen to maintain acid base balance.

Muscle Activity

Potassium plays a significant role in the activity of skeletal and cardiac muscle. Together with sodium and calcium, potassium regulates neuromuscular stimulation, transmission of electrochemical impulses, and contraction of muscle fibres. This effect is particularly notable in the action of heart muscle. Even small variations in serum potassium concentration are reflected in electrocardiographic (ECG) changes. Variations in serum levels or low serum potassium may cause muscle irritability and paralysis. The heart may even develop a gallop rhythm and finally cardiac arrest.

CARBOHYDRATE METABOLISM

When blood glucose is converted to glycogen for storage, 0.36 mmol of potassium is stored for each 1 g glycogen. When a patient with diabetic acidosis and treated with insulin and glucose, rapid glycogen production draws potassium from the serum. Serious hypokalemia can result unless adequate potassium replacement accompanies treatment.

Protein Synthesis

Potassium is required for the storage of nitrogen in muscle protein and general cell protein. When tissue is broken down, potassium is lost together with the nitrogen. Amino acid replacement includes potassium to ensure nitrogen retention.

Potassium Requirement

As with sodium, no specific dietary requirement is given for potassium. However, based on balance studies of the amount needed to replace losses and maintain normal body stores and plasma levels, the RDA standard estimates a minimum safe daily intake of adult will approximately 1,600 to 2,000 mg. In light of considerable evidence that dietary potassium has a beneficial effect on hypertension, in its report *Diet and health: Implications for reducing chronic disease risk*, the National Research Council has recommended an increase in potassium by eating more fruits and vegetables. The RDA has stated a safe and adequate range of daily potassium intake for adults of 1875 to 5625 mg. The usual diet contains about 2,000 to 4,000 mg/day which is ample for common need.

Food Sources

Legumes, whole grains, fruits such as orange and bananas, leafy green vegetable, broccoli, potatoes and meats supply considerable amount. People who eat large amount of fruits and vegetable have a high potassium intake of about 8 to 11 g/day, well about the minimum safe level of 2 g/day.

Hypokalemia: When serum potassium content is below normal, the condition is said to be hypokalemia. Prolonged hypokalemia is likely to cause injury to myocardium and kidneys.

The clinical conditions cause hypokalemia are:
- Prolonged diarrhoea and vomiting resulting in continued loss of digestive juices.
- Intravenous administration of potassium-free fluid to replace digestive juice loss by prolonged vomiting.
- Overactivity of adrenal cortex (cushing's syndrome) which causes increased excretion of body potassium in urine and thereby causing potassium deficiency.
- Prolonged use of diuretics.
- Hypokalemia may be developed during treatment of heart failure with digitalis.

- Hypokalemia may be developed during treatment of diabetic coma with insulin, since during the synthesis and storage of glycogen and of protein stimulated by insulin; potassium is quickly withdrawn from ECF and retained in tissues.
- Hypokalemia is a characteristic feature of rare disease called "Familial periodic paralysis". In this condition K is withdrawn from ECF and retained in the cells.

Symptoms: The symptoms of hypokalemia include muscular weakness, irritability, paralysis, tachycardia and dilation of the heart with gallop rhythm and changes in ECG of the heart.

Hyperkalemia: The signs and symptoms of hyperkalemia are cardiac and central nervous system (CNS) depression. The heart signs include bradycardia and low heart sounds followed by peripheral vascular collapse, leading to cardiac arrest. The other symptoms are mental confusion, weakness, numbness and flacid paralysis of extremities. Marked elevation of serum K occurs in patients in the following conditions

- Renal failures
- Severe dehydration
- Addison's disease due to decreased excretion of potassium by kidney
- Intravenous administration excessive amount of potassium salts (Table 5.8).

Table 5.8: Sodium, potassium and magnesium contents of some foods (mg/100 g)

Foodstuffs	Sodium	Potassium	Magnesium
Cereals:			
Barely	4	179	127
Maize (corn)	6	290	144
Rice, raw milled	3	110	48
Rice, parboiled milled	9	161	68
Wheat flour, refined	14	101	55
Wheat, whole	18	349	139
Cereal products:			
Bread (without salt)	10	64	38
Bread (with added NaCl)	420	46	27
Biscuits (with added NaCl)	520	67	42
Cornflakes (with added NaCl)	870	120	80
Pulses:			
Black gram dhal	75	643	185
Chick pea dhal	72	386	139
Cowpea	95	323	230

Contd.

Table 5.8: Sodium, potassium and magnesium contents of some foods (mg/100 g)
(Contd.)

Foodstuffs	Sodium	Potassium	Magnesium
Field bean	89	402	196
Green gram dhal	49	643	189
Lentil	29	402	94
Peas, dry	20	640	124
Oilseeds and nuts:			
Almonds	6	856	257
Cashew nut, roasted	41	425	126
Cashew nut, salted	428	422	129
Groundnut, roasted	24	686	156
Groundnut, salted	420	675	152
Milk and milk products:			
Butter, unsalted	4	25	10
Butter, salted	840	25	10
Cheese, processed	740	100	48
(with added salt)			
Milk, cow's	50	140	13
Milk, dried	420	1260	102
Eggs, meat and fish:			
Egg, hen (whole)	122	129	11
Meat (lamb)	70	290	21
Fish	61	304	24
Pork, raw	65	390	24
Pork, cured (with	930	326	200
NaCl added)			
Vegetable:			
Cabbage, raw	20	233	13
Carrots, raw	47	341	23
Cauliflower, raw	13	295	24
Potato, raw	4	503	22
Radish	18	322	15
Spinach	71	470	88
Fruits:			
Apple, raw	1	110	8
Cherries	2	191	12
Cranberry juice	1	60	9
Grapes	3	158	13
Grape fruit	1	136	12
Lemon	1	104	11
Orange	1	200	11
Papaya	3	234	12
Pears	2	130	7

COPPER

This trace element has frequently been called the iron twin. The two elements are metabolized in much the same way and share function as cell enzyme components. Heart and Elvehjem (1928) showed that copper is essential along with iron for curing iron deficiency anaemia.

ABSORPTION, METABOLISM, STORAGE AND EXCRETION

Copper absorption occurs in small intestine. Entry at the mucosal surface is facilitated by diffusion, and exit across the basolateral membrane is primarily by active transport, but facilitated transfer may also occur within the intestinal absorbing cells, copper ions are bound to metallothionein, with greater affinity than zinc or other ions. Some evidence suggests that the amount of copper absorbed is regulated by the amount of metallothionein in the mucosal cells. Net absorption of copper varies from 25% to 60%.

Approximately 90% of the copper in serum is incorporated into ceruloplasmin; the rest is bound loosely to albumin, transcuperin, and other proteins; free amino acids; and possibly histidine. Copper is transported in the blood to other tissue; primarily bound to albumin. It also exists in blood as ceruloplasmin, a functional protein that acts as an enzyme at the erythrocyte forming cells of the bone marrow. Serum copper and immunoreactive ceruloplasmin levels tend to be higher in women than in men; the serum copper concentration is greatest in the neonate and decreases gradually during the first year of life.

Copper bound to albumin in blood may serve as a temporary storage site for copper. In the liver copper binds to metallothionein, this serves as storage form, and is incorporated into ceruloplasmin and secreted into the plasma for the transport of copper to cells. Copper is also secreted from the liver as a component of bile, the major route of excretion of copper, once in the GI tract, copper become part of the pool that may be reabsorbed or excreted; depending on the body's need for copper. Biliary excretion increases in response to excessive intake of copper but may not be able to keep up with intake, allowing it to reach toxic levels. Small amount of copper are found in urine sweat and menstrual blood. Copper can be conserved by the kidney if necessary when substantial amounts are filtered through the glomeuruli and reabsorbed in the tubules.

Functions

Copper in blood exists in the form of copper protein complex, hemocuprin in red blood cells and ceruloplasmin in plasma. The role of copper in preventing anaemia may be due to an ability to assist the absorption of iron, stimulate the synthesis of the non-protein haeme or globin parts of haemoglobin or to release stored iron from ferritin in the liver. As part of a multi-functional enzyme called ceruloplasmin copper is involved in the oxidation of ferrous ions to ferric ions.

Copper plays an important role in the metabolism of fatty acids and in the formation of ribonucleic acid. Copper in the body is capable of binding bacterial toxins and increase the activity of antibiotics.

Copper is necessary for the maintenance of normal haemoglobin status and is also a part of many enzyme systems. Many physiological functions in mammals such as erythropoiesis, skeletal mineralization, connective tissue formation, myelin formation, and melanin pigments synthesis, oxidative phosphorylation and others are dependent on the availability of copper. These functions are accomplished by enzymes that either have copper as prosthetic groups or require the participation of copper for their activity. A few of the copper metallo enzymes and their respective physiological roles are as follows:

1. Tyrosine (required for melanin formation)
2. Uricase (in purine metabolism)
3. Cytochrome oxidase (electron transport)
4. Ferroxidase I (cerulo plasmin)
5. Ferroxidase II present in intestine, plasma bone marrow and liver (involved in the oxidation of ferrous iron to ferric form)

DEFICIENCY

Copper is widely distributed in natural foods, so a general dietary deficiency is rare. The only signs of copper deficiency found in adults are neutropenia and microcytic anaemia, but deficiency is very rare in adults; probably because copper accumulates in the liver throughout life in most individuals. Copper is stored in the liver, therefore, deficiency develops slowly as copper stores become depleted. Premature infants are likely to have copper deficiency unless given a copper supplement, because most of the copper is normally transferred across the placenta during the last few months of a full-term pregnancy.

Copper deficiency is characterized by anaemia, neutropenia, and skeletal abnormalities, especially demineralization. Other changes may also develop, including subperiosteal haemorrhages, hair and skin depigmentation and defective elastin formation. The failure of erythropoiesis as well as cerebral and cerebellar degeneration may lead to death. Neutropenia and leukopenia are the best early indicators of copper deficiency in children.

Menkes syndrome, also know as kinky-hair syndrome, results in copper malabsorption, increased urinary copper transport, all of which cause an abnormal distribution of copper among organs and within cells. Affected infants have retarded growth, defective keratinization and pigmentation of the hair, hypothermia, degenerative changes in aortic elastin, abnormalities of the metaphyses of long bones, and progressive mental deterioration. These infants typically do not survive first few months. Many defects exist in connective tissue in patients with Menkes syndrome.

TOXICITY

Copper poisoning occurs from contamination of foods with copper from containers or ingestion of higher quantities of copper salt. Symptoms of acute copper poisoning include excessive salivation, epigastric pain, nausea, vomiting and diarrhoea, consumption of milk based formula foods or weaning foods stored in brass containers may prove harmful. Liver failure is often associated with massive accumulation of liver copper.

Chronic copper toxicity is relatively rare but occurs in the hereditary condition called Wilson's disease. In this disease, failure to excrete copper in bile leads to accumulation of copper in the liver, brain, and kidneys.

CHROMIUM

Chromium content of adult body is estimated to be 6 mg. It is in all organic matter and appears to be an essential nutrient.

ABSORPTION, TRANSPORT, STORAGE AND EXCRETION

As with other minerals organic and inorganic forms of chromium are absorbed differently. Organic chromium is readily absorbed but quickly passes out of the body. Less than 2% of trivalent chromium consumed is absorbed. Chromium absorption is increased by oxalate and is higher in iron deficient animals than in animals with adequate iron, suggesting that it shares some similarities with the iron absorption pathway.

With dietary intake of 40 µg or more per day, chromium absorption reaches and remains at a plateau, at such high intakes urinary excretion increases to maintain balance. The type of dietary carbohydrate consumed modifies absorption from chromium chloride, whose absorption efficiency is 2% or less.

Chromium and iron are carried by transferrin, however, albumin is also capable of assuming this role if iron transferrin saturation is high. In addition, α and β globulin and lipoproteins can also bind chromium. Primarily the kidneys excrete inorganic chromium with small amount being excreted through hair, sweat and bile. (Organic chromium is excreted through bile.) Strenuous exercise, physical trauma, or as increased intake of simple sugar results in increased chromium excretion.

FUNCTION

Chromium potentiates insulin action and as such influences carbohydrate, lipid and protein metabolism. Although the chemical nature of the relationship between chromium and insulin activity has not been clearly identified, chromium may have a beneficial effect on serum triglyceride levels in patients with non-insulin dependent diabetes mellitus.

The proposed role of chromium with a so-called Glucose Tolerance Factor (GTF) is controversial. A possible chromium nicotinic acid (chromium polynicotinase) complex has been identified, but its structure has not been established by modern chemical techniques. Another possible role for chromium similar to that of zinc is in the regulation of gene expression.

DEFICIENCY

Chromium deficiency results in insulin resistance and a few lipid abnormalities, which can be ameliorated by chromium supplementation. Chromium was not accepted as an essential nutrient until 1977 however, when patients received TPN exhibited abnormalities of glucose metabolism (impaired glucose tolerance or hyperglycemia glycosuria) that were reversed by chromium supplementation.

TOXICITY

When chromium picolinate takes as a supplement on high doses by athletes and power lifters has resulted in some adverse effects, primarily skin lesions (Table 5.9).

Table 5.9: Summary of some macro minerals

Mineral	Metabolism	Physiologic function	Clinical application	Food source
Magnesium	Absorption according to intake load, hindered by excess fat, phosphate calcium, protein, excretion regulated by kidney.	Constituent of bones and teeth, coenzyme in general metabolism, smooth muscle action, neuro muscular irritability, cation in intracellular fluid.	Low serum level following gastrointestinal losses, tremor, spasm in deficiency induced by malnutrition, alcoholism.	Milk, cheese, meat seafood, whole grains, legumes, nuts.
Sodium	Readily absorbed, excretion chiefly by kidney, controlled by aldosterone.	Major cation in extracellular fluid, water balance, acid base balance. Cell membrane permeability, problems, muscle absorption of glucose.	Losses in gastrointestinal disorders, diarrhoea. Fluid electrolyte and base balance problems, muscle action, losses in tissue catabolism. Treatment of diabetic acidosis, rapid glycogen production reduces.	NaCl—salt sodium compounds in banking and processing milk, cheese meat, egg, carrots, beats, spinach, celery

Contd.

Table 5.9: Summary of some macro minerals (*Contd.*)

Mineral	Metabolism	Physiologic function	Clinical application	Food source
			serum potassium level. Losses with diuretic therapy.	
Potassium	Readily absorbed, secreted and reabsorbed in gastrointestinal circulation, excretion chiefly by kidney, regulated by aldosterone.	Major cation in intracellular fluid, water balance, acid-base balance, normal muscle irritability, glycogen formation, protein synthesis.	Losses in gastrointestinal disorder, diarrhoea, fluid electrolyte acid-base balance problems, muscle action.	Fruits, vegetables, legumes, nuts, whole grains, meat. Especially heat action.
Chlorine	Readily absorbed excretion controlled by kidney.	Major anion in extracellular fluid, water balance, acid-base balance, chloride-bicarbonate shift, gastric hydrochloride digestion.	Losses in gastrointestinal disorder, vomiting diarrhoea, tube drainage hypochloremic alkalosis.	NaCl—Salt
Sulphur	Elemental form absorbed as such, split from amino acid sources (Methionine and cystine in digestion and absorbed into portal circulation). Excreted by kidney in relation to protein intake and tissue catabolism.	Essential constituent of protein structure. Enzyme activity and energy metabolism through free sulphahydryl group (-SH). Detoxification reactions.	Cystine renal calculi, cystinuria	Meat, egg, milk, cheese, legumes, nuts

Source: Williams Sue Rodwell, 1985, nutrition and diet therapy, times mirror/mosby college publishing St. Louis.

IRON

Healthy adult men have about 3.6 g of total body iron, whereas women have about 2.4 g. Adult women have much lower amount of iron in storage than men do. Iron is highly conserved by the body. Approximately 90% is recovered and reused everyday. The rest is excreted, primarily in the bile. Dietary iron must be available to maintain iron balance to meet this 10% gap or else iron deficiency results.
* Forms of iron in the body
* Iron distribution in the body is given in Table 5.10.

Table 5.10: Distribution and turnover of iron in adult human body

Type of iron	Quantity (mg)	As % of total iron in the body
Total iron in the body	4000	100
Haemoglobin iron	3000	75
Ferritin iron (storage iron)	750	20
Transferrin (transport iron)	3 (normal) 9 (max. capacity)	–
Myoglobin (in muscle) iron	150	4
Cytochrome and other iron containing enzymes	6	–
Iron turnover in the body per day	20–25	–
Iron absorption from the intestines per day	2–3	–

TRANSPORT IRON

A trace of iron 0.05 to 0.18 mg/day, is in plasma bound to its transport carrier protein transferrin (2 Fe + globulins).

IRON PORPHYRIN COMPOUNDS (HAEME COMPOUNDS)

Most of body's iron is about 70%, occurs in red blood cells as a vital constituent of the haeme portion of haemoglobin. Another 5% is a part of the muscle oxygen carrying haemoglobin, and myoglobin.

STORAGE IRON

About 20% of the body iron is stoned as the protein iron compound ferritin (4 FeOOH n + globulin) mainly in liver, spleen and bone marrow. Excess iron as stored in the body as haemosiderin (ferric hydroxide + non-nitrogenous compound) interchanging with ferritin as needed.

CELLULAR TISSUES IRON

The remaining 5% of body iron is distributed throughout cell as major component of oxidative enzyme system for the production of energy. Haeme enzyme: Mithochondrial cytochromes, microsomal cytochrome, catalase, peroxidase. Flauin enzymes: Suceinic dehydrogenase, xanthine oxidase, DPNH-cytochrome C reductase, iron chelate enzyme acconitase.

ABSORPTION, TRANSPORT AND STORAGE

The main control of the body's iron balance is at the point of intestinal absorption dietary iron enters the body in 2 forms—haeme and non-haeme. By far the large portion is non-haeme—all plant sources plus 60% of animal sources. But it is absorbed at the much slower rate than the smaller haeme portion, because non-haeme iron is highly bound in its food sources to organic moleculer in the form of ferric iron (Fe^{+++}). In the acidic medium of the stomach, it must be dissociated and reduced to the more soluble ferrous iron (Fe^{++}). This is a source of nutritional concern because of non-haeme's greater quantity in the diet (Fig. 5.7).

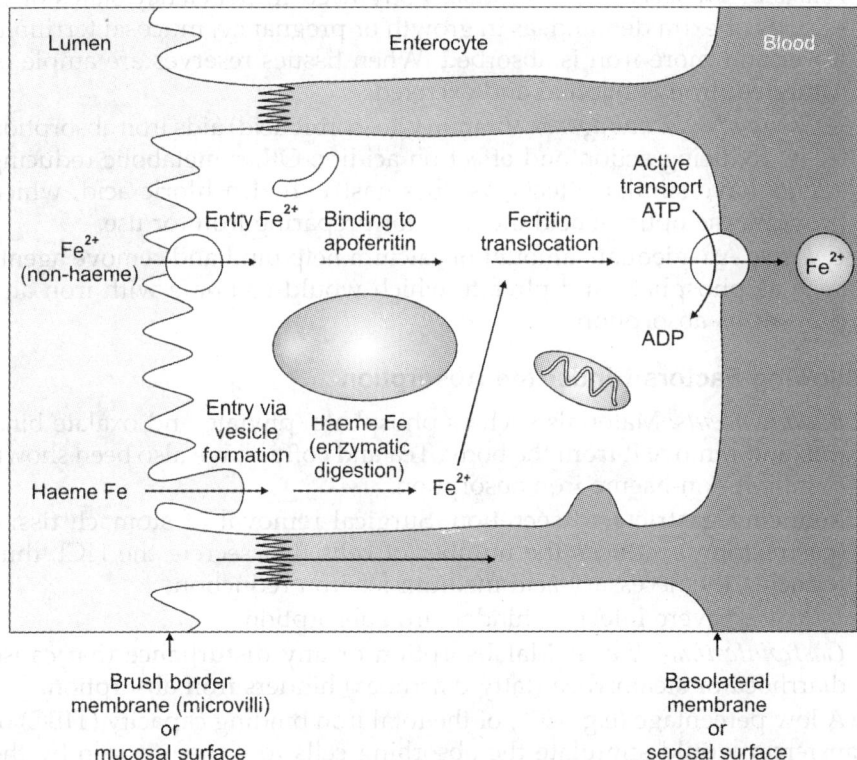

Fig. 5.7: Intestinal absorption of iron from haeme and non-haeme sources by an intestinal absorbing cell or enterocyte. Enterocytes contain two membranes—the brush border membrane and the basolateral membrane. The entry step of non-haeme iron at the brush border membrane is different from that of haeme iron. Haeme iron enters by vesicle formation around the haeme, whereas non-haeme iron (ionic iron) enters by facilitated diffusion down a concentration gradient. Absorbed ions combine with apoferritin to form ferritin complexes that move across the cell by diffusion to the basolateral membrane for the exit step of absorption by active transport. The iron of haeme iron is enzymatically removed, and these ions exit at the basolateral membrane by an unknown mechanism. (*ATP*, Adenosine triphosphate; *ADP*, adenosine disphosphate.)

Haeme iron (i.e. the intact ferroporphyrin ring) is absorbed areas the brush border (mucosa) of intestinal absorbing cells (enterocytes) after it is digested from animal sources. After haeme enters into cytosol, the ferrous iron is enzymatically removed from the ferroporphyrin complex. The free iron ions combine immediately with apoferrtin to form ferritin in the same way that free non-haeme iron combine with apoferritin. Ferritin is an intracellular store and a ferry that carries bound iron from the brush border to the basolater membrane of the absorbing cell. The final step of absorption by which iron ions are moved into the blood occurs at basolateral membrane of the absorbing cell and involves an active transport mechanism.

FACTORS AFFECTING ABSORPTION

1. *Following are favouring absorption:* Body need in deficiency states or in periods of extra demand, as in growth or pregnancy, mucosal ferritin is lower and more iron is absorbed. When tissues reserves are ample or saturated, iron is rejected and excreted.
2. *Acidity and reduction agents:* Vitamin C (ascorbic acid) aids iron absorption by its reducing action and effect on acidity. Other metabolic reducing agents have similar effects, as does gastric hydrochloric acid, which provides the optimal acid medium for preparing iron for use.
3. *Calcium:* An adequate amount of calcium help bind and remove agents such as phosphate and phytate which would combine with iron and prevent its absorption.

Following Factors Hinder the Absorption

1. *Binding agents:* Materials such as phosphate, phytate and oxalate bind iron and remove it from the body. Tea and coffee have also been shown to inhibit non-haeme iron absorption.
2. Reducing gastric acid secretion: Surgical removal of stomach tissue (gastrectomy) reduces the number of cells that secrete the HCl, thus reducing the necessary acid medium for iron reduction.
3. *Infection:* Severe infection hinders iron absorption.
4. *Gastrointestinal disease:* Malabsorption or any disturbance that cause diarrhoea or steatorrhea (fatty diarrhoea) hinders iron absorption.

A low percentage (e.g. 15%) of the total iron binding capacity (TIBC) of transferrin would stimulate the absorbing cells to transport iron by the exit step at the basolateral membrane to the blood. Some researchers suggest that the amount of transferrin receptors on the basolateral membranes of the absorbing cells can be increased (i.e. up-regulated) to permit more transport of iron to awaiting transferrin molecules, each of which has the capacity to bind two iron ions (atoms). At low saturations, more vacancies are available on the transferrin molecules to take up iron and carry it to the bone marrow and other tissues to meet their needs. Conversely, if the iron concentration in the body is excessive, the TIBC may approach 40% to 50%, in which case the absorbing cells would be down-regulated, and less iron would be allowed to be absorbed. The latter situation occurs during iron overload to protect the body against toxicity.

Transport

As we seen in the mucosal cells of the duodenum and proximal jejunum, iron is oxidized and bound with the plasma transferrin for transport of body cells. Normally only about 20 to 35% of the iron binding capacity of transferrin filled. The remaining capacity forms an unsaturated plasma reserve for handling variances in iron intake.

Storage

Bound to plasma transferrin, iron is delivered to its storage sites in bone marrow and to some extent in the liver. Here it is transferred to apoferritin again to form ferritin for storage and use as needed in synthesizing haemoglobin for red blood cells. This binding with apoferritin provides a stable exchangeable storage form for the body needs. Between 200 and 1,500 mg of iron is stored in the liver, 30% is in bone marrow and the rest is found in the spleen and muscle up to 20 mg is used in haemoglobin synthesis for storage.

Excretion

Iron is only lost from the body through bleeding and in very small amount through defecation, sweat and the normal exfoliation of hair and skin. Most of iron lost in the faeces could not be absorbed from food. The remainder comes from bile and the cells exfoliated from the GI epithelium. Almost no iron is excreted in the urine. Daily iron loss is approximately 1mg for men and slightly less for nonmenstruating women. The loss of iron accompanying menstruation over ages about 0.5 mg/day. However, wide variations exist among individuals, and menstrual losses of more than 1.4 mg of iron daily have been reported in approximately 5% of normal women (Fig. 5.8).

Function

The function of iron is related to its ability to participate in oxidation and reduction reaction chemically, iron is a highly reactive element that can interact with oxygen to form intermediates with the potential of damaging cell membranes or degrading DNA. Iron must be tightly bound to proteins to prevent these potentially destructive oxidative effects.

CO-FACTOR OF ENZYMES AND OTHER PROTEINS

It is an active component of the cytocromes (enzymes) involved in the process of cellular respiration and energy (ATP) generation. Iron also seems to be involved in immune function and congenitive performance,

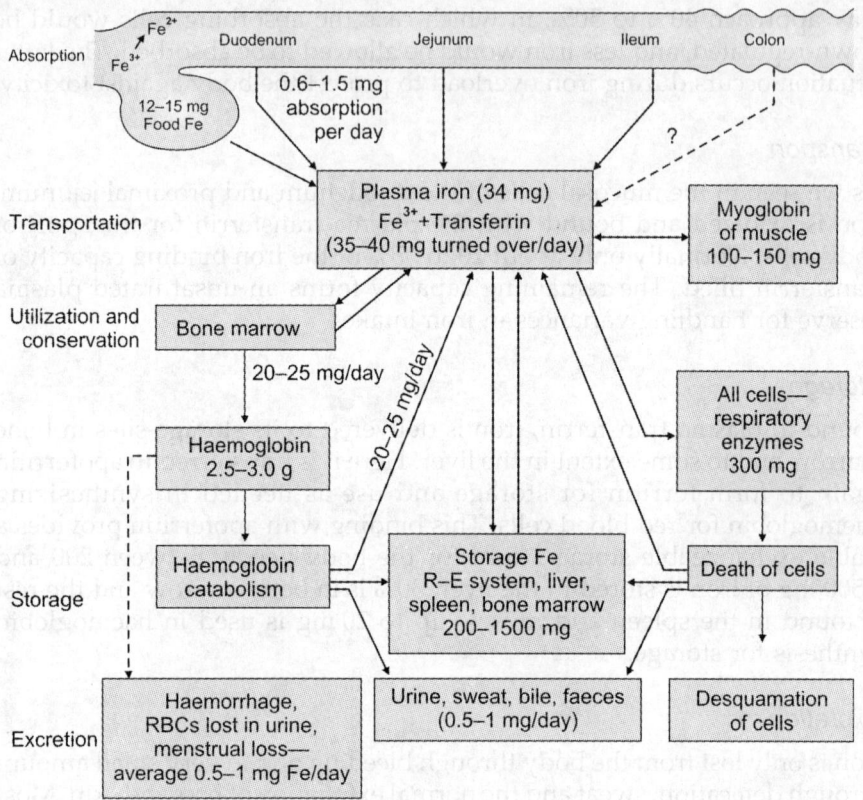

Fig. 5.8: Iron metabolism in adults. Most iron is absorbed from the duodenum and jejunum, after which it is transported as plasma iron or bound to transferrin. (*RBCs*, Red blood cells; *R-E system*, reticuloendothelial system)

Oxidative production of ATP within the mitochondria involves many haeme and non-haeme iron containing enzymes. The cytocromes present in almost all cells, function in the mitochondrial respiratory chain in the transfer of eletrons and the storage of energy through the alternative oxidation and reduction (redox) of iron ($Fe^{2+++} \leftrightarrow Fe^{3+++}$).

ACTIVITIES OF IRON CONTAINING ENZYMES

1. Conversion of β carotene to active form of vitamin A.
2. Synthesis of purines, which form an integral part of deoxyribonucleic acid and ribonucleic acid.
3. Synthesis of carnitine like substance needed for tansport of fatty acids.
4. Synthesis of collagen, one of the proteins of the body.
5. Detoxification of drugs and other toxic compounds in the liver and intestine.
6. Synthesis of the neurotransmitter dopamine, serotonin and norepinephrine.
7. Essential for catecholamine metabolism.

TRANSPORT AND STORAGE OF OXYGEN

Due to iron oxidation reduction (redox) properties iron has a role in blood and respiratory transport of (O_2) and CO_2. Haemoglobin works in two ways:

1. The iron containing haeme combines with oxygen in the lungs and
2. The haeme releases the oxygen in tissues, where it picks up carbon dioxide and the releases it in the lungs after its return from the tissue. Myoglobin also a haeme containing protein serves as an oxygen reservoir within muscle.

FORMATION OF RED BLOOD CELLS

Bone marrow produces immature cells known as erythroblasts. As erythroblasts in the bone marrow, many synthesise the iron containing haeme growth in a process requiring the help of vitamin B_{12} and copper. The haeme group becomes bound to globin moleclules, also synthesised by the erythroblasts, to form completed haemoglobin molecules. The haemoglobin containing cells are known as reticulocytes and are released from the bone marrow into the blood. Within 24 to 36 hours after their release, the nuclei of the reticulocytes disintegrate and the cells become mature erythrocytes ready to being the transport of O_2 to the tissues and that of CO_2 away from the tissues (Fig. 5.9).

Because a red blood cell has no nuclei, it cannot produce the enzyme and protein necessary for long term survival. The life of RBC is 120 days. When RBC die, they are removed from blood by cells of the liver, bone

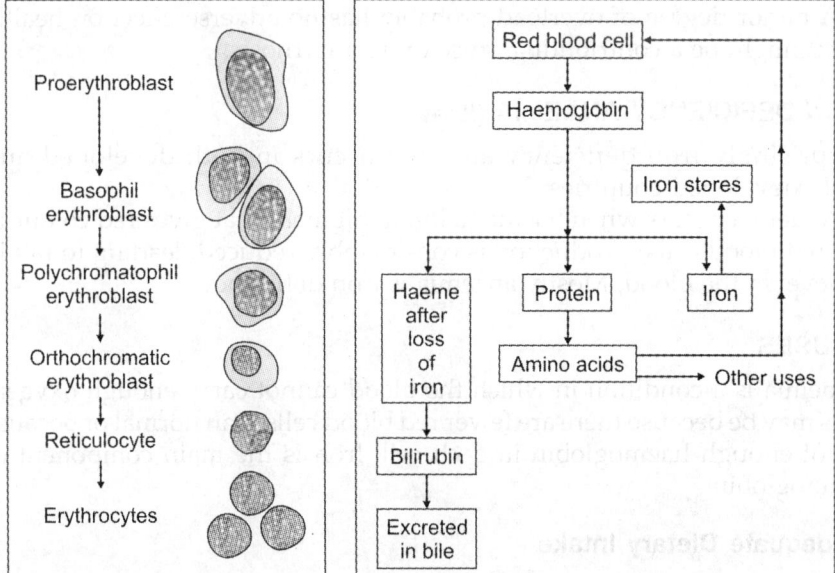

Fig. 5.9: Genesis and destruction of red blood cell

marrow and spleen which are part of the reticuloendothelial system. In the spleen, the iron and amino acid derived from haemoglobin are slavaged recycled. The iron is stored as haemosiderin and ferritin in the liver and spleen or is returned to the bone marrow for incorporation into new haemoglobin molecules. In this way iron is effectively conserved and reused. The amino acids are released to the blood, where they are available to all cells for the synthesis of new proteins or for the oxidative release of bilirubin, which is transported to the liver and then excreted in bile.

Toxicity

Haemochromatosis

It is an inborn error of metabolism. There is a failure to control iron absorption from the small intestine. The excess iron is then deposited in the tissues. The characteristic features are an enlarged and cirrhotic liver, pancreatic diabetes, as slate gray discolouration of the skin and hypogonadism probably secondary to iron deposition in the pituitary. The disease is fatal if the iron content in the body is not reduced.

Siderosis

In siderosis nutritional iron overload occurs due to high iron intake usually over 100 mg/day. Such intakes are usually not by iron originally present in food due to adventitious iron from iron vessels used in cooking and more frequently in the preparation of alcoholic beverages. The condition is common in Bantu population of Johannesburg who drink bear brewed from maize or sorghum in iron vessels. Siderosis is common among people who drink cheap wines made from iron vessels.

A minor degree of overload probably has no adverse effect on health, but it might be a contributing cause of liver cirrhosis.

IRON DEFICIENCY ANAEMIA (IDA)

Surprisingly iron deficiency anaemia occurs in both developed and underdeveloped countries.

Anaemia occurs when haemoglobin (a pigment that gives red colour to the red blood cells) production is considerably reduced, leading to fall in its level in the blood. Mostly anaemia is iron deficiency.

CAUSES

Anaemia is a condition in which the blood cannot carry enough oxygen. This may be because there are fewer red blood cells than normal or because is not enough haemoglobin in each cell. Iron is the main component of haemoglobin.

Inadequate Dietary Intake

The most cause of anaemia is dietary inadequacy of iron. In Indian communities such as vegetarian lifestyle with insufficient haeme iron causes iron deficiency anaemia. Studies have shown that iron absorption range 2–6%, depending upon the type of cereals in the diet. Phytates and tannins present in Indian diet interfere with iron absorption to a significant extent. The chemical determined iron content of the Indian diets is apparently high (15 mg/1000 calories), but 30% is unabsorbable contaminant iron. The true dietary iron content is, therefore, only 10 mg/1000 calories, which can meet the iron requirement of adult men and children less than 6 years, provide their dietary intake meets the energy requirements.

BLOOD LOSS

When you lose blood, you lose iron. If you do not have enough iron stored in your body to make up for the lost iron, you will develop iron-deficiency anaemia.

In women, long or heavy menstrual periods or bleeding fibroids in the uterus may cause low iron levels. Blood loss that occurs during childbirth is another cause of low iron levels in women.

Internal bleeding (bleeding inside the body) also may lead to iron-deficiency anaemia. This type of blood loss is not always obvious, and it may occur slowly. Some causes of internal bleeding are:

- A bleeding ulcer, colon polyp, or colon cancer
- Regular use of aspirin or other pain medicines, such as non-steroidal anti-inflammatory drugs (for example, ibuprofen and naproxen)
- Urinary tract bleeding

Blood loss from severe injuries, surgery, or frequent blood drawings also can cause iron-deficiency anaemia.

Inability to Absorb Enough Iron

Even if you have enough iron in your diet, your body may not be able to absorb it. This can happen if you have intestinal surgery (such as gastric bypass) or a disease of the intestine (such as Crohn's disease or celiac disease).

Prescription medicines that reduce acid in the stomach also can interfere with iron absorption.

Inadequate Utilization

This can take place secondary to chronic gastrointestinal disturbances, defective release of iron from stores into the plasma and defective iron utilization owing to a chronic inflammation or other chronic disorder.

Increased Demand

An increased iron requirement and increased red blood cell production is required when the body is going through changes such as growth spurts in children and adolescents, or during pregnancy and lactation. The body needs more iron when a large amount of cell divisions occur in pregnancy and during periods of rapid childhood growth.

Prevalent People

Infants and Young Children

- Infants and young children need a lot of iron to grow and develop. The iron that full-term infants have stored in their bodies is used up in the first 4 to 6 months of life.
- Premature and low-birth-weight babies are at even greater risk for iron-deficiency anaemia. These babies do not have as much iron stored in their bodies as full-term infants.
- Iron-fortified baby food or iron supplements, when used properly, can help prevent iron-deficiency anaemia in infants and young children.
- Young children who drink a lot of cow's milk may be at risk for iron-deficiency anaemia. Milk is low in iron, and too much milk may take the place of iron-rich foods in the diet. Too much milk may also prevent children's bodies from absorbing iron from other foods.
- Children who have lead in their blood also may be at risk for iron-deficiency anaemia. Lead can interfere with the body's ability to make haemoglobin. Lead may get into the body from breathing in lead dust, eating lead in paint or soil, or drinking water that contains lead.

Teens

- Teens are at risk for iron-deficiency anaemia if they are underweight or have chronic illnesses. Teenage girls who have heavy periods also are at increased risk for the condition.

Women

- Women of childbearing age are at higher risk for iron-deficiency anaemia because of blood loss during their monthly periods. About 1 in 5 women of childbearing age has iron-deficiency anaemia.
- Pregnant women also are at higher risk for the condition because they need twice as much iron as usual. The extra iron is needed for increased blood volume and for the fetus' growth.
- About half of all pregnant women develop iron-deficiency anaemia. The condition can increase a pregnant woman's risk for a premature or low-birth-weight baby.

Adults Who Have Internal Bleeding

Adults who have internal bleeding, such as intestinal bleeding, can develop iron-deficiency anaemia due to blood loss. Certain conditions, such as colon cancer and bleeding ulcers, can cause blood loss. Some medicines, such as aspirin, also can cause internal bleeding.

Other At-Risk Groups

- People who get kidney dialysis treatment may develop iron-deficiency anaemia. This is because blood is lost during dialysis. Also, the kidneys are no longer able to make enough of a hormone that the body needs to produce red blood cells.
- People who have gastric bypass surgery also may develop iron-deficiency anaemia. This type of surgery can prevent the body from absorbing enough iron.

Certain eating patterns or habits may put one at higher risk for iron-deficiency anaemia. This can happen if one:

- Follows a diet that excludes meat and fish, which are the best sources of iron. However, vegetarian diets can provide enough iron if you eat the right foods. For example, good nonmeat sources of iron include iron-fortified breads and cereals, beans, tofu, dried fruits, and spinach and other dark green leafy vegetables.
- Eats poorly because of money, social, health, or other problems.
- Follows a very low-fat diet over a long time. Some higher fat foods, like meat, are the best sources of iron.
- Follows a high-fibre diet. A large amount of fibre can slow the absorption of iron.

Diagnosis

Diagnostic Tests and Procedures

Many tests and procedures are used to diagnose iron-deficiency anaemia. They can help confirm a diagnosis, look for a cause, and find out how severe the condition is.

Complete Blood Count

Often, the first test used to diagnose anaemia is a complete blood count (CBC). The CBC measures many parts of blood. This test checks haemoglobin and haematocrit levels. Haemoglobin is an iron-rich protein in red blood cells that carries oxygen to the body. Haematocrit is a measure of how much space red blood cells take up in blood. A low level of haemoglobin or haematocrit is a sign of anaemia.

The normal range of these levels varies in certain racial and ethnic populations. The CBC also checks the number of red blood cells, white blood cells, and platelets in blood. Abnormal results may be a sign of infection, a blood disorder, or another condition.

Finally, the CBC looks at mean corpuscular volume (MCV). MCV is a measure of the average size of red blood cells. The results may be a clue as to the cause of anaemia. In iron-deficiency anaemia, for example, red blood cells usually are smaller than normal.

Other Blood Tests

If the CBC results confirm anaemia, need other blood tests to find out what is causing the condition, how severe it is, and the best way to treat it.

Reticulocyte count: This test measures the number of reticulocytes in blood. Reticulocytes are young, immature red blood cells. Over time, reticulocytes become mature red blood cells that carry oxygen throughout the body. A reticulocyte count shows whether bone marrow is making red blood cells at the correct rate.

Peripheral smear: If iron-deficiency anaemia presents, red blood cells will look smaller and paler than normal.

Tests to measure iron levels: These tests can show how much iron has been used from body's stored iron. Tests to measure iron levels include:

- Serum iron: This test measures the amount of iron in blood. The level of iron in blood may be normal even if the total amount of iron in body is low. For this reason, other iron tests are also done.
- Serum ferritin: Ferritin is a protein that helps store iron in body. A measure of this protein helps doctor find out how much of body's stored iron has been used.
- Transferrin level or total iron-binding capacity: Transferrin is a protein that carries iron in blood. Total iron-binding capacity measures how much of the transferrin in blood is not carrying iron. If iron-deficiency anaemia presents, then it shows a high level of transferrin that has no iron.

Clinical Findings

The signs and symptoms of iron-deficiency anaemia depend on its severity. Mild to moderate iron-deficiency anaemia may have no signs or symptoms. When signs and symptoms do occur, they can range from mild to severe. Many of the signs and symptoms of iron-deficiency anaemia apply to all types of anaemia.

Signs and Symptoms of Anaemia

- The most common symptom of all types of anaemia is fatigue (tiredness). Fatigue occurs because body does not have enough red blood cells to carry oxygen to its many parts. Also, the red blood cells that body makes have less haemoglobin than normal. Haemoglobin is an iron-rich protein in red blood cells. It helps red blood cells carry oxygen from the lungs to the rest of the body.
- Anaemia also can cause shortness of breath, dizziness, headache, coldness in hands and feet, pale skin, and chest pain.
- If don't have enough haemoglobin-carrying red blood cells, heart has to work harder to move oxygen-rich blood through body. This can lead to irregular heartbeats called arrhythmias (ah-RITH-me-ahs), a heart murmur, an enlarged heart, or even heart failure.

- In infants and young children, signs of anaemia include poor appetite, slow growth and development, and behavioural problems.

Signs and Symptoms of Iron Deficiency

- Signs and symptoms of iron deficiency may include brittle nails, swelling or soreness of the tongue, cracks in the sides of the mouth, an enlarged spleen, and frequent infections.

- People who have iron-deficiency anaemia may have an unusual craving for nonfood items, such as ice, dirt, paint, or starch. This craving is called pica.

- Some people who have iron-deficiency anaemia develop restless legs syndrome (RLS). RLS is a disorder that causes a strong urge to move the legs. This urge to move often occurs with strange and unpleasant feelings in the legs. People who have RLS often have a hard time sleeping.

- Iron-deficiency anaemia can put children at greater risk for lead poisoning and infections.

- Some signs and symptoms of iron-deficiency anaemia are related to the condition's causes. For example, a sign of intestinal bleeding is bright red blood in the stools or black, tarry-looking stools.

- Changes in structure and function of epithelial tissue: Mostly tongue, nails, mouth, and stomach are affected. The skin may appear pale and thin inside the lower eye lid, may be light pink instead of red. Finger nails can become thin and flat and eventually koilonychias (spoon-shaped nails) develops. Mouth changes include atrophy of the lingual papillae, burning redness and in severe cases a completely smooth waxy and glistening appearance to the tongue (glossitis). Angular stomatitis and dysphagia may occur. Gastritis occurs frequently and may result in achloryhydria. A progressive untreated anaemia results in cardiovascular and respiratory changes that can eventually lead to cardiac failure.

A heavy menstrual bleeding, long periods, or other vaginal bleeding may suggest that a woman is at risk for iron-deficiency anaemia.

Treatment

- Treatment for iron-deficiency anaemia will depend on its cause and severity. Treatments may include dietary changes and supplements, medicines, and surgery.

- Severe iron-deficiency anaemia may require a blood transfusion, iron injections, or intravenous (IV) iron therapy. Treatment may need to be done in a hospital.

- The goals of treating iron-deficiency anaemia are to treat its underlying cause and restore normal levels of red blood cells, haemoglobin, and iron.

Supplements

Iron

- May need iron supplements to build up iron levels as quickly as possible. Iron supplements can correct low iron levels within months. Supplements come in pill form or in drops for children. Oral administration of inorganic iron in the ferrous form—ferrous sulphate 50–200 mg (60 mg elemental iron) 3 times daily for adults and 6 mg/kg for children.
- A large amount of iron can be harmful, so should take iron supplements only as doctor prescribes. Keep iron supplements out of reach from children. This will prevent them from taking an overdose of iron.
- Iron supplements can cause side effects, such as dark stools, stomach irritation, and heartburn. Iron can also cause constipation, so doctor may suggest to use a stool softener.
- The body tends to absorb iron from meat better than iron from nonmeat foods. However, some nonmeat foods also can help to raise iron levels.
- An improvement in riboflavin status may stimulate iron absorption and turnover to affect an increase in iron store and help in the release of iron from ferritin.

Vitamin C

- Vitamin C helps the body absorb iron. Good sources of vitamin C are vegetables and fruits, especially citrus fruits. Fresh and frozen fruits, vegetables, and juices usually have more vitamin C than canned ones.
- If taking medicines, ask doctor or pharmacist whether can eat grapefruit or drink grapefruit juice. Grapefruit can affect the strength of a few medicines and how well they work.

Treatment to Stop Bleeding

- If blood loss is causing iron-deficiency anaemia, treatment will depend on the cause of the bleeding. For example, if one has a bleeding ulcer, doctor may prescribe antibiotics and other medicines to treat the ulcer.
- If a polyp or cancerous tumor in intestine is causing bleeding, may need surgery to remove the growth.
- If one has heavy menstrual flow, doctor may prescribe birth control pills to help reduce monthly blood flow. In some cases, surgery may be advised.

Treatments for Severe Iron-deficiency Anaemia

Blood Transfusion

- If iron-deficiency anaemia is severe, one may get a transfusion of red blood cells. A blood transfusion is a safe, common procedure in which blood is given through an IV line in blood vessels. A transfusion requires careful matching of donated blood with the recipient's blood.

- A transfusion of red blood cells will treat anaemia right away. The red blood cells also give a source of iron that body can reuse. However, a blood transfusion is only a short-term treatment. Doctor will need to find and treat the cause of anaemia.

Iron Therapy

- If one has severe anaemia, doctor may recommend iron therapy. For this treatment, iron is injected into a muscle or an IV line in blood vessels.
- IV iron therapy presents some safety concerns. It must be done in a hospital or clinic by experienced staff. Iron therapy usually is given to people who need iron long-term but cannot take iron supplements by mouth. This therapy also is given to people who need immediate treatment for iron-deficiency anaemia.

Prevention

Dietary changes: The absorption of haeme iron is better than that of non-haeme iron.

- The best source of iron is red meat, especially beef and liver. Chicken, turkey, pork, fish, and shellfish also are good sources of iron. Examples of nonmeat foods that are good sources of iron include:
  - Iron-fortified breads, cereals, and whole grains.
  - Peas; lentils; white, red, and baked beans; soybeans; and chickpeas
  - Tofu
  - Dried fruits, such as dates, raisins, and apricots
  - Spinach and other dark green leafy vegetables
  - Prune juice
  - Jaggery
- The nutrition facts labels on packaged foods will show how much iron the items contain. The amount is given as a percentage of the total amount of iron need everyday.
- Vitamin C rich foods increase iron absorption. Citrus fruits include oranges, grapefruits, guava, amla and similar fruits.
- Other fruits rich in vitamin C include kiwi fruit, strawberries, and cantaloupes.
- Vegetables rich in vitamin C include broccoli, peppers, Brussels sprouts, tomatoes, cabbage, potatoes, and leafy green vegetables like turnip greens and spinach.

Supplementation

- Under Reproductive and Child Health Programme (1997), young children and adolescent girls are given iron and folic acid.
- Children 6–24 months old are at the high risk of the irreversible long-term consequences of iron deficiency, namely impaired physical and mental development. They are given 20 mg of elemental iron and 100 µg of folic acid.

- Adolescent girls on attaining menarche should consume weekly dosage of one IFA tablet containing 100 mg elemental iron and 500 µg of folic acid.
- All pregnant mothers are given 60 mg of elemental iron and 500 µg of folic acid.

Fortification

- Iron fortification is done for many items made from refined grains as iron is lost in processing. Pasta, white rice, enriched breads, ready-to-eat breakfast cereals, oatmeal and enriched grits are typically iron-fortified. Iron-enrichment levels vary from brand to brand, but most products contain at least 25% of the recommended dietary allowance for iron.
- Fortification with iron has been successfully tried for wheat flour, sugar, milk, fish sauce and curry powder too.

Salt is considered as an eminently suitable vehicle for iron fortification in India as it satisfies all the criteria for an ideal vehicle. Salt is consumed in India by all segments of population, rich as well as poor, perhaps more by the poor. Salt consumption lies within a narrow range and one gets 1 mg of iron per gram of fortified salt.

6   Vitamins

In 1912 Hopkin found there is an unknown substances in all natural foods which are essential for growth. He called it "accessory food factors". In the same year Funk coined the unknown substances as vitamin.

i. Vitamins are an organic compound that is not an energy producing substance made of carbon, hydrogen, oxygen and sometimes nitrogen and other elements.

ii. It facilitates biochemical reactions within cells to help regulate body process such as growth and metabolism.

iii. These are natural components of foods, usually necessary in very small quantities.

iv. It is not manufactured by the body in adequate amount to meet normal physiological needs.

CLASSIFICATION

Vitamins are usually grouped and distinguished according to their solubility in either fat or water.

i. Vitamins A, D, E and K are fat soluble.

ii. The B group of vitamins and vitamin C are water soluble vitamins.

FAT SOLUBLE VITAMINS

1. Fat soluble vitamins closely associated with lipids in their fate in the body. They are absorbed with fat in chylomicrons that enter the lymphatic system before circulating in the bloodstream. Whenever fat absorption is impaired, in the case of cystic fibrosis or pancreatic insufficiency, deficiencies of fat soluble vitamins occur.

2. When consumed in excess amount, it gets stored in liver and adipose tissues, therefore do not have to be eaten everyday.

3. Toxicity can be developed if consumed in large dosage over a prolonged period.

VITAMIN A

McCollum and Davis (1917) and Osborne and Mendel (1913) showed that a fat soluble factor present in butter was essential for the growth of animal.

117

The term vitamin A refers to retinoid with the biologic activity of retinol, and also includes retinal, the aldehyde, and retinoic acid.

CHEMISTRY AND PROPERTIES

The chemical structure of vitamin A (retinol) is given in Fig. 6.1. Vitamin A contains a β-ionone ring. The side chain contains 2 isoprene units;

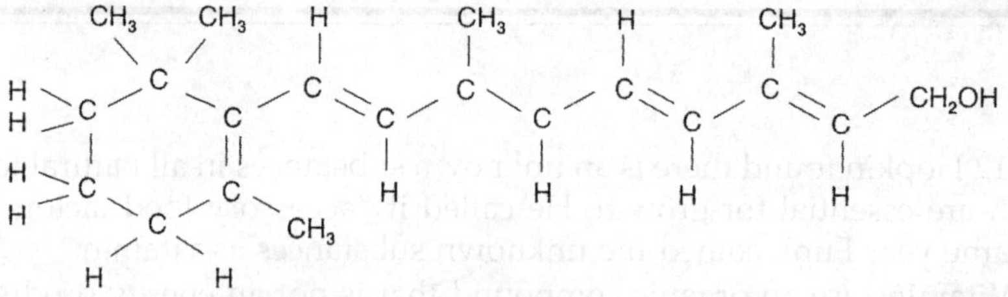

Fig. 6.1: Chemical structure of vitamin A (retinol)

4 double bonds and one alcoholic group. Due to the presence of four double bonds, vitamin A is destroyed easily by oxidation. Due to the presence of alcoholic group, it forms esters such as palmitate, acetate, succinate, etc.

Vitamin A_2 differs from vitamin A in having one more double bond in the β-ionone ring. Vitamin A_2 present in livers of fresh water fish. Vitamin A is oxidized to vitamin A aldehyde in the retina of eyes.

Retinoic Acid

Provitamin vitamin A, carotenoids are found in plants. Carotenoids, of which β-carotene, lutein and lycopene are among the most common, are found in deep yellow and orange fruits and vegetables and most dark-green leafy vegetables. Carrots, cantaloupe, broccoli, peas and spinach are major contributors to β-carotene intake.

Functions

The important functions of vitamin A are as follows.

Vision (Fig. 6.2)

Rhodopsin is the light-sensitive pigment in the rod cells of the retina. It is comprised of 11-cis retinal (the chromophore) and a protein called opsin. Within the eye, all-trans retinol (vitamin A) is converted by enzymes to 11-cis retinal and this binds spontaneously with opsin to form rhodopsin. Light induces isomerization of the 11-cis retinal in rhodopsin to all-trans retinal and this causes the opsin and retinal to dissociate and the pigment to become bleached. It is this light-induced cis to trans isomerization that generates the nervous impulses that we perceive as vision. Enzymes in the eye then regenerate 11-cis retinal and the rhodopsin. Rhodopsin is the

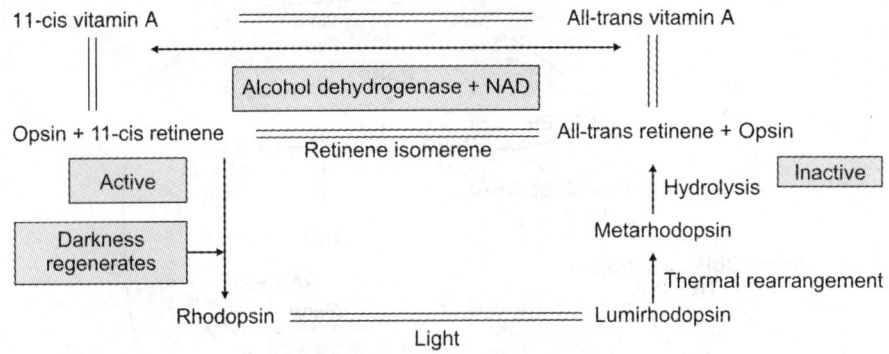

Fig. 6.2: Vitamin A visual cycle

most light sensitive of the human visual pigments and is responsible for our night vision. In bright light rhodopsin is completely bleached and other less sensitive pigments in the cones of the eye are responsible for day vision. During dark adaptation, rhodopsin is being regenerated. Vitamin A maintains the integrity of epithelial tissues in the eye, respiratory tract, gut, etc.

Epithelial Tissues

Vitamin A is essential for the normal formation of epithelial tissues. Vitamin A helps in maintaining the integrity of epithelial tissue in eye, respiratory track, gut and elsewhere. Due to deficiency in vitamin A there are pathological changes in the integrity of epithelial tissues. Normal epithelial tissue columnar or cuboidal cells or goblet cells produce mucus, which moistens the epithelial surface. Retinoic acid acts as a hormone, which binds to specific receptors within the epithelial cells and controls the expression of numerous genes; these receptors are similar to those that mediate the actions of steroid and thyroid hormones. This control of gene expression and protein synthesis regulate the proliferation and differentiation of epithelial cells. Retinol also has a role in the synthesis of cell surface glycoproteins which contains the sugar mannose.

Gene Expression

Vitamin A (specifically, retinoic acid) acts as a hormone to affect gene expression. Within the cell, CRABP transports retinoic acid to nucleus. In the nucleus, retinoic acid 9-cis-retinoic acid binds to retinoic acid receptors or retinoid receptors on the gene. Subsequent interaction allows stimulation or inhibition of transcription of specific genes, thus affecting protein synthesis and many body processes. Only a few of these processes are known, and they include morphogenesis (including differentiation and production of keratin proteins) (Fig. 6.3).

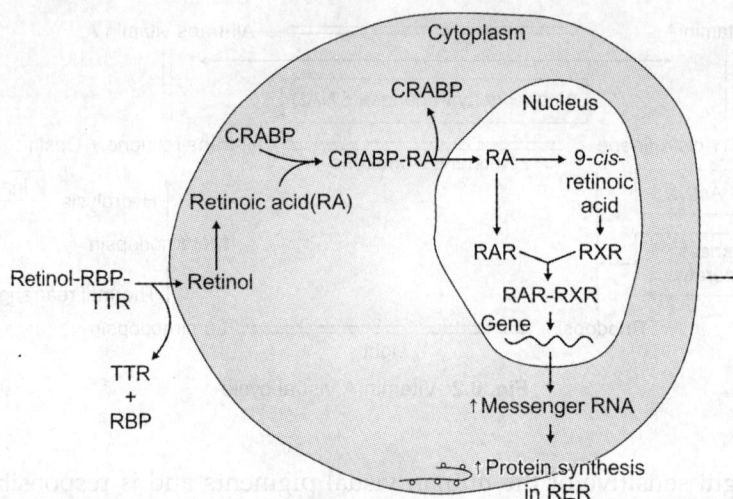

Fig. 6.3: Role of vitamin A in gene expression. CRABP, cellular retinoic acid-binding protein; RAR, retinoic acid receptor; RBP, retinol-binding protein; RXR, retinoid X receptor; TTR, transthyretin

Immunity

Vitamin A is responsible for proper functioning of the immune system. It is associated with reduced resistance to infection and increased child mortality. Due to deficiency in vitamin A there is reduced antibody production, reduced numbers of natural killer cells in the circulation and neutrophils show a reduced ability to ingest and kill pathogens and tumour cells. In children there is evidence to indicate that vitamin A supplements are beneficial for reducing morbidity and mortality among HIV infected children.

REPRODUCTION AND FOETAL DEVELOPMENT

Due to deficiency in vitamin A, reproduction does not take place through:
1. Infertility in the males
2. Failure of the females to conceive or resorption or abortion of the foetus, if conceived

Vitamin A is necessary for normal foetal development. Foetal abnormalities occur both in vitamin A deficiency and overload and this has been conformed by experimental studies on animal. These effects on development are mediated by the effects of retinoic acid on gene expression in the foetus resulting in the prevention of some forms of neoplastic transformation.

Absorption, Transport and Storage

Absorption

Vitamin A enters the body as retinol (preformed vitamin A) from animal sources and as the carotene (precursor of vitamin A) from plant sources.

Retinoid and carotenoids are incorporated into micelles along with other lipids for passive absorption into the mucosal cells of the small intestine. In the intestinal wall during absorption, some of the carotene is converted to vitamin A. Some fat in the food mix simultaneously absorbed, stimulates bile release for effective absorption of vitamin A. Once in the intestinal mucosal cells, retinol is bound to be a cellular retinol-binding protein (CRBP) and re-esterified (primarily by lecithin retinol acyl transferase [LRAT]) into retinyl esters (Fig. 6.4).

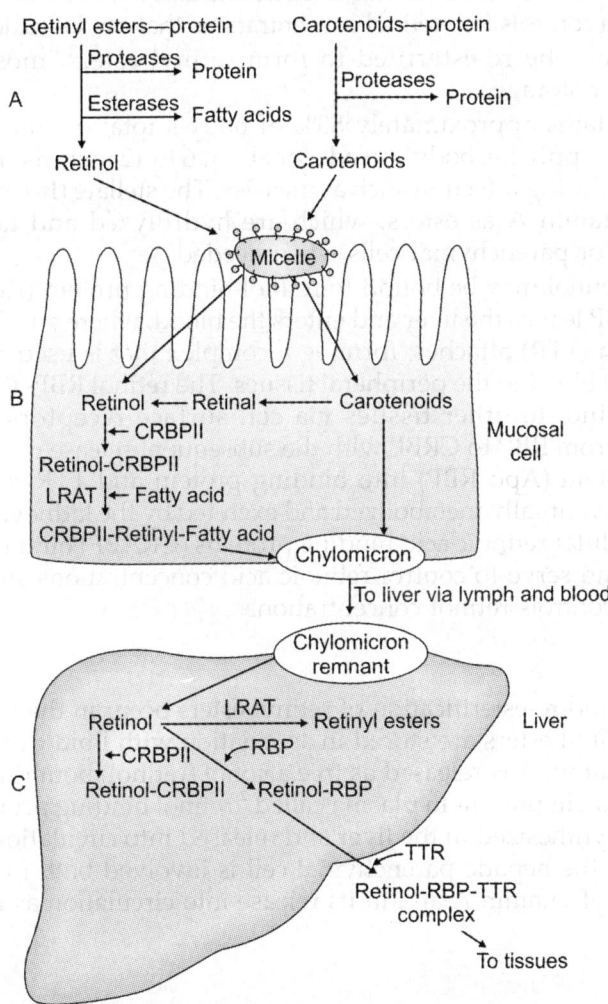

Fig. 6.4: Retinol and carotenoids. A: Digestion. B: Absorption. C: Transport. CRBPII, Cellular retinol binding protein II; RBP, retinol-binding protein; TTR, transthyretin

Transport

Carotenoids and retinyl esters are incorporated into chylomicrons for transport into the lymph and eventually the bloodstream or may be cleaved into retinal, which is then reduced to retinol and re-esterified into retinyl esters. These retinyl esters, like those produced from absorbed retinol, are also incorporated into chylomicrons.

Storage

The liver, by far the most efficient storage organ for vitamin A. Chylomicron remnants deliver retinyl esters to the liver. These esters are immediately hydrolyzed into retinol and free fatty acids.

Retinol in the liver has three major metabolic fats. Retinol may be bound to CRBP, which controls free retinol concentrations that can be toxic in the cell.

Retinol may be re-esterified to form retinyl esters, mostly retinyl palmitate, for storage.

Liver contains approximately 80% of body's total quantity, which is sufficient to supply the body's needs for about 6 to 12 months. These stores are reduced during infection such as measles. The stellate (Ito) cells contain stores of vitamin A as esters, which are hydrolyzed and taken up by hepatocytes or parenchymal cells when needed.

Finally, retinol may be bound to retinol-binding protein (RBP). Retinol bound to RBP leaves the liver and enters the blood, where another protein-transthyretin (TTR) attaches, forming a complex that is used to transport retinol in the blood to the peripheral tissues. The retinol RBP-TTR complex delivers retinol to other tissues via cell surface receptors. Retinol is transferred from RBP to CRBP with the subsequent release of Apo retinol-binding protein (Apo RBP) into binding protein and TTR to the blood. Apo RBP is eventually metabolized and excreted by the kidney. In addition to CRBP, cellular retinoic acid binding proteins (CRABP) bind retinoic acid in the cell and serve to control retinoic acid concentrations similar to the way CRBP controls retinol concentrations.

Metabolism

Hydrolysis and re-esterification of retinyl esters occur in the liver and the resulting retinyl esters are stored in association with lipid droplets. From this store vitamin A is released as free alcohol (retinol) bound to a specific transport protein present in plasma called "retinol binding protein" (RBP). The RBP is synthesized in the liver and released into circulation. Thus it is evident that the hepatic parenchymal cell is involved both in the uptake and storage of vitamin A and in its release into circulation as retinol-RBP complex.

Toxicity

Only preformed vitamin A is toxic in high doses. Although high intakes of naturally occurring and fortified preformed vitamin A can produce toxicity, the risk of toxicity is much more likely when supplements of vitamin A are consumed. At levels of daily intake above 4,000 IU per kg (especially 5, 00,000 IU per day) hyper vitaminosis A can develop.

In children with acute hyper vitaminosis A (>10 times the RDA), vomiting and bulging fontanelles are noted. In older children, growth failure, pseudo tumour cerebri, sixth nerve paresis, and optic atrophy develop. At all ages, nonspecific findings such as irritability, skin dryness, desquamation of skin over the palms and soles, myalgia, arthralgia, abdominal pain, and hypoplastic anaemia may be present.

Hepatosplenomegaly also occurs. In chronic hyper vitaminosis, cortical thickening of bones of the hands and feet develops with tenderness and weakness. Premature closer of the epiphyses has been observed.

In adults, early symptoms of overdose include nausea, vomiting, anorexia, malaise, cracking of skin and lips, headache and irritability. Long-term use of vitamin A by the elderly can lead to increased plasma level of retinol and biochemical evidence of liver damage. Hepatic fibrosis has been associated with excessive ingestion of vitamin A in a few cases. In adult receiving 50,000 to 1,00,000 IU per day, nausea, vomiting, skin desquamation, fatigue, hair loss, bone pain and hepatomegaly can occur. One case-control study has shown that a high intake of dietary retinol is associated with an increased risk for osteoporosis.

Deficiency (Tables 6.1 – 6.5)

The only unequivocal clinical signs of deficiency in humans occur in the eye. These changes have been classified in five stages, listed in order of increasing severity:

X0—effect on the retina: poor dark adaptation.

X1—effect on the conjunctive: xerosis (dryness) detected by dullness of the conjunctiva in bright light; frequent presence of bitot spots, an

Table 6.1: Recommended daily dietary intakes of vitamin A

Life stage group Infants[a]	Vitamin A (µg/day)	Life stage group Females	Vitamin A (µg/day)
0–6 months	400	9–13 years	600
7–12 months	500	14–18 years	700
		19–>70 years	700
Children			
1–3 years	300	Pregnancy	
4–8 years	400	14–18 years	750
		19–50 years	770
Males			
9–13 years	600	Lactation	
14–18 years	900	14–18 years	1200
19–>70 years	900	19–50 years	1300

[a]Estimate based on adequate intake (AI). All others based on recommended daily allowance (RDA). Adapted from standing committee on the Scientific Evaluation of Dietary Reference Intakes, Food and Nutrition Board, Institute of Medicine. Dietary reference intakes for vitamin A, vitamin K, arsenic, boron, Washington, DC: National Academies Press, 2001

accumulation of foamy white debris and fatty material near the limits of the eye, especially laterally.

X2— effect on the cornea: xerosis along with superficial erosion.

X3—effect on the cornea: irreversible corneal ulceration.

X4—effect on the cornea: scaring and softening.

Table 6.2: Approximate vitamin A content of selected foods

Food	Portion	RE As retinol	As pro-vitamins	Percentage of RDI (1,000 RE)
Grains				
Corn bread	1 muffin	16	16	1–5
Wheat bread	1 slice	0	0	0
Meats				
Salmon	3 oz	43		1–5
Liver, beef	3 oz	9,119		>100
Chicken, roasted	1 cup	22		1–5
Shrimp	1 oz	6		>1
Tuna, fresh broiled	3 oz	642		>40
Tuna, canned, water	4 oz	62		5–12
Fruits and vegetables				
Apple	2.75 in		7	1–5
Orange	2.6 in		27	<1
Strawberries	1 cup		5	>40
Cantaloupe	1 cup		516	>40
Watermelon	1 cup		59	5–12
Green beans, fresh	1 cup		83	5–12
Spinach, cooked, fresh	1 cup		1,750	>100
Corn, cooked, fresh	1/2 cup		18	1–5
Potatoes, white	8.75 in		0	0
Potatoes, sweet	1 each		24,50	>100
Carrots, cooked	1/2 cup		1,292	>100
Tomatoes	1 each		139	10–24
Dried apricots	16 halves		676	>40
Dried prunes	7 halves		187	10–24
Dairy				
Milk				
Whole	1 cup	76		5–12
Skim, enriched	1 cup	149		10–24
Eggs, large	1 each	97		5–12
Butter	1 tbs	106		5–12
Ice cream	1 cup	133		10–24

RE, retinol equivalents; RDI, recommended dietary intake.

Data from hands ES. Food finder, 2nd ed. OR: ESHA research, 1990.

Table 6.3: Relative content of carotenoids in food sources

Food	β-Carotene	α-Carotene	Lutein/zeaxanthin	Lycopence
Apricots	4+	–	–	1+
Beet greens	1+	tr	–	–
Broccli, cooked	1+	–	1+	–
Carrot, cooked	3+	2+	–	–
Corn	tr	–	–	1+
Mango	1+	tr	–	–
Spinach, raw	2+	–	3+	–
Tomato juice, canned	1+	–	–	1+

1+, 8–25 mg/3.5 oz; 2+, 25–60 mg/3.5 oz; 3+, 60–110 mg/3.5 oz; 4+, >110 mg/3.5 oz; tr, trace. Adapted from sauberlich HE. Laboratory tests for the assessment of nutritional status, 2nd ed. Boca raton, FL: CRC press, 1999. Other good sources of β-carotene include red palm oil, herbs and greens, peaches, sweet potatoes, pumpkin, squash, and tomato ketchup; of α-carotene, pumpkin and banana; of lutein, beets, egg yolk, and kiwi fruit of zeazanthin, egg yolk and potato; and of lycopene, watermelon.

Table 6.4: Guidelines in interpreting serum vitamin and carotene levels

	Vitamin A		Carotene	
Interpretation	(μg/dL)	(μmol/L)	(μg/dL)	(μmol/L)
Normal	>20	>0.7	>40	>1.4
Normal, not ingesting vegetables	>20	>0.7	<40	<1.4
Low intake, marginal stores	10–19	0.35–0.66	20–39	0.7–1.34
Deficient stores	<10	<0.35	Variable	
Severe liver disease	<20	<0.7	>40	>1.4
Excess vitamin A ingestion	>65	>2.28	>40	>1.4
Excess carotene ingestion (also, hypothyroidism, hyperlipidemia, anorexia nervosa, hypercholesterolemia of diabetes)	>20	>0.7	>300	>10.5

Adapted from sauberlich HE. Laboratory texts for the assessment of nutritional status, 2nd ed. Boca raton, FL: CRO press, 1999.

Table 6.5: Vitamins, vitamers, and their functions

Group	Vitamers	Provitamins	Physiologic functions
Vitamin A	Retinol Retinal Retinoic acid	β-carotene Cryptoxanthin	Visual pigments; cell diff-erentiations; gene regulation
Vitamin D	Cholecalciferol (D$_3$) Ergocalciferol (D$_2$)		Ca homeostasis; bone metabolism
Vitamin E	α-tocopherol γ-tocopherol Tocotrienols		Membrane antioxidant

Contd.

Table 6.5: Vitamins, Vitamers, and their functions (*Contd.*)

Group	Vitamers	Provitamins	Physiologic functions
Vitamin K	Phylloquinones (K_1) Menaquinones (K_2) Menadione (K_3)		Blood clotting; Ca metabolism
Vitamin C	Ascorbic acid		Reductant in hydroxylations in biosynthesis of collagen and carnitine and in the metabolism of drugs and steroids
	Dehydroascorbic acid		
Vitamin B_1	Thiamine		Coenzyme for decarboxylations of 2-keto acids and transketolations
Vitamin B_2	Riboflavin		Coenzyme in redox reactions of fatty acids and the TCA cycle
Niacin	Nicotinic acid Nicotinamide		Coenzymes for several dehydrogenases
Vitamin B_6	Pyridoxol		Coenzymes in amino acid metabolism
	Pyridoxal Pyridoxamine		
Folate	Folic acid		Coenzymes in single-carbon metabolism
	Pteroylmonoglutamate Polyglutamyl folacins		
Biotin	Biotin		Coenzyme for carboxylations
Pantothenic acid	Pantothenic acid		Coenzyme in fatty acid metabolism
Vitamin B_2	Cobalamin		Coenzyme in metabolism of propionate, amino acids, and single carbon fragments

TCA, Tricarboxylic acid

VITAMIN A DEFICIENCY DISORDERS

The most obvious effects of vitamin A deficiency are on the eye. Dietary vitamin A deficiency is often associated with protein energy malnutrition, causing problems, most from South Asia, had clinical eye disease (xerophthalmia) caused by vitamin A deficiency. Two-third of those newly diagnosed die within months of going blind because of enhanced susceptibility to infections. Even subclinical vitamin A deficiency increases childhood morbidity and mortality.

Vitamin A, we know, is essential for maintenance of healthy epithelium and normal vision. Deficiency symptoms show up after liver reserve of the vitamin has been depleted. These symptoms can also be the result of a deficiency of protein or zinc, either of which reduces the amount of vitamin A released from liver stores. Symptoms may result from low dietary intakes, interference with absorption and storage or interference with the conversion of carotene to vitamin A. Deficiency of vitamin 'A' manifests in the form of eye lesions, which are grouped under 'xerophthalmia', can be either mild leading to night blindness and changes in conjunctiva (white of the eye) or in severe form causing damage to cornea (black of the eye) leading to irreversible blindness.

SIGNS AND SYMPTOMS OF VITAMIN A DEFICIENCY

Clinical features of vitamin A deficiency:

a. *Night blindness (XN):* Night blindness is the earliest symptoms of vitamin A deficiency. This is the state that reduction in the supply of vitamin A aldehyde, i.e. retinal to the rod cells of the retina results in impairment of dark adaptation. The speed with which the eye recovers its full powers after exposure to bring light is directly related to the amount of vitamin A that is available to form rhodopsin. The recovery process is known as dark adaptation.

People with vitamin A deficiency may find it difficult to see the way to their seats in the movie theatre, whereas those with sufficient of vitamin A manage without difficulty. Those deficient in vitamin A usually cannot see in dim light, either at dusk or dawn. It is treatable in this stage.

b. *Xeropthalmia:* This condition refers to xerosis of conjunctiva and cornea.

   i. *Conjunctival xerosis:* Conjunctiva in normal children is bright white, smooth and glistening, conjunctival xerosis is characterized by dryness of the conjunctiva, after exposure to air for 10–15 seconds by keeping eyelids drawn back, which also become thick, rough and wrinkled. This is due to the keratinization of the epithelial cells. The pigmentation gives the conjunctiva a smoky appearance.

   ii. *Corneal xerosis:* This follows conjunctival xerosis the surface of the cornea has a "rough, pebbly, appearance and lacks lustre". The breaking up time of the tear film is shortened to less than 10 seconds. The cornea appears lazy, bluish and milky.

Bitot's Spots

This is a small, irregularly shape silver-grey plaque with a foamy surface on the bulbar conjunctiva. It is only connected with vitamin A deficiency, it occurs together with conjunctiva xerosis in young children. However, ketatomalacia due to vitamin A deficiency can also be precipitated without Bitot's spots.

Corneal Ulcer

Corneal xerosis, if not treated promptly, leads to ulceration of the cornea. Initially, the ulcer may be shallow, and if it becomes deep, it may lead to perforation resulting in prolapse of contents of the eye ball. These lesions are more common in the lower central cornea.

Keratomalacia

This is a condition of rapid destruction and liquefaction of full thickness of cornea, leading to prolapse of iris, resulting in permanent blindness. Usually keratomalacia consists of characteristic softening of the entire thickness of a part or more often the whole of the cornea leading to deformation or destruction of the eyeball. It is painless but the corneal structure just melts into cloudy gelatinous mass, dead white or dirty yellow in colour. Extrusion of the lens and loss of the vitreous may occur. In infective conditions, the eye will be red and swollen.

FOLLICULAR HYPERKERATOSIS

The normal human skin contains pores which are the opening of follicles and reach the surface through the pores. Hairs emerge from the roots through the same follicles. In follicular hyperkeratosis, the follicles become blocked with plugs of keratin derived from their epithelial lining which has undergone squamous metaplasia. Because of the roughness in appearance, the condition has been called toad skin or Phrynoderma. It is characterized by horny papular eruptions on the posterior and lateral aspects of limbs and on the back and buttocks.

INCREASED SUSCEPTIBILITY TO INFECTION

The action of the cilia of the epithelial cells is involved in protecting the body against infection by sweeping the cell surface clear of invading micro organisms. In vitamin A deficient keratinized cells, the cilia are lost and the body is more vulnerable to infection.

In vitamin A deficiency, both specific and non-specific protective mechanisms are impaired. The humoral response to bacterial, parasitic and viral infections; cell mediated immunity mucosal immunity; natural killer cell activity and phagocytosis are impaired. Once an infection has taken hold, it can aggravate a preexisting vitamin A deficiency, placing the individual at even greater risk of further infections and perhaps eventual death. Carotenoids which do not act as a source of vitamin A also stimulate immune response. This may be due to their role as antioxidants. Children with mild xerophthalmia are known to be at increased risk of respiratory infection and diarrhoea.

Aetiology

Some of the causes of vitamin A deficiency are given below.

Inadequate Diet

Child is born with poor stores of vitamins and minerals due to maternal malnutrition. Diets of pregnant women are deficient in several nutrients, including vitamin A. The concentration of vitamin A in breast milk is low among undernourished mothers and most poor mothers delay complementary feeding beyond the age of one year and foods containing vitamin A are seldom given. The daily intake of vitamin A is about 100 mg while the recommended intake is 400 mg of retinol. The exclusively vegetable-based diets, therefore, contain β-carotene and a little or none of performed vitamin A except from breast milk.

Poverty and Ignorance

Low purchasing power of the communities and their consequent inability to meet nutrient requirements and traditional wrong beliefs and ignorance are also important causes. β-carotene rich sources like green leafy vegetable and papaya are avoided with the belief that these are deleterious to the health of children.

Infections

During acute infections, vitamin A intake in preschool children is reduced due to impaired appetite and impaired vitamin A absorption as in acute diarrhoea and respiratory infection and consequently, serum levels of vitamin A are significantly reduced during acute infections. Vitamin A deficiency is often associated with ascariasis and giardiasis.

Increased Excretion

Vitamin A excretion is increased in cancer, urinary tract infections and chronic infectious disease.

Treatment

All forms of vitamin A deficiency are treated with a massive oral dose of vitamin A in oil (2,00,000 IU), immediately after diagnosis. In the case of those with persistent vomiting and diarrhoea and intramusculary injection of 1,00,000 IU of water miscible vitamin A can be substituted for the oral dose.

This followed by another dose of 2, 00,000 IU one to four weeks later. In the case of infants and children weighing less than 8 kg, the same schedule may be followed casing half the dose of vitamin A. Acute corneal lesions should be considered as medical emergency and should be referred to the nearest hospital for treatment of the general condition in addition to the treatment of the eye disease.

However, xerophthalmic children with severe PEM need to be carefully monitored and given additional doses as needed, usually every 4 weeks, until their nutritional, especially protein, status improves.

Children suffering from vitamin A deficiency will most often be suffering multiple micronutrient deficiencies and this should be considered when giving the dietary advice and nutrition education that should always accompany treatment (Table 6.6).

Table 6.6: Treatment of xerophthalmia and measles in all age groups

Timing of dose[a]	Children aged 0–5 months	Children aged 6–12 months	Children over 12 months, male adolescents and male adults[b]
Immediately on diagnosis	50,000 IU	100,000 IU	200,000 IU
The following day (give to mother to administer at home on the next day, if necessary)	50,000 IU	100,000 IU	200,000 IU
At a subsequent contact (at least 2 weeks later)	50,000 IU	100,000 IU	200,000 IU

Source: WHO (1997).
[a]All vitamin A to be given orally and as an oil-based preparation.
[b]Unless in a medical emergency, women of reproductive age should not receive this supplement.

In women of reproductive age with night blindness or Bitot's spots, a daily dose of 10,000 IU or a weekly dose of 25,000 IU of vitamin A for at least 4 weeks is the recommended treatment schedule.

Prevention

The main causes of vitamin A deficiency in the developing world are insufficient dietary intake of vitamin A, poor bioavailability of provitamin A sources, especially in vegetable and the lack of vitamin A in the cereal staple (such as rice), other important contributory factors include the increased requirements at certain stages in the lifecycle, increased utilization of vitamin A during infection, especially measles, and sociocultural factors such as intra household distribution and gender.

The public health significance of vitamin A deficiency was recognized and acknowledged globally in December 1992, at the Food and Agriculture Organization (FAO/WHO) International Conference on Nutrition (ICN), where representatives of 159 countries agreed to eliminate vitamin A deficiency (and the iodine deficiency disorders) as public health problem by the end of the twentieth century and to reduce substantially the prevalence of iron deficiency anaemia. In 1990 the World Summit for Children, sponsored by UNICEF, had established broader goals for the health and well-being of children and the nutrition goals, including those for the micronutrients, agreed to at this forum were echoed at the ICN.

- Food-based approaches, including dietary diversification, nutrition education and fortification of staple and value added foods.
- Supplementation with vitamin A capsules with increasing interest in a multi-micronutrient supplement and weekly low dose supplements.
- Public health interventions such as immunization adding vitamin A supplementation to national immunization days, promotion of breast feeding and treatment of infectious disease.

- Change in the possibilities that are available to people by modification of the political, socio-economic and physical environment as with so much of public health, the most vulnerable are those who are the poorest.
- *Food-based approaches:* Improving dietary diversification through increasing the variety and frequency of micronutrient rich food sources through nutrition education and horticultural approaches have been shown to be effective in many settings.
- *Nutrition education:*
  - A need to increase the awareness of the community about the significance of proper diet in the prevention of vitamin A deficiency and also about the all health and nutrition programmes.
  - Nutrition education should target vulnerable groups such as pregnant woman, lactating mother and preschoolers.
  - Pregnant woman should be made aware that they must include adequate amount of vitamin A from the initial stage of pregnancy for optimum stores for both mother and foetus.
  - Colostrum is rich in vitamin A, hence nutrition education should be given to pregnant woman regarding colostrum.
  - It should be made mandatory, regular intake of vitamin A, and β-carotene rich foods should be given to infants and preschool children.
  - For infants foods such as carrot, pumpkin, spinach, and other dark green leafy vegetables can be given in boiled and mashed forms and also fruits such as banana, papaya and mango can be given in weaning period.
  - The health functionaries can approach with a proper multimedia communication and experts for success of nutrition education.
  - Food and Nutrition Board has been imparting education and training in nutrition, as well as, on home scale preservation of fruits and vegetables.
- *Horticultural interventions:*
  - Horticultural approach has been shown effective in many settings. Horticultural approach such as home garden, and improved methods of food preparation, preservation and cooking that conserve the micronutrients content.
  - Home gardening has been found to be a feasible long-term strategy, to increase production and consumption of leafy and other vegetables and fruits.
  - Home gardening has important outcome such as empowerment of poor, preparation of recipe based on locally available nutritious food, so that there is a successful increase in micronutrient intake.
  - The Indian Council of Agricultural Research (ICAR) has established 101 Krishi Vignan Kendras or Farm Science Centres so far in various parts of the country impart training in agricultural technologies to farmers.

- Knowledge about importance of locally available food and its cultivation can be promoted.

NUTRITIONAL SUPPLEMENTATION

The rational of supplementation with high dose of vitamin A rest on the fact that these fat soluble nutrients can be stored in the body particularly in the liver. The national prophylaxis programme against nutrition blindness is being implemented. This involves oral administration of massive dose of 2,00,000 IU of vitamin A every 6 months to a preschool children. This approach found to be feasible by extensive field trials carried out by NIN and it has a significance reduction in prevalence of ocular sign of vitamin A deficiency among preschool children.

Fortification

- Fortifications have been identified as most cost effective and a major factor to control micronutrient deficiency. Vanaspathi was the first food fortified in India.
- Low cost processed foods for supplementary feeding of infants, preschool children and school children (ICDS and mid-day meal programme) to be fortified with vitamin A.
- Both toned and double toned milk are fortified with vitamin A.

Vitamin K

The studies of biochemical by Dam and Schonhyeder (1934) at the University of Copenhagen working with a hemorrhagic disease in chicks that were fed a fat-free diet led to the discovery of vitamin K. They found that the absent factor responsible was a fat soluble blood clotting vitamin. Because of its blood clotting function, they called it coagulations vitamin, or vitamin K. Later they succeeded in isolating and identifying the compound from alfalfa.

Vitamin K, is a group of compounds derived from 2-methyl-1, 4-nophthoquinone. Naturally occurring forms include

- Vitamin K_1 (phylloquinone, synthesized by plants and present in food)
- Vitamin K_2 (menaquinones, synthesized in humans by intestinal bacteria)

Synthetic water soluble forms of vitamin K include menadione (vitamin K_3) and menadiol (vitamin K_4), which does not require bile for absorption and goes directly into the portal blood system (Fig. 6.5) (Table. 6.7).

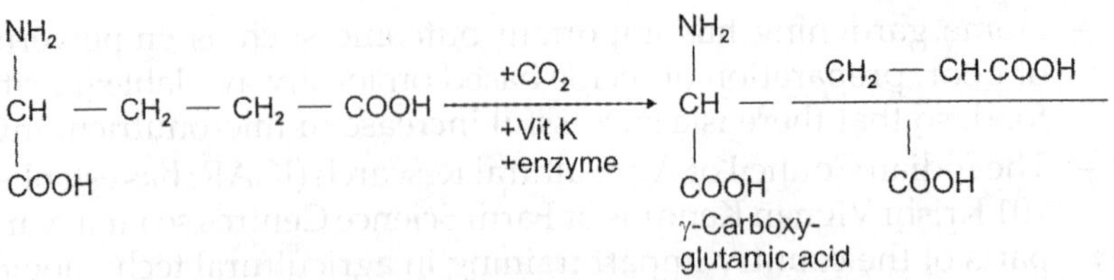

Fig.6.5: Formation of 3-carboxy glutamic acid

Table 6.7: Chemistry of vitamin K

S.No	Name of vitamin	No. of carbon atoms in side chain	Chemical structure
1.	Vitamin K_1 (phylloquinone)	20	2-methyl-3-phytyl-1, 4 napthoquinone
2.	Vitamin K_2 (menaquinone-7)	35	2-methyl-1, 4 naphthoquinone containing isoprene units
3.	Menadione (synthetic) (vitamin K substitute) (menaquinone-0)	0	2-methyl 1, 4 napthoquinone
4.	Menaquinone-4	20	Formed in the body from menadione by the attachment of a geranyl-geranyl group and from vitamin K_1 by replacement of phytyl side chain, by geranyl-geranyl side chain.

ABSORPTION, TRANSPORT AND STORAGE

The phylloquinone (K_1) are absorbed by energy dependent process in the small intestine. However, the menaquinones (K_2) and menadione (K_3) are absorbed in the small intestine and colon by passive diffusion.

Like the other fat soluble vitamins, absorption depends on a minimum amount of dietary fat and on bile salts and pancreatic juices. The absorbed vitamer K is packaged in the intestinal chylomicrons and travel via the abdominal lacteals into the lymphatic system and then into the portal blood for transport to the liver. In liver they are incorporated into VLDLs and subsequently delivered to the peripheral tissues of LDLs.

Vitamin K is found in low concentrations in many tissues, where it is localized in cellular membranes. Because of the metabolism of the vitamin, tissues show mixtures of vitamer K even when a single form is consumed. Most tissues contain phylloquinone and menaquinones.

Metabolism

Phylloquinone can be converted to menaquinones by successive bacterial dealkylation and realkylation before absorption. Side-chain shortening and oxidation produce metabolites that are excreted in the faeces via the bile, frequently as glucoronic acid conjugates, and catabolize phylloquinone and menaquinones. Menadione is metabolized more rapidly; it is excreted primarily in the urine as a phosphate sulfate, or glucoronide derivative.

Function

Vitamin K is required for blood clotting. It is co-factor for the carboxylation of glutamate residues in the post synthetic modification of proteins to form the unusual amino acid γ-carboxy glutamate, abbreviated to gla.

The first step in the reaction is oxidation of vitamin K hydroquinone to the epoxide. The epoxide then activates a glutamate residue in protein substrate to a carbanion that reacts non-enzymatically with carbon dioxide to form γ-carboxyglutamate. Vitamin K epoxide is then reduced to quinone by a warfarin sensitive reductase, and the quinone is reduced to the active hydroquinone by either the same warfarin sensitive reductase or a warfarin insensitive quinone reductase.

In the presence of warfarin, vitamin K epoxide cannot be reduced back to the active hydroquinone, but accumulates, and is excreted as variety conjugates.

The only function of vitamin K is its use by the liver in the synthesis of various substances needed for blood clotting. Among these substances the most important are prothrombin factor II, proconverting factor III, plasma thromboplastin component IX and stuart factor, factor X. Each contains 4–6 γ-carboxyglutamate residues per mol. γ-carboxyglutamate chelates calcium ions, and so permit the binding of the blood clotting proteins to membrane. Vitamin K appears to be necessary to catalyze the conversion of the precursor of prothrombin to prothrombin in the liver; it does this by helping to convert the glutamic acid of the protein to a new amino acid, γ carboxyglutamate acid. In turn prothrombin in the blood catalyze the conversion of fibrinogen into fibrin, another factor involved in blood coagulation. Prothrombin levels in the blood determine the rate at which blood will clot. For blood to clot, fibrinogen, a soluble protein must be converted into fibrin. Thrombin catalysis the proteolysis of fibrinogen (Figs 6.6 and 6.7).

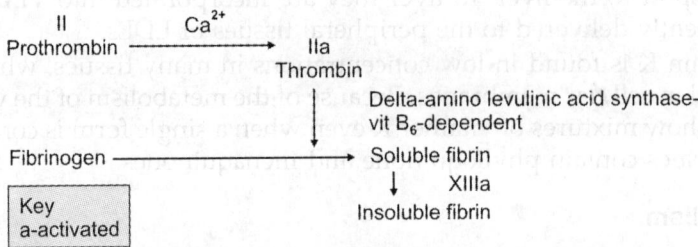

Fig. 6.6: The activation of prothrombin

Deficiency

Acute deficiency of vitamin K may occur in new born infants if not given synthetic vitamin K at birth. Deficiency in healthy adults is rare since vitamin K is widely available from the diet and is also synthesized by gut bacteria. However, secondary deficiency resulting in prolonged blood clotting time can occur in people with fat malabsorption, especially due to biliary obstruction or hepatic disease, or following intestinal resection or prolonged antibiotic use.

The effects of vitamin K may be antagonized by the excessive intake of vitamins A and E.

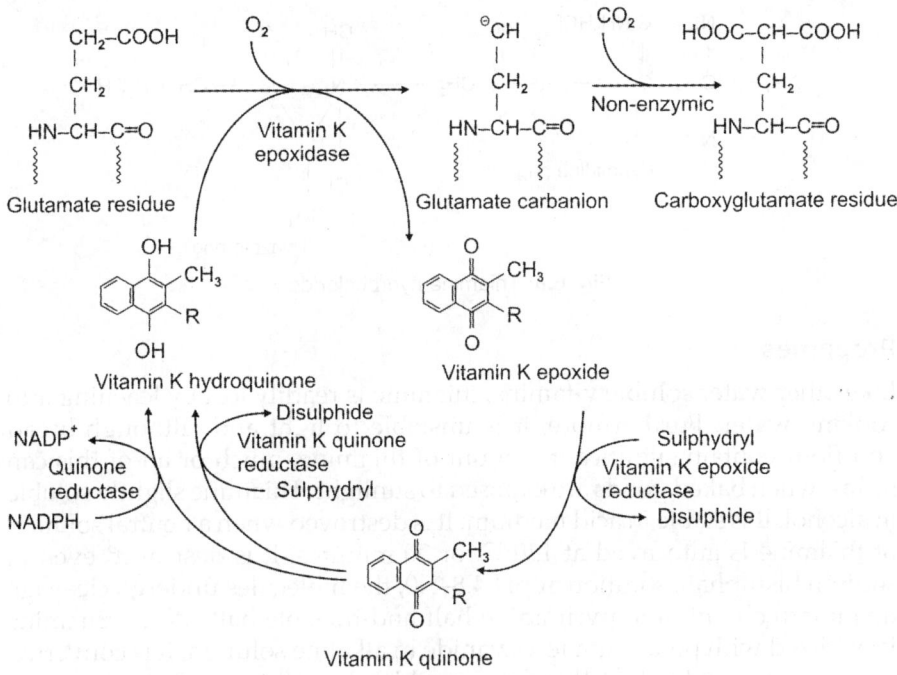

Fig 6.7: The role of vitamin K in γ-carboxyglutamate synthesis

Toxicity

Vitamin K_1, (phylloquinone), the form naturally occurring in food, appears to be relatively safe. Limited human studies suggest that a daily supplementary intake of 1mg/day would be unlikely to result in adverse effects (EVM 2003). However, supplemental intakes are usually contraindicated in people taking anticoagulant therapy. The synthetic water soluble forms of vitamin K, particularly K_3 (menadione), are more toxic. High doses of water soluble vitamin K_3 (menadione) may result in oxidative damage, red cell fragility and the formation of methaemoglobin and its use for non-medical purposes are not recommended. Excessive doses in premature infants have also caused serious liver problems and brain damage.

WATER SOLUBLE VITAMINS

1. *Thiamine (vitamin B_1):* Historically, thiamine deficiency affecting the peripheral nervous system (beriberi) was a major public health problem in south East Asia following the introduction of the stem powered mill that made highly polished (thiamine-depleted) rice widely available.

   Takkai (1885) prevented the occurrence of beriberi in the Japanese navy by changing the diet. Its basic nature and metabolic function were then clarified in the early 1930s.

   Chemical structure: Thiamine contains pyrimidine ring and thiazole ring (Fig. 6.8).

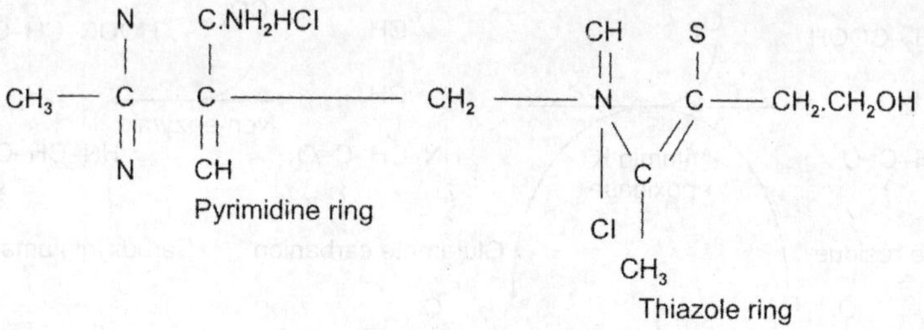

$$CH_3 - \overset{\overset{\displaystyle N}{|}}{\underset{\underset{\displaystyle N}{||}}{C}} \quad \overset{\overset{\displaystyle C.NH_2HCl}{|}}{\underset{\underset{\displaystyle CH}{||}}{C}} ------- CH_2 ------ N \quad C - CH_2.CH_2OH$$

Pyrimidine ring

Thiazole ring

Fig. 6.8: Thiamine hydrochloride

Properties

Like other water soluble vitamins, thiamine is readily lost by leaching into cooking water. Furthermore, it is unstable to light and, although bread and flour contain significant amount of thiamine, much or all of this can be lost when baked goods are exposed to sunlight. Thiamine slightly soluble in alcohol. It is stable in acid medium. It is destroyed when a neutral solution of thiamine is autocaved at 120°C for 30 minutes. It is destroyed even in sodium bisulphate solution at pH 4.8–5.0, the molecules undergo cleavage quantitatively into the pyrimidine half and thiazole half. When thiamine is oxidized with potassium ferricyanide in alkaline solution, it is converted into a compound called thiochrome which has a strong fluorescence in ultraviolet light.

Absorption and Transport

Most dietary thiamine is present as phosphates, which are readily hydrolysed by intestinal phosphatases, and free thiamine is readily absorbed in the duodenum and proximal jejunum and then transferred to the portal circulation as free thiamine or thiamine mono phosphate. This is an active transport process and is inhibited by alcohol, which may explain why alcoholics are especially susceptible to thiamine deficiency.

Tissues take up both free thiamine and thiamine monophosphate, and then phosphorylate them further to yield thiamine diphosphate (the active coenzyme) and thiamine triphosphate.

Thiamine is not stored in large quantities in the tissues. The tissue content is highly relevant to increased metabolic demand, as in fever, increased muscular activity, pregnancy and lactation.

Some of free thiamine is excreted in the urine, increasing with diuresis and a significant amount also is lost in sweat.

Metabolic Functions of Thiamine

The main function of thiamine as a metabolic control agent relates to energy metabolism. When actively combined with phosphorus as the coenzyme thiamine pyrophosphate (TPP), thiamine serves as a coenzyme in key reactions that produce energy from glucose or that convert glucose to fat for tissue energy storage.

Functions of TPP

Thiamine pyrophosphate (TPP) is essential as a coenzyme for the enzyme catalyzing the following reactions:
1. Decarboxylation of pyruvic acid and α-ketoglutaric acid.
2. Ketol formation as in the formation of sedoheptulose from xylulose and ribose in the hexose monophosphate (HMP) shunt pathway.

DECARBOXYLATION OF PYRUVIC ACID

This reaction takes place mainly in yeast during alcoholic fermentation. It does not take place in animal tissues.

$$\text{Pyruvic acid} \xrightarrow[\text{+ TPP}]{\text{carboxylase}} \text{acetaldehyde} + CO_2$$

Oxidative Decarboxylation of Pyruvic Acid

The reaction involved in the oxidative decarboxylation of pyruvic acid is described below. The enzyme involved is called pyruvic dehydrogenase complex and the coenzymes required are TPP and lipoic acid.

$$\text{Pyruvic acid} \xrightarrow[\substack{\text{Complex} \\ \text{+ TPP}}]{\substack{\text{Pyruvic} \\ \text{dehydrogenase}}} \text{hydroxyethyl TPP} + CO_2 \text{ (active acetaldehyde)}$$

$$\text{Hydroxyethyl TPP+ lipoic acid} \xrightarrow[\substack{\text{dehydrogenase} \\ \text{complex}}]{\text{Pyruvate}} \text{acetaldihydrolipoic acid} + \text{TPP}$$

Oxidative Decarboxylation of α-ketoglutoric Acid

$$\text{α-ketoglutaric acid} \xrightarrow[\substack{\text{dehydrogenase} \\ \text{complex + TPP}}]{\text{α-ketoglutaric}} \text{succinic semi-aldehyde TPP} + CO_2$$

α-Ketol Formation in HMP Shunt Pathway

The enzyme transketolase requires TPP as a coenzyme and brings about the following reaction in the HMP pathway.

$$\text{Xylulose-5 phosphate + ribose-5 phosphate} \xrightarrow[\text{+TPP}]{\text{transketolase}} \text{Sedoheptulose-7 phosphate + glyceraldehyde 3 } PO_4$$

$$\text{Xylulose-5 phosphate + erythrose-4 phosphate} \xrightarrow[\text{+TPP}]{\text{transketolase}} \text{Fructose 6 phosphate + glyceraldehyde 3 } PO_4$$

Deficiency (Causes)

I. Deficiency may develop from a decrease in intake, an increase in tissue utilization (e.g. pregnancy) or combination of 2 factors.

II. The clinical setting most commonly associates with thiamine deficiency include chronic alcoholism, malabsorption syndromes, nausea and vomiting of pregnancy.

III. *Anti-thiamine factors:* These factors in food can alter thiamine activity and be a cause of vitamin deficiency. The thermolabile factor found in the fresh water fish and shellfish and thermostable factor in the leaves have both been reported to cause of deficiency when coupled with low thiamine intake.

Symptoms

I. *Dry beriberi:* Chronic deficiency of thiamine, especially associated with a high carbohydrate diet results in beriberi; which is symmetrical ascending peripheral neuritis. Initially the patient complaints of weakness, stiffness and cramps in the leg and is unable to walk more than short distance. Initially its numbness in feet and ankle, as progresses, the ankle jerk reflex is lost, spreads to leg fully.

In this stage patient is unable to keep either the toe or the whole foot extended off the ground. When arms are affected, there is a similar inability to keep the hand extended wrist drop.

II. *Wet beriberi:* The heart may also affected in beriberi, with dilation of arterioles, rapid blood flow, increased pulse rate and pressure and increased jugular venous pressure leading to right sided of heart failure and oedema, so called wet beriberi. The signs of chronic heart failure may be seen without peripheral neuritis. The arteriolar dilation and possibly also the oedema, probably result from high circulation concentration of lactate and pyruvate as a result of impaired activity of pyruvate dehydrogenase.

III. *The Wernicke-Korsakoff syndrome:* In alcohol abuse the Wernicke-Korsakoff syndrome occurs due to central nervous system lesions. Initially there is a confused state, Korsakoff psychosis, which is characterized by confabulation and loss recent memory, although memory for past events may be unimpaired. This is characterized by nystagmus and extraocular palsy. It occurs acutely.

Treatment

Thiamine hydrochloride is available in tablets form (5 to 1,000 mg), in injectable form (100 or 200 mg per ml) and as an elixir (2.25 mg per 5 ml). Mild deficiency may be treated with 15 mg per day parenterally (or 25–50 mg orally) for 1 week, followed by a maintenance oral dose. For severe deficiency one may require large dose up to 100 mg twice daily for 3 days followed by oral supplementation of 5 to 30 mg/day until a normal diet is resumed.

Prevention

As per the Indian government regulations, the extent of rice polishing should not exceed 5%. If rice is milled beyond 10%, then most of the thiamine is lost, avoiding excessive milling and polishing of cereal grains can increase the thiamine intake from cereal diets. Traditional family cooking practices need to be encouraged. Alcoholic drinks should be discouraged, fortification of vitamin in bread can be done.

Sources

Although thiamine is abundant in all foods, they are easily removed during processing of grains or destroyed during heating. Whole wheat, hand pounded raw or parboiled rice contain adequate amount of thiamine. If this rice is milled more than 10%, most of the thiamine is lost. Because thiamine is water-soluble, much of the content of the vitamin (up to 80%) is extracted in cooking liquid. Therefore, method of food preparation is also considered. Electronic cooking may reduce the loss of thiamine. Using baking powder or if soda is added during cooking, almost all thiamine is lost.

Thiamine deficiency occurs even when the ratios of thiamine with energy is very less. Pulses and most whole cereals have a ratio of about 1.2 mg/1,000 kcal and are actively protective against beriberi. Raw polished rice has a value of about 0.15 mg/1,000 kcal and is beriberi producing.

Niacin (Vitamin B_3)

Niacin is also called nicotinic acid and is designated as vitamin B_3. In 1937, Elvehgem and co-workers isolated nicotinic acid from liver and made the important discovery that it cured black-tongue in dogs. Three groups of workers in 1937, independently and simultaneously, reported that nicotinic acid was effective in curing pellagra in human beings.

Humans are not entirely dependent on dietary niacin as it can also be synthesized from the amino acid tryptophan (60 mg of tryptophan are required to produce 1 mg of niacin).

CHEMISTRY AND PROPERTIES

The chemical structure of nicotinic acid and nicotinamide are given in Fig. 6.9.

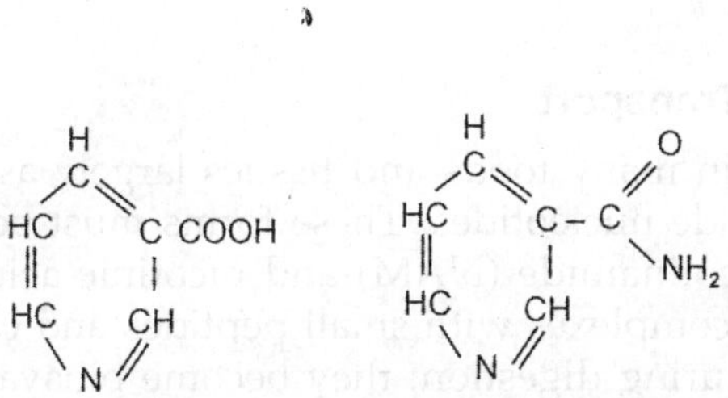

Fig. 6.9: Chemical structure of nicotinic acid and nicotinamide

Nicotinic acid is sparingly soluble in water. It is freely soluble in alkalinhydroxides and carbonates forming salts. It is stable to heat and not destroyed by autoclaving at 120°C for 20 minutes in acid or alkaline medium, when heated or autoclaved in a strong alkaline or acid solution. It is converted into nicotinic acid.

Precursor Role of Tryptophan

Curious observations were made by early investigations why did milk which is low in niacin cure or prevent pellagra and why pellagra to common in groups subsisting on diet high in corn. In 1945 scientist at the University of Wisconsin finally made the key discovery, tryptophan can be used by the body to make niacin and it is precursor of niacin.

Conversion of Tryptophan to Niacin

Synthesis of niacin from tryptophan (Fig. 6.10).

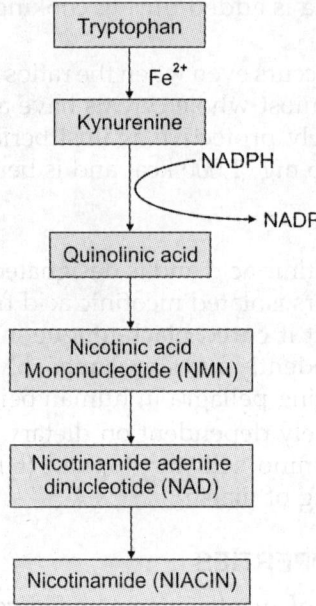

Fig. 6.10: Synthesis of niacin from tryptophan. NADPH, nicotinamide adenine dinucleotide phosphate in the reduced form.

Absorption and Transport

Niacin is present in many foods and tissues largely as coenzyme forms such as nicotinamide nucleotides. These forms must be digested to give absorbed form nicotinamide (NAM) and nicotinic acid (NA). Niacin is covalently bound complexes with small peptides and carbohydrates that are not released during digestion; they become bioavailable by alkaline hydrolysis.

Nicotinic acid and nicotinamide are rapidly absorbed from the intestine through the portal vein into the general circulation, by a sodium dependent saturable process.

METABOLISM OF THE NICOTINAMIDE NUCLEOTIDE

The nicotinamide nucleotide coenzymes can be synthesized from either of the niacin vitamers, and from quinolinic acid, an intermediate in the metabolism of tryptophan. In the liver, the oxidation of tryptophan results in a considerably greater synthesis of NAD than is required and this is catabolized to form nicotinic acid and nicotinamide, which are taken up by tissues for synthesis of coenzymes.

NAD and NADPH can be produced from NA and NAM. The NAM is deaminated to yield NA. Then two ribose phosphates are attached to the nitrogen in the pyridine ring. Next adenosine is attached to the ribose. Finally an amino group is added to the acid group, forming an amide yield NAD. NAD can be phosphorylated in the HMP shunt to yield NADPH.

NAD and NADPH is catabolized by hydrolysis to yield NAM, which can be deaminated into NA or methylated to yield 1-methylnicotinamide (mNAM). Dietary protein deficiency changes the profile of urine metabolites, presumably because of change in the amount of tryptophan converted to niacin.

Functions

Nicotinamide is a component of two coenzymes NAD and NADP which take part in several enzyme reactions.

I. *Glycolysis:*

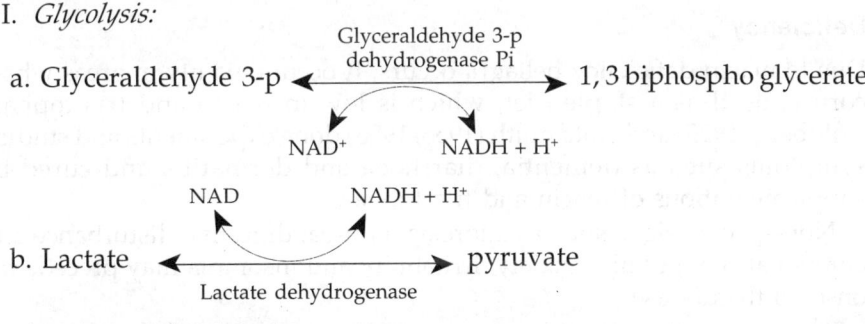

a. Glyceraldehyde 3-p $\xleftrightarrow{\text{Glyceraldehyde 3-p dehydrogenase Pi}}$ 1, 3 biphospho glycerate

NAD⁺   NADH + H⁺

NAD   NADH + H⁺

b. Lactate $\xleftrightarrow{}$ pyruvate

Lactate dehydrogenase

II. *Krebs cycle/TCA cycle:*

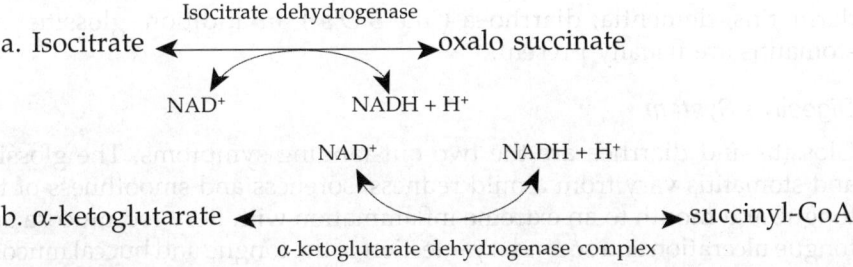

a. Isocitrate $\xleftrightarrow{\text{Isocitrate dehydrogenase}}$ oxalo succinate

NAD⁺   NADH + H⁺

NAD⁺   NADH + H⁺

b. α-ketoglutarate $\xleftrightarrow{}$ succinyl-CoA

α-ketoglutarate dehydrogenase complex

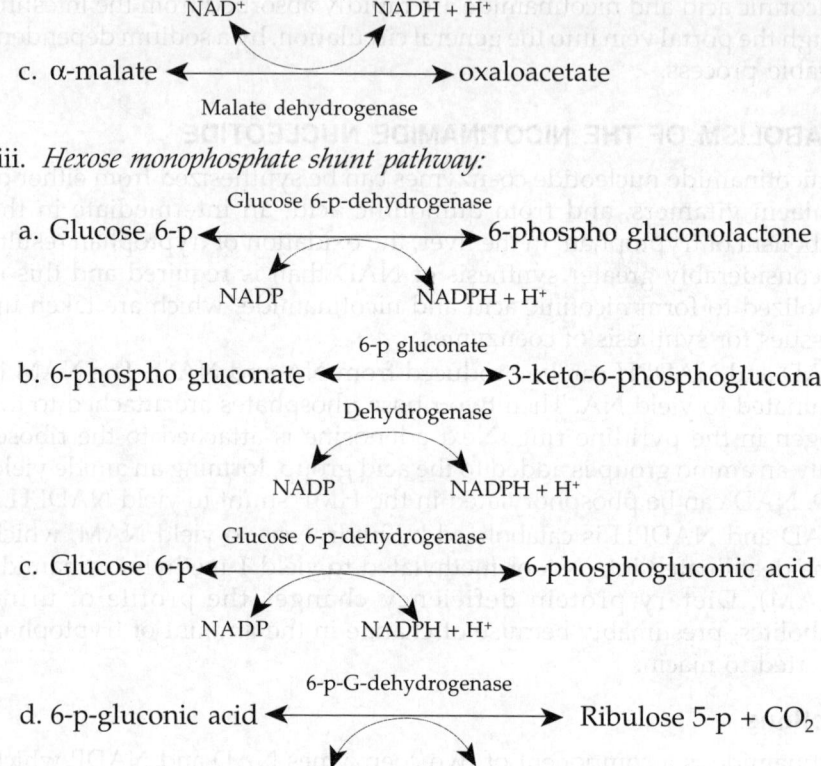

iii. *Hexose monophosphate shunt pathway:*

Deficiency

Due to niacin deficiency pellagra occurs. It occurs mainly in areas where corn is used as a staple diet, which is low in niacin and tryptophan. Goldberg (1925) and Goldsmith (1956, 1958) done experiments and studied symptoms such as dementia, diarrhoea and dermatitis and cured by supplementations of niacin and tryptophan.

Non-specific signs such as anorexia, nausea, digestive disturbance and emotional changes like anxiety, irritability and insomnia may precede the onset of the disease.

The typical clinical features are muscular weakness and skin eruptions, severe deficiency of niacin leads to pellagra, which is characterised by dermatitis, dementia, diarrhoea ("the 3 D's"), in addition, glossitis and stomatitis are usually present.

Digestive System

Glossitis and diarrhea are the two outstanding symptoms. The glossitis and stomatitis vary from a mild redness, soreness and smoothness of the tongue and mouth to an extreme inflammation with fiery red mucosa and tongue ulceration and secondary infection of the tongue and buccal mucosa.

Nausea and vomiting are seen in most cases. The diarrhoeas may range from a few to several loose stools a day with blood and mucus.

Skin

The dermatitis is the most characteristic of the disease. It is symmetrical in distribution. In early stage a bright red erythremia resembling sunburn occurs over the exposed parts of the body. The commonest sites are the back of the fingers and hands, the forearms, dorsum of the feet and ankles and the neck. In the beginning, the skin is red and slightly swollen. The lesions may worsen by the formation of vesicles and bullae with cracking of the skin. Secondary infection is always present with improvement, the skin becomes dry, less red and the surface desquamates. The dermatitis is precipitated by exposure to sunlight.

Nervous System

Delirium is the commonest severe mental disturbance in acute pellagra. Dementia is more frequently seen in the chronic cases. Milder mental disturbances consisting of irritability, change in disposition, depression, inability to concentrate, poor memory are more common in the mild cases. The symptoms of posterolateral degeneration, ataxia, spasticity and the involvement of the bladder and rectal sphincters are seen in chronic cases.

Untreated pellagra can cause death (which is often referred to as "the fourth D").

Treatment

Pellagra can be cured by a good diet containing adequate amount of protein, tryptophan and /or niacin as well as other members of B-complex group of vitamins. Glossitis, dermatitis, diarrhoea, mental symptoms of pellagra respond to oral doses of 100–500 mg/day, depend on the severity of the symptoms.

In regions pellagra is common, nicotinamide tablets (30 mg/tablet), should be distributed to the people. The staple food, usually corn or sorghum flour, should be fortified with nicotinic acid. People should encourage to consume peanuts, meat and liver which are rich sources of niacinamide.

Sources

Nicotinic acids present in most foods except in fats and oils, mainly as the pyridine nucleotides NAD and NADP. It is removed during grain processing; sometime it is present in form that is not absorbed (e.g. in corn).

They are found in many foods, lean meats, poultry, fish, peanuts and yeasts are particularly rich sources. Niacin exists predominantly as protein bond NA in plant tissues. Milk and eggs contain small amount of niacin, but they are excellent source of tryptophan giving them significant niacin equivalent contents.

PANTOTHENIC ACID

Pantothenic acid was isolated and synthesized between 1938 and 1940. Because it occurs in all forms of living things and is an acid it was named pantothenic acid. It was isolated in a pure form as its calcium salt, by Williams and co-workers.

CHEMICAL STRUCTURE AND PROPERTIES

Pantothenic acid

Pantothenic acid is a pale viscous oil. It has not been obtained so for in a crystalline form but its sodium, potassium or calcium salt crystalline readily. They are highly soluble in water. Pantothenic acid is stable to autoclawing at 120°C for 30 minutes in neutral solution but is destroyed rapidly in acid or alkaline medium.

Pantothenic acid exists in tissues as coenzyme A. A compound containing pantothenic acid stimulates the growth of *lactobacillus bulgaricus* [*lactobacillus bulgaricus* factor]. LBF exists in 2 forms called pantothenic and pantothine.

Absorption and Metabolism

About 85% of dietary pantothenic acid occurs as CoA or phosphopantetheine. In the intestinal lumen these are hydrolysed to pantetheine; intestinal mucosal cells have a high pantethinase activity and rapidly hydrolyse pantetheine to pantothenic acid. The absorption of pantothenic acid is by diffusion and occurs at a rate throughout the length of the small intestine; intestinal bacterial synthesis may contribute to pantothenic acid nutrition.

The first step in pantothenic acid utilization is phosphorylation. Pantothenate kinase is rate limiting, so that, unlike many vitamins, which are accumulated by metabolic trapping, there can be significant accumulation of the pantothenic acid in tissue.

Function

All tissues are capable of forming coenzyme A from pantothenic acid, coenzyme A discovered by Lupimann in 1947. Coenzyme A participates in a large number of enzyme reactions:
1. In the metabolism of carbohydrates,
2. Fatty acid synthesis and metabolism,

3. Propionate metabolism and
4. The metabolism of branch chain fatty acid in acetylation reaction.

Acetyl CoA (acetyl derivative of coenzyme A) is formed in the oxidation of pyruvic acid and fatty acids.

It involved in many acetylation and condensing and transfer reactions as indicated below:

   i. Choline + acetyl CoA $\longrightarrow$ acetylcholine + CoA

   ii. Succingl CoA + acetoacetate $\longrightarrow$ succinate + acetoacetyl CoA

   iii. Methylmalonyl CoA + pyruvate $\longrightarrow$ propinonyl CoA + oxaloacetate

   iv. Acetyl CoA + oxaloacetate $\longrightarrow$ citrate + CoA

Deficiency

Pantothenic acid is widely distributed in all foodstuffs, as a result, deficiency has not been unequivocally reported in human being except in specific depletion studies which have generally used the antagonist ω-methyl–pantothenic acid results in the following signs and symptoms after 2–3 weeks.

1. Neuromotor disorders including paraesthesia of the hands and feet, hyperactive tendon reflexes and muscle weakness. These can be explained by the role of acetyl CoA in the synthesis of the neurotransmitter acetylcholine and impaired formation of threonine acylesters in myelin. Demyelination may explain the persistence and reccurence of neurological problems many years after nutritional rehabilitation in people who had suffered from burning foot syndrome.
2. Mental depression, which again may be related to either acetylcholine deficit or impaired myelin synthesis.
3. Gastrointestinal complaints include severe vomiting and pain, with depressed gastric acid secretion in response to gastrin.
4. Decreased serum cholesterol and decreased urinary excretion of 17-ketosteroids, reflecting the impairment of steroidogenisis.
5. Decreased acetylation of p-aminobenzoic acid, sulphonamides and other drugs, reflecting reduced availability of acetyl CoA for these reactions.

Dietary Sources (Table 6.8)

Table 6.8: Pantothenic acid content of foods

Foodstuffs	Pantothenic acid (mg/100 g)
Rich sources	
Dried yeast	10–11
Liver (ox, sheep and goat)	7–8
Rice polishing	3–4
Wheat germ	2–3

Contd.

Table 6.8: Pantothenic acid content of foods (*Contd.*)

Foodstuffs	Pantothenic acid (mg/100 g)
Good sources	
Whole cereals	0.6–1.5
Legumes	0.6–2.2
Nuts and oilseeds	0.6–2.1
Egg	1.5–1.6
Meat	0.3–0.4
Milk	0.3–0.4
Fish	0.5–0.6
Fair sources	
Milled cereals	0.5–0.7
Vegetables	0.2–1.0
Fruits	0.1–0.3

Treatment

If deficiency is suspected, it is treated by the oral administration of 10 mg/day. This vitamin has been used to treat paralytic ileus, with 50 to 100 mg/day given parentally. Tablets of 25 and 500 mg are available as calcium pantothenate.

VITAMIN B$_{12}$

Vitamin B$_{12}$ was isolated in 1948 from liver, as a red crystalline compound containing cobalt. It has derived the names of cobalamine and cyanocobalamin because of the presence of cobalt and cynide (CN) group respectively in its structure. Other names of vitamin B$_{12}$ are antipernicious anaemia factor and extrinsic factor of castle.

CHEMICAL STRUCTURE AND PROPERTIES

It has complicated chemical structure. It contains cobalt (4–5%). It has a molecular weight of 1355 and an empirical formula $C_{63}H_{88}N_{14}O_{14}PCO$.

1. Exposure of an aqueous solution vitamin B$_{12}$ to sunlight results in the destruction of the vitamin.
2. B$_{12}$ occurs in liver and tissues in (2) forms (1) cyanocobalamin (vitamin B$_{12}$) and (2) hydroxycobalamin (vitamin B$_{12}$). Both the forms have the same biological activity in the experimental animals and for the micro-organisms. When cyanobalamin in solution is autoclaved, it is converted partly to hydroxyl cobalamin since hydroxyl cobalamin is heat labile, it is destroyed autoclaving at 120°C for 30 minutes (Fig. 6.11).

Absorption, Transport and Metabolism

A very small amount of vitamin B$_{12}$ can be absorbed by passive diffusion across the intestinal mucosa, but under normal conditions this is insignificant, accounting for less than 1% of large oral doses. The major

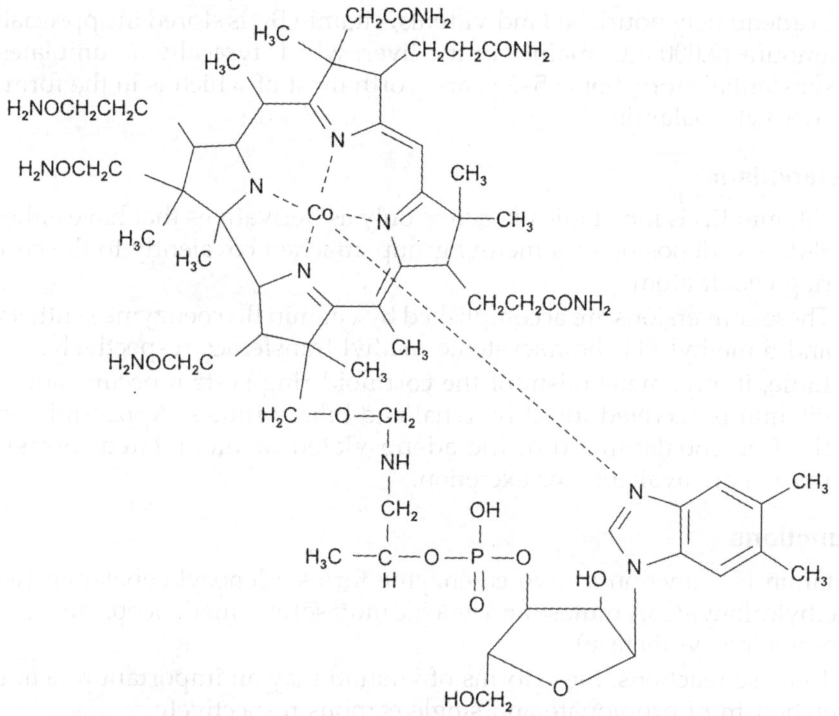

Fig. 6.11: Vitamin B_{12}. Four coordination sites on the central cobalt atom are chelated by the nitrogen atoms of the corrin ring, and one by the nitrogen of the dimethylbenzimidazole nucleotide. The sixth coordination site may be occupied by: CN^- (cyanocobalamin), OH^- (hydroxocobalamin), H_2O (aquocobalamin), $-CH_3$ (methylcobalamin) or 5'-deoxyadenosine (adenosylcobalamin)

route of vitamin B_{12} absorption is by way of attachement to a specific binding protein in the intestinal lumen.

1. In the stomach vitamin B_{12} binds to cobalophilin, a binding protein secreted in the saliva.
2. In the duodenum cobalophilin is hydrolysed, releasing the vitamin B_{12} for binding to intrinsic factor.
3. This intrinsic factor is a small glycoprotein secreted by the parietal cells of the gastric mucosa, which also secrete hydrocholoric acid
4. Vitamin B_{12} is absorbed from the distal third of the ileum, there are intrinsic factor vitamin B_{12} binding sites on the brush border of the mucosal cells in this region. Neither free instinsic factor nor free vitamin B_{12} interacts with these receptors.
5. In plasma, vitamin B_{12} circulates and bounds to transcobalmins I, which is required for tissue uptake of the vitamin, and transcobalamin II, which seems to be a storage form of the vitamin.
6. TC III (transcobalamin III) is the main transporter protein for newly absorbed cobalamins as they circulate to peripheral tissues.

7. In adequately nourished individuals, vitamin B_{12} is stored in appreciable amount (2,000 mg) mainly in the liver, which typically accumulates a substantial store. Some 5–7 years worth most of which is in the form of adeoxylcobalamin.

Metabolism

1. Vitamin B_{12} is metabolically active only as derivatives that have either a 5'-deoxyadenosine or a methyl group attached covalently to the corrin ring cobalt atom.
2. These conversions are accomplished by vitamin B_{12} coenzyme synthetase and 5-methyl FH_4 homocysteine methyl transferace respectively.
3. Little, if any, metabolism of the corrinoid ring system occurs, and the vitamin is excreted intact by renal and biliary routes. Apparently only the free cobalamins (not the adenosylated or methylated forms) in plasma are available for excretion.

Functions

Vitamin B_{12} function in two co-enzyme forms adenosyl cobalamin (with methylcalonyl-CoA mutase and leucine mutase) and methylcobalanin (with methionine synthetase).

In these reactions, these forms of vitamin play an important role in the metabolism of propionate and single carbons respectively.

Vitamin B_{12} is involved in the conversion of methylmalanyl-CoA to succinyl-CoA, which is involved in the degradation of fatty acids containing an odd number of carbon atoms.

In the bone marrow, where the erythroblast precursors of red blood cells are formed, both vitamin B_{12} and folate are needed. $N^{5,10}$ methylene tetrahydrofolate provides the methyl groups needed for the synthesis of DNA. If DNA cannot be produced in adequate amounts, the erythroblasts cannot divide and mature properly.

Vitamin B_{12} is also required for the synthesis of myelin, the white sheath of lipoprotein that surrounds many nerve fibres.

VITAMIN B_{12} DEFICIENCY

Causes

1. Vitamin B_{12} must be bound to intrinsic factor, produced by the parietal cells of the stomach, before it is absorbed in the terminal ileum. Inability to produce intrinsic factor results in pernicious anaemia.
2. Antibodies against gastric mucosa can probably be responsible for destroying the mechanism of producing instrinsic factor. The disease thus arises as an autoimmune disorder.
3. In the stomach, vitamin B_{12} binds to cobalophilin, a binding protein secreted in the saliva, it has to be hydrolyzed in duodenum for binding to instrinsic factor, further pancreatic insufficiency can therefore be a

factor in the development of vitamin B_{12} deficiency as failure to hydrolyse as cobalophilin will result in the excretion of cobalophilin-bound vitamin B_{12} rather than transfer to intrinsic factor.

4. Inadequate ingestion like a poor diet lacking in microorganisms and animal foods which are the sole source of vitamin B_{12} can lead to pernicious anaemia.

5. Increased requirements during infancy and pregnancy for nucleic acid synthesis may cause anaemia.

The most important deficiency disease occurring in human being due to vitamin B_{12} deficiency is pernicious anaemia.

Signs and Symptoms

Blood

The RBC count is low 1.5–2.5 million per mm^3 (normal 4.5 to 5.5 million). The average diameter of the cell is well above normal about 8.2 μ as compared to normal diameter of 7.3 μ. There is evidence that the abnormal circulating red cells are undergoing excessive destruction with consequent increase in the serum bilirubin content. The Hb% content is low (8–9%).

Bone Marrow

The nucleated red cells of the marrow are greatly increased. If the successive nucleated cell stage in erthropoisis are called stages I, II, III and IV, then in pernicious anaemia cells of stages I and II constitute 70%, and of stages III and IV 30%, while in normal persons the reverse is the case. The cells of stage I are peculiar and different from the normal cells and are called megaloblastic hyperplasia.

Stomach

The cells which secreted acid and enzymes are atrophied. The gastric secretions are devoid of acid, pepsin and intrinsic factor (IF).

Mouth

Soreness and inflammation of the tongue commonly seen.

Nervous System

In about 80% of the cases, parasthesia (numbness and tingling) occurs in fingers and toes. Occasionally there are objective signs of involvement of the spinal cord (vitamin B_{12} neuropathy). In advanced cases, demyelination of the white fibres of the spinal cord occurs affecting first dorsal column and later, the lateral column (combined sub-acute degeneration of the cord).

Treatment

If the haemoglobin level is under 4 g/dl, blood transfusion should always be given. Physical activity should be at a minimum until the haemoglobin is above 7 g/dl.

Vitamin B_{12} should be given in a dosage of 1,000 mcg intramuscularly twice during the first week, then 250 mcg weekly until the blood count is normal. Then 1,000 mcg every six weeks is given. Folic acid should never be used alone in the treatment of pernicious anaemia as it does not prevent the development of neurological complications and may precipitate them.

To cope up with regeneration of blood, 200 mg ferrous sulphate is given thrice daily. Vitamin B_{12} levels in maternal milk and serum are low in pernicious anaemia. The clinical picture gets corrected administering a single dose of 50 μg of vitamin B_{12} to the mother or to the infant.

Dietary Sources (Table 6.9)

Table 6.9: Important dietary sources of vitamin B_{12}

Foodstuffs	Vitamin B_{12} (μg/100 g)
Rich sources	
Liver, goat	120
Liver, ox	118
Liver, pig	59
Liver, sheep	133
Good sources	
Meat, goat	11
Meat, sheep	30
Fish	23
Egg, hens	11
Egg, ducks	9
Fair sources	
Whole milk powder	2.4
Skimmed milk powder	3.2
Cow's milk, fresh	0.5
Buffalo milk, fresh	0.4
Goats milk, fresh	0.1
Human milk	0.02

VITAMIN D

Vitamin D is unique in that under optimal conditions the body can synthesize all the vitamin D it needs. Vitamin D_2 (ergocalciferol) is produced during ultraviolet (UV) irradiation of ergosterol, a plant sterol. Vitamin D_3 (cholecalciferol) is formed from 7-dehydrocholesterol in the skin by the action of UV light. About 100 IU is produced per day from endogenous sources in persons living in temperate zone. Sunscreens (protections) can reduce production of vitamin D_3 by >95%.

Vitamins D_2 and D_3 require further metabolism to yield the metabolically active form of 1, 25-dihydroxyvitamin D (calcitriol) (Fig. 6.12).

Absorption, Transport and Storage

Dietary vitamin D is absorbed from the small intestine with lipids by passive diffusion. Vitamin D into chylomicrons enters the lymphatic system and enters the plasma. Later, it gets delivered to the liver by chylomicron remnants or to the specific carrier vitamin D binding protein (DBP), or transcalciferin.

Metabolism

Vitamin D from the skin is bound to a plasma binding protein, so that its uptake by the liver is limited. Dietary vitamin D is absorbed by incorporation into mixed micelles and enters very-low-density lipoproteins or chylomicrons, which are take up by the liver. Thus, hepatic uptake is not limited by the plasma binding protein, and toxic levels of metabolites can be reached after oral ingestion. The liver adds a 25-hydroxyl group, whereas the kidney adds hydroxyl groups at positions 1 and 24. Adipose tissue is the major storage site of vitamin D metabolites. Both 1,25-dihydroxyvitamin D_3 and other polar metabolites of vitamin D are excreted in bile and participate in an enterohepatic circulation, although the quantitative importance of this in humans is not clear. Deficiency of either calcium or phosphorus results in the formation of 1,25-dihydroxyvitamin D_3, but some other metabolites are also functional. The production of 24, 25 dihydroxyvitamin D_3, in the kidney is not closely regulated. The biologic importance of this metabolite is not established, but it may alleviate bone disease in uremic patients.

Function

Calcium and Phosphate Absorption

Calcium and phosphate absorption is increased by 1,25-dihydroxyvitamin D_3 to maintain blood levels of calcium and phosphorus. Bone mineralization results because the plasma is supersaturated with both minerals. In addition, the vitamin mobilizes calcium (and phosphate) from bone and increases the renal reabsorption of calcium. A decline in calcium concentration leads to reduction of calcium binding to the calcium censing G-protein coupled transporter system found in the parathyroid gland. All these effects result in increased serum levels of calcium and phosphate and normal mineralization. Evidence for an independent effect of the vitamin (especially 25-hydroxyvitamin D) on bone mineralization is limited. 1, 25-Dihydroxy vitamin D produced in the kidney under regulation by PTH plays an important role in mobilizing calcium from bone to maintain serum calcium and phosphorus levels within a normal range. PTH also binds to receptors on the osteoblast, stimulating increased bone turnover and calcium/phosphorus mobilization. Both PTH and 1, 25 dihydroxy vitamin D_3 enhance distal tubular calcium reabsorption, retaining most of the 7 g of calcium filtered each day (Fig. 6.12).

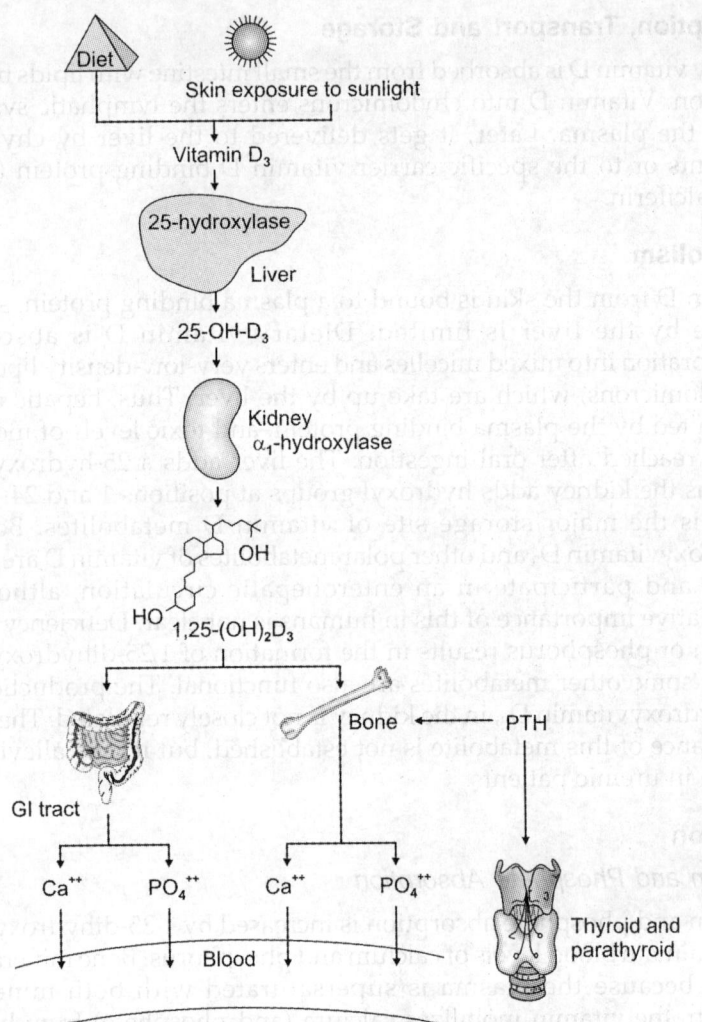

Fig. 6.12: Metabolism and function of vitamin D. Vitamin D_3 (cholecalciferol) changes into its biologically active forms: 25-$(OH)D_3$ and 1,25-$(OH)_2D_3$ (calcitriol). Calcitriol increases calcium and phosphate absorption in the intestine, increases calcium and phosphate resorption in bone, and acts on the kidney to decrease calcium loss in urine.

Muscle Function

Vitamin D improves muscle function and corrects decreased phosphate concentrations in muscle in deficiency states. Some vitamin D metabolites, especially 25-hydroxyvitamin D, may have a direct effect on bone to improve calcium deposition.

Cellular Function

Vitamin D has been implicated in many general cellular functions, such as cell proliferation and myocardial function. 1,25 dihydroxyvitamin D_3

downregulates hyperproliferative cell growth. Cancer cells have 1-hydroxylase activity, and low exposure to sunlight is associated with increased mortality from breast cancer. Vitamin D also induces 24-hydroxylase activity, which acts on 1,25 dihydroxyvitamin D_3 to form the inert metabolite calcitroic acid.

Deficiency

Oral vitamin D maintains vitamin D status less effectively than skin derived vitamin D. Nevertheless, oral supplements are sometimes needed. Indications for supplementation include breast-feeding in infancy, fat malabsorption, advanced age, institutionalization (especially if the patient is not exposed to the sun), uremia and long term use of corticosteroids.

Vitamin D deficiency results in the disease rickets among infants and children and osteomalacia in adults.

Rickets

Rickets is caused by a failure of osteoid to calcify in children. It leads to softening and weekening of the bones. Rickets is characterized by structural abnormalities of the weight-bearing bones like tibia, ribs, humers radius, ulna.

In rickets, the calcification of newly formed bone and epiphyseal cartilage is decreased. Decreased amounts of calcium are deposited in the collagen elaborated by cartilage cells. Wide osteoid seams are found most often in the long bones because they grow the fastest. Craniotabes, chest deformity, bending of long bones, enlarged epiphyses of long bones, greenstick fractures, swollen wrists, muscle weakness, seizures, tetany, inability to initiate walking and decreased growth are noted. The tetany is associated with vitamin D deficiency results from hypocalcemia. Muscle weakness will be due to decrease in muscle phosphate.

The risk factors are usually:
1. Inadequate exposure to sunlight.
2. Following strict vegetarianism (totally excluding animal food).
3. Prolonged exclusive breast food from vitamin D deficient mother.
4. When melanin is abundant in skin.

In the shafts of the long bones and in the membranous bones, there is produced instead of endosteal and periosteal bone, an excessive amount of uncalcified bone, called osteoid. This osteoid is the framework of bone, without limesalt addition, so that it is both soft and radiotranslucent. The amount of osteoid laid down varies at different points, increasing at areas of stress and strain, but decreasing at points of tension.

Treatment

Calcium absorption is only about one-third of normal when vitamin D is deficient. Vitamin D when taken with calcium, increases serum

25-hydroxyvitamin D levels, minimizes bone loss and may reduce to incidence of fractures.

To avoid deficiency a healthy subjects without exposure to sunlight requires 1,000 IU per day (for infants 0 to 12 months) and 2,000 IU per day (for older children and adults).

Dietary sources rich in vitamin D are fatty fish (e.g. mackerel, salmon), fish liver and oils, egg yolk and fortified foods. The content in cow's milk varies with the season from ten times less in winter than in summer. Vitamin D in milk may be more biologically available than from other dietary sources.

Osteomalacia

In adults, the endochondral growth of long bones has ceased; consequently, decreased calcification of cartilage is not a factor. Osteoblast mediated mineralization is affected by vitamin D deficiency, but changes occur over a longer period of time, and the clinical presentation is not as fulminant as in children. Subclinical bone disease occurs with normal blood calcium levels. By the time bone disease has become severe, hypocalcemia and hypophosphatemia are often present. Skeletal pain and muscle weekness occur anywhere in the body, but the long bones are less affected than bones in the shoulders, hips and spine.

The risk factors are:

i. Aging

ii. Renal disease (lack of 1-α-hydroxylase)

iii. Severe hepatic disease (decreased 25-hydroxylase activity)

iv. Intestinal resection/gastrointestinal disease

v. Celiac disease (decreased absorption)

vi. Gastric surgery (possibly because of decreased uptake)

vii. IBD (multifactorial)

viii. Pancreatic insufficiency/cystic fibrosis (malabsorption due to steatorrhea which leads to calcium-fatty acid complex formation)

ix. After use of anticonvulsant medication (which may cause inactive metabolites to form)

x. Decreased sunlight exposure and dietary intake.

Treatment

When it comes to treatment, it is the same as for rickets, when osteomalacia is primarily due to a defective intake of vitamin D. Supplementation of 1,000 to 2,000 IU per day is recommended. If there is evidence of malabsorption, a single massive dose of 50,000 IU should be given intramuscularly once at the beginning of 6 months. After 6 months, the patient should consume daily 400 IU of vitamin D.

Osteoporosis

Osteoporosis is defined by a low bone mass. Etiology are
- Early postmenopausal
- Late postmenopausal (after 70 years of age)
- During induced
    - A decline in renal 1-α-hydroxylase activity with age may result in decreased calcium adsorption and increased secretion of parathyroid hormone.
    - Chronic vitamin D deficiency may be a factor in osteoporosis in elderly patients in nursing homes due to poor dietary intake and decreased outdoor activity.
    - Chronic abuse of alcohol is a frequently overlooked cause of osteoporosis in men. Chronic pancreatitis and small bowel injury resulting from alcohol abuse may impair calcium and amino acid absorption.
    - Decreased intake of vitamin D, lack of sunlight, and altered vitamin D metabolism (in cirrhotics) are probably important (Table 6.10).

Table 6.10: Differential diagnosis of osteomalacia and osteoporosis

Clinical Features	Osteomalacia	Osteoporosis
Skeletal pain	A major complaint and usually persistent.	Usually associated with a fracture
Fractures	Occurs occasionally; healing delayed.	Very common; heals normally
Skeletal deformity	Common	Absent
Radiographic features:		
Loss of density of bone	Widespread	Irregular and most often marked in the spine
Loss of bone detail	Characteristic	Not characteristic
Loser's zones	Diagnostic	Absent
Biopsy:		
Histological changes	Excess osteoid tissue with bone present in normal quantity.	Bone reduced in quality but fully mineralized
Biochemical changes:		
Serum Ca and P	Often low	Normal
Serum alkaline Phosphatase	Often high	Normal
Urinary calcium	Often low	Normal/high
Response to treatment:		
Vitamin D	Dramatic	None

Treatment

Some evidence has been found that short-term therapy with low-dose 1,25-dihydroxyvitamin D_3 relieves osteoporosis, improvement is not maintained.

Toxicity

Hypervitaminosis D occurs because of excessive intake of vitamin D, since it is stored in adipose tissue and released slowly. Although serum 1,25-dihydroxyvitamin D concentrations are regulated by calcium levels, 25-hydroxyvitamin D levels are not become 25-hydroxyvitamin D_3 which itself has physiologic effects, albeit less potent than those of 1,25-dihydroxyvitamin D, hypercalcemia and hypercalciuria can ensue.

Acute hypercalcemia causes nausea, anorexia, itching, polyuria, abdominal pain, constipation, bone pain, metallic taste, and dehydration. In chronic cases, nephrocalcinosis, metastatic calcification, renal failure and kidney stone may develop. Weight loss, irritability, psychosis, pancreatitis, photophobia, hypertension, cardiac arrhythmias and elevated levels of blood urea nitrogen, aspartate aminotransferase, calcium, and alanine aminotransferase have been reported.

Treatment

Prednisone, diuresis, and a low calcium may be required along with withdrawal of vitamin D.

VITAMIN E

Vitamin E is composed of a number of tocopherols and tocotrienols, each with different levels of activity. The naturally occurring vitamin E produced by plants includes at least 8 different forms α, β, γ and δ plus the corresponding tocotrienols.

CHEMISTRY AND PROPERTY

All tocopherols differ from one another in the number and position of methyl groups on the chroman ring that is the first ring of tocol nucleus.

Only α-tocopherol is considered the active form of vitamin E so the RDA for vitamin E is based only on alpha-tocopherol. It is a pale yellow oil, stable to acids and heat and insoluble in water.

Tocopherols are very susceptible to oxidation and these lead to loss of vitamin activity. As tocopherols are extremely susceptible to oxidation, they protect less susceptible compounds by breaking up the chain of oxidation reations. This property is make use in commercial use of tocopherols as antioxidants.

Absorption, Transport and Storage

Unlike any other fat soluble vitamins, it is also absorbed through oil solutions. Absorption requires biliary (bile salt micelles) and pancreatic (esterase) secretions.

Less than 40% of an oral dose is absorbed, and this amount is decreased by excess unsaturated fatty acids in the lumen.

Only free α-tocopherol is found in the intestinal lymph. In serum, two-thirds of the vitamin is bound to and hydrolyzed on LDL, and the remnants are transferred to HDL.

- Some vitamins are transferred to extrahepatic tissues (adipose and muscle), with the rest taken up by liver.
- No carrier is specific for vitamin E; therefore, its serum level is proportional to the total lipid level.
- Under normal conditions a very little vitamin is excreted through urine or faeces.

Functions

The primary function of vitamin E in body is that it acts as an antioxidant, protecting polyunsaturated fatty acids (PUFAs) and other lipid molecules from oxidative damage. By this, it helps

i. To maintain the integrity of PUFA-rich cell membranes

ii. Protects red blood cells against hemolysis

iii. Protects vitamin A from oxidation.

Food Source

It is found in green leafy vegetables, seeds and oils, eggs, liver and muscle meats.

Toxicity

A little evidence of toxicity even at very high intake is seen. Symptoms of hypervitaminosis E are muscle weakness, fatigue, headache, nausea. It may impair the absorption of other fat-soluble vitamins.

WATER-SOLUBLE VITAMINS

Water-soluble vitamins dissolve in water and directly absorbed in the blood stream. We need a continuous supply of them in our diets because there is no reserved in storage; they are eliminated in urine when consumed in excess amounts. The water-soluble vitamins are the B-complex group and vitamin C.

Vitamin B Complex

B-complex group of vitamins comprises eight water-soluble vitamins which are nutritionally essential.

Riboflavin

In 1926, Goldberger and co-workers showed that pellagra was cured by autoclaved yeast which was devoid of thiamine. This factor was called

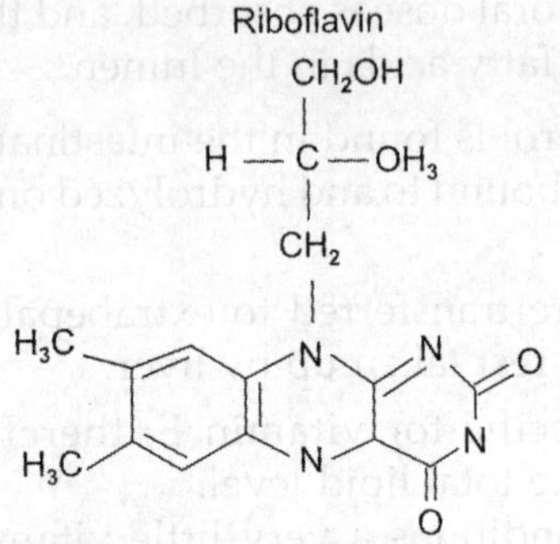

Riboflavin

Fig. 6.13: Structure of riboflavin

vitamin B_2 (riboflavin). Riboflavin was the first component to be isolated in a pure state from milk, eggs, liver.

Riboflavin is slightly soluble in water and alcohol, but insoluble in fat solvents. Riboflavin is heat stable but unstable in UV light (Fig. 6.13).

Function

Riboflavin forms a part of the two coenzymes flavin mononucleotide (FMN) and flavin adenine dinucleotide (FAD). The prosthetic group is bound to the enzyme, accepts on H^+ ion, and then it is reoxidized by interacting with another H^+ acceptor, usually a cytochrome of the mitochondrial electron transport chain. Flavin participates in both one- and two-electron transfers.

It functions as coenzymes for succinic dehydrogenase; oxidases of fatty acid, glucose and glycine; and xanthine oxidases. Thus, the richest sources of the vitamin are metabolically active tissues, not storage tissues (Table 6.11).

Table 6.11: Some flavin-linked dehydrogenases

Enzyme	Coenzyme	Reaction
NADH dehydrogenase	FMN	NADH $\rightarrow$ NAD
Succinate dehydrogenase	FAD, Fe	Succinate $\rightarrow$ furmarate
L-α-Glycero-p-dehydrogenase	FAD	Glycerol-P $\rightarrow$ Dihydroxyacetone-P
Choline dehydrogenase	FAD	Choline $\rightarrow$ Betaine aldehyde
Acetyl-CoA-dehydrogenase	FAD (ETF)	Acetyl-CoA $\rightarrow$ Dehydroacyl–CoA
Sarcosine dehydrogenase	Flavin (ETF), Fe	Sarcosine $\rightarrow$ Glycine + HCHO
Dimethylglycine dehydrogenase	Flavin (ETF), Fe	Dimethylglycine $\rightarrow$ Sarcosine + HCHO
Aerobic dehydrogenase		
L-amino acid oxidase	FMN	Amino acid $\rightarrow$ Keto acid + NH_3 + H_2O_2
D-amino acid oxidase	FAD	Amino acid $\rightarrow$ Keto acid + NH_3 + H_2O_2
Xanthine oxidase	FAD	Xanthine $\rightarrow$ Hypoxanthine + H_2O_2
		Xypoxanthine $\rightarrow$ Uric acid + H_2O_2

ABSORPTION, TRANSPORT AND METABOLISM

Riboflavin is absorbed rapidly in the intestine. More riboflavin is absorbed, when it is taken with meals (about 70%) than when it is taken alone (about 15%); however, the capacity for absorption is limited to ~30 mg per day. The vitamin enters plasma as free flavin mononucleotide, is bound to albumin and immunoglobulin, and then is excreted as riboflavin or its metabolites.

It is secreted in the milk and excreted in urine and faeces. Urinary excretion is increased by a negative nitrogen balance and by large amount of thiamine. Excretion is decreased by low-carbohydrates diets, exercise and pregnancy.

SOURCES

Colonic bacteria produce riboflavin, but this is not available for absorption in sufficient quantity to fulfil, daily need. The bacteria must be lysed or killed for the vitamin to be available.

Riboflavin is widely distributed, especially in flesh of mammals and in all leafy vegetable. Tender parts of the plants like the tender leaves and buds contain more riboflavin than older ones. The best sources are yeast, milk, egg whites, kidney, liver, and leafy vegetable. Fish, meat and poultry are good sources. Other vegetables and legumes are not rich source of riboflavin.

Deficiency

Problems associated with riboflavin deficiency include ariboflavinosis which covers orolingual, dermal, hematological and corneal manifestations.

Orolingual Manifestations

Early symptoms are soreness and burning of lips, mouth and tongue. Angular stomatitis is a lesion characterized by maceration and bilateral transverse fissures of the mucocutaneous junction at the angle of the mouth.
- Lesions of the vermilion of the lips, termed cheilosis, will frequently occur.
- The tongue with swollen and abnormally red, magenta coloured, having large flattened papillae called glossitis occur in severe cases.

Dermal Lesions

- Desquamation of the skin and seborrheic dermatitis may be seen, especially in the nasolabial fold ears and scrotum.
- In riboflavin deficiency, there is biochemical defect of rise in homocysteine which may impair the process of collagen cross-linking.

Ocular Mainfestation

Photophobia, tearing, burning and itching of the eyes develop. Corneal vascularization develops around the entire circumference.

Neurological Manifestations

Development of neuropathy is studied in this deficiency.

Haematological Manifestation

Normocytic and normochromic anaemia will be developed.

Some of these symptoms also occur with vitamin B_6 deficiency because the oxidase required to produce the functional form of vitamin B_6 is riboflavin dependent. Riboflavin is required for the metabolism of vitamin B_6, folate, niacin and vitamin K. Thus, multiple other deficiencies often accompany riboflavin deficiency.

Hemodialysis, poor intake, alcoholism, malabsorption may develop the deficiency conditions. Drugs like chlorpromazine, imipramine, amitriptyline and quinacrine can prevent conversion to the active coenzyme.

Treatment

Oral intake of 5 to 10 mg per day, help in treating the deficiency status. When malabsorption is present, prophylactic use of the vitamin at a dose of about 3 mg per day is useful.

PYRIDOXINE (VITAMIN B_6)

Pyridoxine was first isolated in a pure form by Lepkorsky, Kerseztesy and Stevens, Gyorgy, Kuhn and Wendt in the year 1938. It was synthesised in 1939 by Kuhn, *et al.* and Kerseztesy, *et al.*

The term vitamin B_6 encompasses three naturally occurring pyridines— pyridoxine, pyridoxal, and pyridoxamine (Fig. 6.14).

All the three are converted to the metabolically active coenzyme form pyridoxal phosphate, which is primarily involved in the metabolism of amino acids. Pyridoxine is water soluble, heat stable and sensitive to light and alkalis.

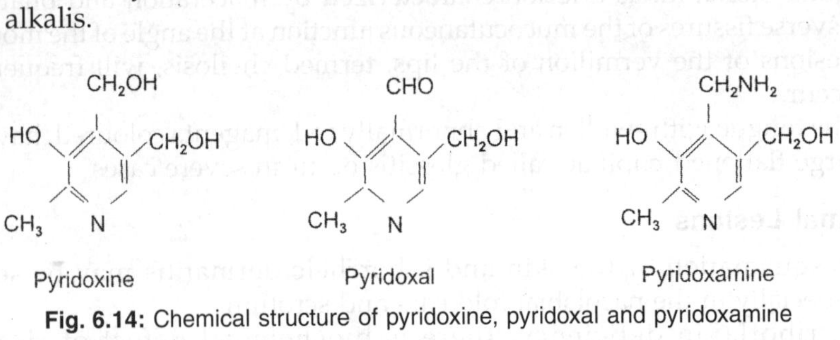

Fig. 6.14: Chemical structure of pyridoxine, pyridoxal and pyridoxamine

All the three are interrelated functionally, the estimates of requirement are based on production or care of clinical signs of deficiency or, more often, on production or reversal of abnormal biochemical test results (e.g. excretion of tryptophan metabolites after a tryptophan load). Requirements are increased during intake of a large amount of protein.

ABSORPTION, TRANSPORT AND METABOLISM

Pyridoxine is absorbed in the upper portion of the small intestine by passive diffusion of the dephosphorylated forms pyridoxine, pyridoxal and pyridoxamine. Absorption is driven by phosphorylation to form pyridoxal phosphate and then by protein binding of each of these metabolites in the intestinal mucosa and blood.

Most of the absorbed vitamin is taken up by the liver and it is metabolized by hepatic flavoenzymes. Pyridoxal phosphate and some pyridoxal are exported from the liver bound to albumin. Free pyridoxal remaining in the liver is rapidly oxidized to 4-pyridoxic acid, which is the main excretory product.

Extrahepatic tissues take up both pyridoxal, and pyridoxal phosphate from the plasma. The phosphate is hydrolysed to pyridoxal, which can cross cell membranes, by extracellular alkaline phosphatase, then trapped intracellularly by phosphorylation.

Some 80% of the body's total vitamin B_6 is pyridoxal phosphate in muscle, mostly associated with glycogen phosphorylase. This does not function as a reserve of the vitamin and is not released from muscle in times of deficiency; it is released into the circulation (as pyridoxal) in starvation, when glycogen reserves are exhausted and there are fewer requirements for phosphorylase activity. Under these conditions it is available for redistribution to other tissues, and especially liver and kidney, to meet the increased requirement for gluconeogenesis from amino acids (Fig. 6.15).

Function

Pyridoxal phosphate is the metabolically active form of vitamin B_6. It is a coenzyme for metabolism of amino acids and in several aspects of the metabolism of neurotransmitters, glycogen, sphingolipids, haeme and steroids.

1. Transaminase system: The transaminases represent a large number of enzymes. Two important systems are the following:

   Glutamic acid + oxaloacetate $\longrightarrow$ α-ketoglutarate + aspartate.

   Alanine + α-ketoglutarate $\rightarrow$ Glutamic acid + Pyruvic acid

2. Amino acid decarboxylase: These enzymes convert amino acids to the corresponding amines.

   Histidine $\rightarrow$ Histamine + CO_2

   Tyrosine $\rightarrow$ Tyramine + CO_2

3. Conversion of tryptophan to niacin.

4. Muscle phosphorylase: It contains pyridoxal phosphate

5. Helps in dehydrases (hydrolyses) which are important in catabolism of threonine, serine and homoserine.

Deficiency

The vitamin B_6 allowance has been estimated depending upon protein intake. Thus, the estimates for women and men are based on the lower rates of protein intake in women than in men. The protein requirements of pregnant and lactating women are increased, thereby intake of vitamin B_6 is also increased.

Vitamin B_6 deficiency leads to metabolic abnormalities resulting from insufficient production of pyridoxal phosphate. Pyridoxine deficiency often occurs as a side effect of drugs.

Drugs like isoniazid, hydralazine and other hydrazines, oral contraceptives, dopamine and penicillamine act as antagonists. Cycloserine also can act in this way. These compounds increase urinary excretion (e.g. isoniazid) or combine with pyridoxal or pyridoxal phosphate to form inactive drug (e.g. hydrazones are derived from hydrazines and a thiazolidine derivative from penicillamine). These effects can be reversed with vitamin B_6 supplements, usually in the range of 2 to 5 mg per day (Fig. 6.15).

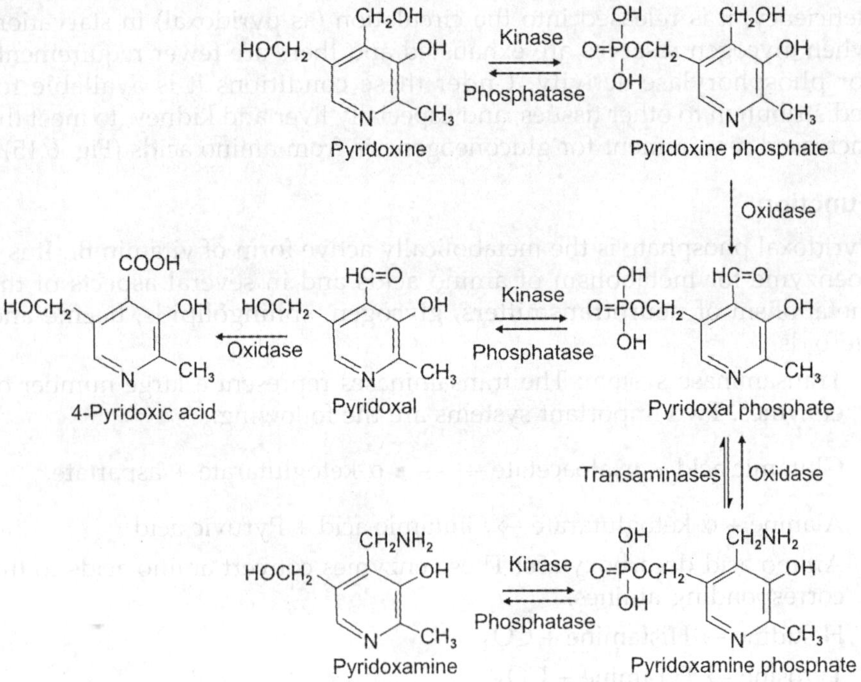

Fig. 6.15: Interconversion of the vitamin B_6 vitamers.

Anaemia

A reversible type of hypochromic microcytic anaemia develops. The anaemia improves after administration of vitamin B_6.

CENTRAL NERVOUS SYSTEM DISTURBANCES

It is reported that epileptiform convulsions occur in infants when vitamin B_6 is deficient. This has been traced to the impairment of the function of B_6 as a code carboxylase in the conversation of glutamic acid to γ-aminobutyric acid (GABA), which further gets metabolised to succinic acid in the brain. It is also reported that GABA, which function as regulator of neuronal activity in normal individuals, is deficient in brain when there is a deficiency of B_6.

$$\text{Glutamic acid} \xrightarrow[\text{Decarboxylase}]{\text{Pyridoxal phosphate}} \text{γ-aminobutyric acid} + CO_2$$

$$\downarrow$$

$$\text{succinic acid}$$

Pyridoxine-dependent Syndromes

These syndromes have been reported, in which tissues levels of the vitamin are normal but binding of the cofactor to the enzyme is impaired. These inherited disorders respond to larger doses of vitamin B_6 than are required to treat deficiency states. (Table 6.12) lists the syndromes.

Table 6.12: Pyridoxine-dependent errors of metabolism

Disorder	Enzyme	Clinical findings	Laboratory findings
Infantile seizures	Glutamic acid decarboxylase	Convulsions	None
B_6-dependent chronic anaemia	δ-aminolevulinic acid (ALA) synthase	Hypochromic anaemia	Increased serum iron
B_6-dependent homocystinuria	Cystathionine β-synthase	Mental retardation, severe collagen disease involving vessels, eye problems, osteoporosis	Homocystinemia homocystinuria, hypermethioninemia
Cystathioninuria	γ-cystathionase	Mental retardation, blood dyscrasia, heart disease	Cystathionuria
Xanthurenic aciduria	Kynureninase	Urticaria, mental retardation	Xanthurenic aciduria
Gyrate atrophy of choroids and retina	Ornithine aminotransferase	Chorioretinal degeneration, blindness	None diagnostic
X-linked sideroblastic anaemia	Erythroid specific δ-ALA synthase	Anaemia	Ringed sideroblasts
Primary hyperoxaluria	Alanine-glyoxylate aminotransferase	Renal stones	Hyperoxaluria

Contd.

Table 6.12: Pyridoxine-dependent errors of metabolism (*Contd.*)

Disorder	Enzyme	Clinical findings	Laboratory findings
Developmental delay	Aromatic-L-amino acid decarboxylase	Hypotonia, oculogyric crises	Elevated 5-hydroxytryptophan in CSF, plasma, and urine
Cohen syndrome	β-alanine α-ketoglutarate transaminase	Hypotonia, obesity, mental retardation, facial/oral/ocular /limb anomalies	None diagnostic

CSF, cerebrospinal fluid.

Adapted from Frank T, Bitsch R, Maiwald J, Stein G. High thiamine phosphate concentrations in erythrocytes can be achieved in dialysis patients by oral administration of benfotiamine. Eur J clin pharmacol 2000; 56: 251.

Oral and Dermal Lesions

Angular stomatitis, glossitis and cheilosis in pregnant and lactating mothers is caused due to pyridoxine deficiency. Riboflavin deficiency impairs pyridoxal phosphate synthesis. Recent study by National Institute of Nutrition, suggests that both riboflavin and pyridoxine deficiencies affect collagen synthesis and maturation which probably results in varying skin lesions in these deficiencies.

Treatment

In treating deficiencies, it is often advisable also to give other B-complex vitamins because multiple deficiencies frequently occur simultaneously. For prophylactic use with isoniazid to prevent peripheral neuropathy, 5 mg per day is probably sufficient, but doses up to 25 mg are used. Treatment of established neuropathy requires 50 to 300 mg per day. Pyridoxine is sometime given to patients with sideroblastic anaemia, dystonia, or Parkinson's disease and to newborns with seizure disorders.

BIOTIN

Biotin was originally known as the "anti-egg white injury factor" because egg white contains a protein called avidin, which combines with biotin in

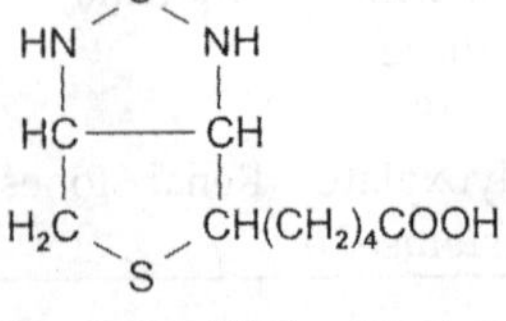

Fig. 6.16: Biotin structure

the intestinal tract and prevents absorption of biotin from intestines. But this is denatured when eggs are cooked.

Biotin is a heterocyclic sulphur containing monocarboxylic acid. The chemical structure of biotin was established by Du vigneaud and colleagues between 1940 and 1942. Biotin is sparkingly soluble in cold water and is freely soluble in hot water. They are heat stable.

The coenzyme of biotin is biocytin. It is a combination of biotin and lysine.

Absorption, Transport and Metabolism

Biotin is synthesized mainly by intestinal bacteria. Most biotin in foods is present as biocytin (ε-aminobiotinyllysine), which is released on proteolysis, then hydrolysed by biotinidase in the pancreatic juice and intestinal mucosal secretions, to yield free biotin.

Free biotin is absorbed by the small intestine and probably colon by the sodium dependent multivitamin transporter (SMVT) that also transports pantothenic acid. Excess biotin is not stored, it is excreted in urine.

Biotin circulates in the blood stream both free and bound to a serum glycoprotein which has biotinidase activity, catalyzing the hydrolysis of biocytin. The incorporation of biotin into enzymes is relatively slow and cannot be considered part of the uptake process. On catabolism of the enzymes, biocytin is hydrolysed by biotinidase, permitting reutilization.

Function

Biotin is a cofactor for carboxylating enzymes. Biotin accepts carbon dioxide to form an intermediated compound and then transfers carbon dioxide to the substrate. It is thus essential as an intermediate of carbohydrate, protein, and fat.

Biotin function to transfer carbon dioxide in a small number of carboxylation reactions. The reactive intermediate is 1-N-carboxybiocytin (Fig. 6.17), formed from bicarbonate in an ATP-dependent reaction. A single holocarboxylase synthetase acts on the apoenzymes of acetyl CoA carboxylase (a key enzyme in fatty acid synthesis), pyruvate carboxylase (a key enzyme in gluconeogenesis), propionyl CoA carboxylase and methylcrotonyl CoA carboxylase to form the active holoenzymes from (inactive) apoenzymes and free biotin (Table 6.13).

Deficiency

Dietary deficiency is rare in humans. High levels of phenylpyruvate, seen in phylketonuria, inhibit pyruvate carboxylase and lead to a functional biotin deficiency.

People who takes a lot of raw eggs, likely to develop biotin deficiency due to impaired biotin absorption. Symptoms like, alopecia maculopapular dermatitis and pallor are noted after many weeks. Depression, lassitude,

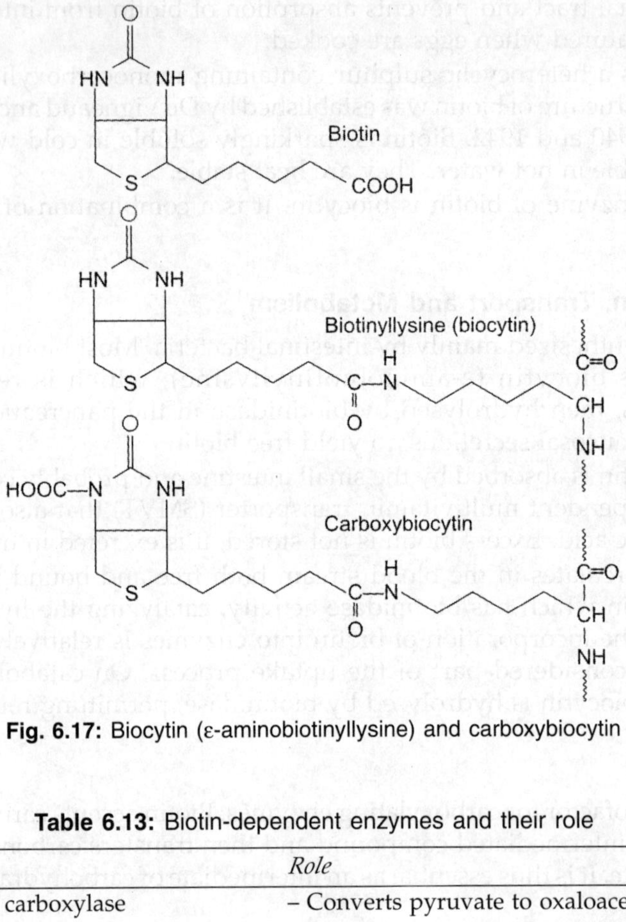

Fig. 6.17: Biocytin (ε-aminobiotinyllysine) and carboxybiocytin

Table 6.13: Biotin-dependent enzymes and their role

Enzyme	Role
• Pyruvate carboxylase	– Converts pyruvate to oxaloacetate
• Acetyl CoA carboxylase	– Converts acetyl CoA to malonyl CoA
• Propionyl CoA carboxylase	– Converts propionate to succinate
• β-methyl crotonyl CoA carboxylase	– Converts β-methyl crotonyl CoA to β-methyl glutanyl CoA

muscle pain, paresthesias, and anorexia with nausea occur. Biotin deficiency produces a scaly dermatitis, whereas zinc deficiency results in the wetter dermatitis.

Sources

Biotin is synthesized by many microorganisms, and it is felt that colonic flora contributes to the available biotin in humans. In food it is present in free and bound forms. In egg yolks, biotin is bound by the protein avidin. Biotin is liberated in the intestine by enzymatic hydrolysis. Rich sources are yeast, liver and other organ meats, fish, soybeans, dairy products, grains, tomatoes and egg yolk.

FOLATE

Folate is the generic name for a group of substances that have similar nutritional properties and chemical structures. Folate is present in foods as a variety of polyglutamates (tetrahydrofolates), with different biological activity. Folic acid (pteroylglutamine acid) refers to the parent compound used fortification of foods and manufacture of supplements but not naturally present in food. Folic acid has higher bioavailability than food folate (Table 6.14).

Table 6.14: Early nomenclature of folic acid

Name	Properties and source	Authors
1. "Wills factor"	Present in autolysed yeast and cures tropical macrocytic anaemia	L. Wills (1933)
2. Vitamin M	Present in liver and cures nutritional cytopenia and diarrhoea in monkeys	Da et al. (1935)
3. Factor U	Chick growth factor present in liver	Stockstad (1938)
4. Vitamin B_c	Present in liver and cures anaemia in chicks	Hogen et al. (1339)
5. Norite eluate factor (L-casei)	Present in liver and essential for growth of L-casei	Snell and Peterson (1940)
6. Folic acid	Present in spinach and essential for growth of L-casei	Mitchell, Snell and Williams (1941)

Folic acid or pteroylmonoglutamic acid is made up of three components:
1. Pteridine
2. Para-aminobenzoic acid (PABA)
3. Glutamic acid (Fig. 6.18).

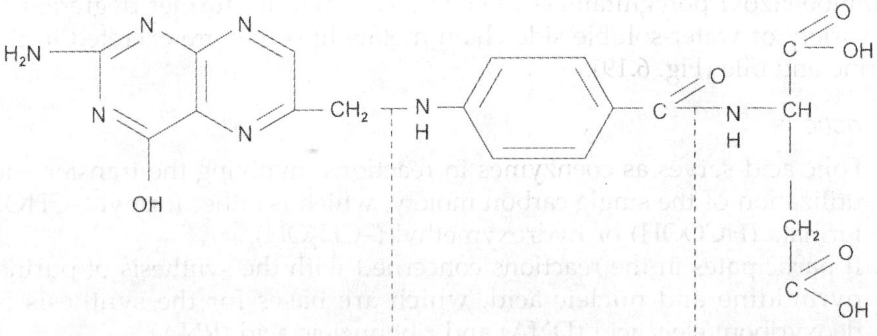

Pteridine   PABA   Glutamic acid

Fig. 6.18: Structure of folic acid

Absorption and Transport

Dietary folates are mostly in the polyglutamate form, which is not quite as available as the unconjugated vitamin.

Folacin is variably available in foods because of the presence of binders, inhibitors and other factors. Dietary folates are absorbed only as the monoglutamate forms of folic acid, 5-methyltetrahydrofolic acid and 5-formyltetrahydrofolic acid. It is absorbed by active transport in small intestine.

The maximum transport occurs after deconjugation to the monoglutamate form. Polyglutamate forms of folate in food are hydrolyzed by folyl poly-γ-glutamate carboxypeptidase; the products of hydrolysis, which contain decreased numbers of glutamate residues, include the monoglutamate form, found in small amount in human salivary, gastric, pancreatic and jejunal juice. The activity of this carboxypeptidase is increased in intestinal mucosa, liver, pancreas, kidney and placenta.

After conversion in the liver to 5-methyltetrahydrofolic acid, the vitamin can enter the plasma as the monoglutamate. Only monoglutamate derivatives found in plasma are taken up by the cells using an energy-dependent process with a specific folate binding protein or a carrier-mediated anion exchange process. They can be stored in tissue as the polyglutamate, or be reexcreted in bile and reabsorbed.

Metabolism

Folate are converted to coenzymes by reduction of pterin ring, elongation of the peptide chain with glutamyl residues, and addition of a one-carbon fragment in position N-5 or N-10 of the pterin ring. Thus, a large variety of folate coenzyme exist. The tetrahydro form is frequently involved, and it is thought that a polyglutamate form is the active coenzyme. These coenzymes function in many reactions involving one-carbon transfers, including purine and thymidylate synthesis, metabolism of several amino acids (especially serine and homocysteine), methylation of biogenic amines, and initiation of protein synthesis by formulation of methionine.

Tissues folates turn over by cleavage of their pteridine and para-aminobenzoyl polyglutamate moieties. The later are further degraded to a variety of water-soluble side-chain metabolites that are excreted in the urine and bile (Fig. 6.19).

Functions

1. Folic acid serves as coenzymes in reactions involving the transfer and utilization of the single carbon moiety, which is either formyl (–CHO), formate (HCOOH) or hydroxymethyl (–CH$_2$OH).
2. It participates in the reactions concerned with the synthesis of purine, pyrimidine and nucleic acid, which are bases for the synthesis of deoxyribonucleic acid (DNA) and ribonucleic acid (RNA).
3. Along with vitamin B$_{12}$, folic acid helps in the transmethylation of homocysteine to methionine, ethanolomine to choline and uracil to thymine.

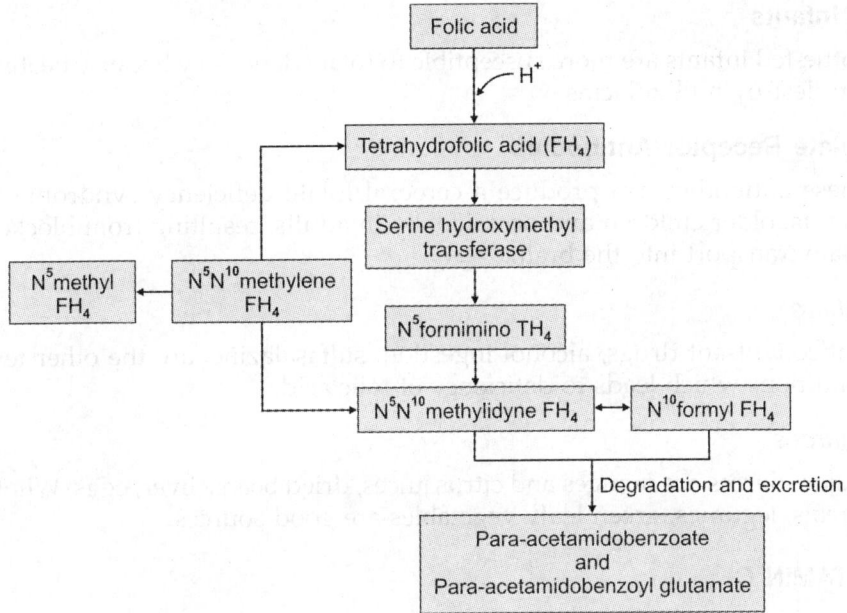

Fig. 6.19: Metabolism of folates

4. Folic acid in conjunction with vitamin B_{12} helps in normal growth and maturation of red blood cells.
5. Folic acid is required for the normal metabolic pathway of histidine, particularly in the conversion of formiminoglutamic acid to glutamic acid.

Deficiency

Anaemia

Megaloblastic or macrocytic anaemia is a symptom of both folic acid and B_{12} deficiency.

Sprue

Sprue is a gastrointestinal disease characterized by intestinal lesions, malabsorption defects, diarrhoea, macrocytic anaemia and general malnutrition.

In Reproductive Health

Requirements of folic acid increases from 100 µg/day during pregnancy for normal foetal growth, since there is a decrease in folate absorption and an increase in urinary excretion during pregnancy.

Neural tube defects could be prevented if women consumed adequate amount of folic acid early in pregnancy. High doses were not recommended because they can mask B_{12} deficiency. It is always recommended to take adequate amount of folic acid before as well as after conception.

In Infants

Bottle-fed infants are more susceptible to folate deficiency because heating can destroy milk folacins.

Folate Receptor Antibodies

These antibodies can produce a cerebral folate deficiency syndrome in infants, older children and occasionally in adults, resulting from blocked folate transport into the brain.

Others

Anticonvulsant drugs, alcohol ingestion, sulfasalazine, are the other few conditions which leads to deficiency of folic acid.

Sources

Major sources are oranges and citrus juices, dried beans, liver, eggs. Whole cereals, legumes, green leafy vegetables are good sources.

VITAMIN C

Vitamin C or ascorbic acid is known as antiscorbutic vitamin, because it has a property to cure the disease called scurvy. Much of the early pioneering work on the isolation of vitamin C was carried out by Zilva during 1917–27.

Ascorbic acid has a structure similar to that of L-glucose and it is a derivative of glucose. It is synthesized from glucose and galactose by plants and animals.

CHEMISTRY

Ascorbic acid is a simple compound containing six carbon atoms, related to the monosaccharide glucose. It is stable to acid but easily destroyed by oxidation, light, alkali and heat especially in the presence of iron or copper.

The oxidised form of ascorbic acid known as dehydroascorbic acid also has vitamin C activity. The oxidation products of dehydroascorbic acid have no vitamin C activity. The structure of vitamin C is shown in Fig. 6.20.

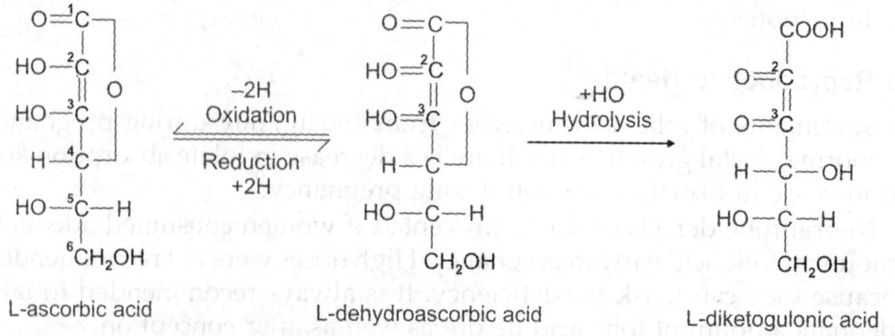

Fig. 6.20: Metabolism of vitamin C

Vitamin C is susceptible to oxidation because it is a reducing agent that function in the body as antioxidant.

Most mammals can synthesise vitamin C from glucose but a few including humans lack the liver enzyme gulonoactone-oxidase, which is required to catalyse one step of the process. It is the lack of the enzyme that forces humans to depend on supplies of vitamin C from their food. Man, monkey, guinea pig, Indian fruit eating bat and red vented bulbul require a supply of vitamin C in their diet. Of the animals that require a supply of the vitamin, guinea pigs and monkeys are most widely used in research. Now fish are also in research of vitamin C. In plant vitamin C accumulates during the ripening process and is presumably synthesised within the plant cells from naturally occurring glucose.

Properties

1. Ascorbic acid readily soluble in water but insoluble in most solvents. It has sour acid taste.
2. Ascorbic acid is extremely unstable and gets easily oxidized to dehydro-ascorbic acid, in the presence of air, light, hydrogen peroxide ferric chloride, iodine and methylene blue.

Absorption, Transport and Metabolism

Species that cannot biosynthesize ascorbic acid absorb it from the diet by active transport and passive diffusion. The oxidized form of the vitamin, dehydroascorbic acid, is better absorbed than the reduced form, ascorbate, or ascorbic acid. The efficiency of enteric absorption of the vitamin is high (80% to 90%) at low intake but declines markedly at intake greater than about 1 g/day, vitamin C is transported in the plasma in the reduced form (ascorbic acid) in free solution. It is taken up by cells through a glucose transporter and a specific active transport system. Each system moves dehydroascorbic acid into cells, where it is readily reduced to ascorbase. The glucose transporter based system of uptake is not as fast as a specific system, but it is stimulated by insulin and inhibited by glucose.

Metabolism

Vitamin C is oxidized to monodehydroascorbic acid. This intermediate can be further oxidized to dehydroascorbic acid, subsequently the oxidized product undergoes irreversible hydrolysis to yield 2,3-diketo-1-gulonic acid, which can be decarboxylated to yield carbon dioxide and several five carbon fragments (xylose, xylonic acid) or oxidized to yield oxalic acid and several 4 carbon fragments (e.g. threonic acid), in addition, the vitamin can be converted to ascorbic acid 2-sulfate.

Functions

Because ascorbic acid easily loose electrons and is reversibly converted to dehydroascorbic acid, it serves as biochemical redox system involved in the synthesis of collagen and carnitine and other metabolic reaction as follows:

1. *Formation of intracellular cement substance:* We require vitamin C to build and maintain body tissues in general, including bone matrix, cartilage, dentin, collagen and connective tissues. When vitamin C is absent, the important ground substances do not develop into collagen. When the vitamin is given, formation of cartilaginous tissue follows quickly. Collagen is a protein substance that exists in many body tissues, such as the white fibres of connective tissues. Blood vessel tissues particularly weakened without the cementing substance from vitamin C's metabolic action that helps provide firm capillary walls.

2. *Absorption of iron and incorporation of plasma iron in ferritin:* Ascorbic acid helps to reduce the ferric iron to ferrous state in the intestine and thus helps in the absorption of iron. Many studies shown that for the incorporation of plasma iron in the tissues as ferritin, ascorbic acid and ATP are required.

3. *Bone formation:* The fundamental pathological changes in ascorbic acid deficiency are the defective formation of bone matrix and ground substance. Calcification is not affected. Vitamin C is necessary for conversion of folic acid to folinic acid, both being required for maturation of erethrocytes. Osteoblasts, that were invading the area of provisional calcification, change histologically into fibroblasts. The matrix they produce is not a gel but a loose connective tissue.

4. *Hydroxylation of aromatic nuclei:* Ascorbic acid plays an important role in (i) hydroxylation of deoxycorticosterone (ii) hydroxylation of tryptophan to 5 hydroxytryptophan and phenylalanine to tyrosine, etc. Ascorbic acid dependent electron transfer in liver microsomes is generally coupled with hydroxylation.

5. *Role cholesterol metabolism:* Vitamin C is required for the synthesis of the carnitine. Carnitine is a small nitrogen containing organic compound involved in the transport of fatty acids into mitochondric to be oxidized to release energy for use by cells.

   Vitamin C is known to be involved in regulating cholesterol metabolism and in maintaining the structure of blood vessels and antioxidant effects of vitamin might prevent tissues damage that leads to cardiovascular disease.

6. *Activation of hormones:* Many peptide hormones and releasing factors are synthesised as precursor molecules that are enzymatically modified into their active forms. Vitamin C is essential for activation of bombesin (human gastrin-releasing peptide) calcitonin, gastrin oxytocin, thyrotropin, corticotropin, vasopression, growth hormone-releasing factor.

7. *General antioxidant:* A variety of damaging oxidizing agents occur in the body, as a result of both normal metabolic processes and exposure to drugs and environmental pollutants. A range of enzymes and

antioxidant reducing agents (including vitamin E, β-carotene and vitamin C) are able to convert these oxidizing agents to harmless substances that can be excreted. Vitamin C can combine with and so "scavenge" many types of oxidizing free radicals. It can also regenerate the reduced form of vitamin E converting the vitamin back into the form in which it can act as an antioxidant.

Deficiency

Acute vitamin C deficiency results in scurvy in individuals unable to synthesize the vitamin.

Blood vessel tissues are particularly weakened without the cementing substance from vitamin C's metabolic action that helps provide firm capillary walls. Thus vitamin C deficiency is characterized by fragile capillaries, easily ruptured by blood pressure or trauma, resulting in tissue bleeding. Deficiency signs including easy bruising, pinpoint haemorrhages of the skin, bone and joint haemorrhages, easy bone fracture, poor wound healing and soft bleeding gums (a condition called gingivitis).

The early symptoms of scurvy are nonspecific include listlessness, fatigue, weakness, shortness of breath, muscle cramps, acting bones, joints and muscle and loss of appetite.

Scurvy can occur in infants who fed with poor enriched vitamin C formulas, characterised as moeller-barlow disease.

In adults it occurs as general weakness, spongy bleeding gums, loose teeth with reabsorped dentine, swallon tender joints and haemorrhages in various tissues.

GENERAL WEAKNESS

The first symptoms reported in experimentally induced scurvy weakness, easy fatigue and listlessness. These are followed by shortness of breath and cramps of extremities.

SWOLLED AND TENDER JOINTS AND HAEMORRHAGES IN VARIOUS TISSUES

Haemorrhages deep in muscle occur particularly in calf thigh and forearm, causing pain in surrounding tissues. Haemorrhages may occur in joints and causing joints to swollen.

BLEEDING GUMS AND LOOSETEETH

In scurvy, gums become swollen blue red spongy and very friable. They may become infected by bacteria. The teeth loosen in the alveolar bone.

Treatment in Infants

Response to the administration of vitamin C is dramatic in acute scurvy. Ascorbic acid (500 to 1,000 mg) has to be given by mouth as a loading dose and repeated daily for a week. In severe cases 1,000 mg ascorbic acid daily should be administered by intravenous drip along with glucose saline for a week followed by 500 mg daily orally for 10 days.

For Adults

Scurvy responds to as little as 10 mg of vitamin C/day. A dose of 60 to 100 mg per day is recommended for repleshing body stores. Tablets are available in doses of 25, 50, 100, 250, 500, 1,000 and 1500 mg. It is available as a syrup at a dose of 500 mg per 5 ml. Parenteral preparations after 500 mg/ml.

Sources

Table 6.15: Ascorbic acid content of foods

Food	Serving	Ascorbic acid per portion (mg)	Percentage of RDI (60 mg)
Fruits			
Banana	One (9 in)	10	10–24
Cantaloupe	1 cup	68	>100
Orange	Whole (2 1/2 in)	70	>100
Grapefruit	Half, red	47	>40
Strawberries	1 cup	85	>100
Pear	One Bartlett	7	10–24
Apple	One (2.75 in)	8	10–24
Fruit juices			
Orange, fresh	1 cup	124	>100
Orange, frozen	1 cup	97	>100
Grapefruit, canned	1 cup	72	>100
Pineapple, frozen	1 cup	30	>40
Vegetables			
Green beans, fresh uncooked	1 cup	18	25–39
Spinach, cooked from fresh	1 cup	40	>40
Cabbage, cooked	1 cup	36	>40
Broccoli, cooked from fresh	1 cup	116	>100
Peas, frozen	1/2 cup	8	10–24
fresh, cooked	1 cup	23	25–39
Potato, baked	1 each	26	>40
Lettuce, iceberg	1cup	2.2	1–5
Tomato, fresh	1 each (2.2 in)	22	25–39
Green pepper, fresh	1/2 cup	44	>40
cooked	1/2	50	>40

Contd.

Table 6.15: Ascorbic acid content of foods (*Contd.*)

Food	Serving	Ascorbic acid per portion (mg)	Percentage of RDI (60 mg)
Dairy products			
Milk, cow, whole	1 cup	2.3	1–5
Milk, human	1 cup	7–12	10–24
Cheese	1 oz	0	0
Egg	1 each	0	0
Meats			
Beef liver, fried	3 oz	19	25–39
Bacon, lunch meat	2 pieces	10	10–24
Fish	3 oz	4	5–12

Table 6.16: Summary of vitamin functions and deficiency states

Vitamin	Function	Results of deficiency	Major food sources
Thiamine B_1	Transketolase coenzyme, muscle tone, appetite	Moderate: Fatigue, apathy, nausea, irritability, numbness	Enriched grains, most animal and vegetable products
Riboflavin/B_2	Part of FAD, FMN that accept/donate [H^+] equivalents	Severe: Beriberi with CHF, polyneuritis, edema	Organ meats, enriched cereals/flours, cheese, eggs, lean meat
Niacin	Part of NAD, NADP that accept /donate [H^+] equivalents	Angular stomatitis, cheilosis, glossitis, seborrheic dermatitis	Meat, nut, dairy products, eggs
Vitamin B_6	Coenzyme in transamination, decarboxylation, transsulfuration	Dermatitis (light-exposed), diarrhoea, swollen tongue, delirium, depression	Grains, seeds, organ meats, lean meats
Pantothenic acid	Part of CoA/acetyl carrier protein	Seborrheic dermatitis, red tongue, irritability, weakness, convulsions, neuritis	Organ meats, cereals/ flours, nuts, eggs
Biotin	Coenzyme in decarboxylation, deamination	Anorexia, nausea, fatigue, numbness, insomnia	Organ meats, eggs, soy flour
Folate	Formation of purines, pyrimidines, haeme, tyrosine, glutamate	Scaly dermatitis, anorexia, glossitis, muscles pain	Organ meats, green vegetables, legumes, eggs, fish, nuts, whole wheat products

Contd.

Table 6.16: Summary of vitamin functions and deficiency states (Contd.)

Vitamin	Function	Results of deficiency	Major food sources
Vitamin B$_{12}$	Transfer of single carbon units, synthesis of CH$_3$-	Megaloblastic anaemia, glossitis, diarrhoea	Organ meats, muscle meats, eggs, dairy products, fish
Vitamin C	Collagen formation, iron absorption, metabolism of folate	Sore tongue, weakness, neuropathy, mental changes, pernicious anaemia	Citrus fruits, other fruits, green peppers, leafy vegetables
Vitamin A	Visual adaptation, body/bone growth, gene expression	Weight loss, fatigue, sore gums/joints, petchiae, bone fractures	Organ meats, eggs, dairy (fortified)
Vitamin D	Calcium/ phosphorus absorption, bone mineralization	Night blindness, xerosis, xero-phthalmia, follicular dermatitis, abnormal teeth	Carotene: yellow vegetable, fruits
Vitamin E	Antioxidant against free radicals	Rickets, osteomalacia, tetany	Vitamin D-fortified foods (cereals, dairy), fish oils
Vitamin K	Synthesis of clotting factors, glutamate	Haemolysis, ophthalmoplegia, peripheral neuropathy Delayed blood clotting, haemor-rhagic disease of the newborn	Vegetable oils, nuts, seeds, eggs, meats Widely distributed (dairy, meat, eggs, fruit, vegetables)

CH$_3$-, methyl groups; CHF, congestive heart failure; FAD, flavin adenine dinucleotide; FMN, flavin mononucleotide; NAD, nicotinamide adenine dinucleotide; NADP, nicotinamide adenine dinucleotide phosphate.

7   Water

Water is essential to life and it is the largest single component of the body. At birth, water accounts for approximately 75% to 85% of total body weight; this proportion decreases with age and level of adiposity. In adults, total body water accounts for about 70% of the lean body mass. Variations observed are mainly due to differences in fat contents. Metabolically active cells of the muscle and viscera have the highest concentration of water, whereas calcified tissue cells have the lowest. Total body water is higher in athletes than in non-athletes and decreases significantly with age because of diminished muscle mass. In normal 70 kg male, total body water is approximately 42 L. This is contained in three major compartments.

- The intracellular fluid (28 L), about 35% of lean body weight.
- The interstitial fluid that bathes the cells (9.4 L, about 12%)
- Plasma (4.6 L, about 4–5%)
- In addition, a small amount of water is contained in bone, dense connective tissue, and epithelial secretions, such as the digestive secretions and cerebrospinal fluid.

WATER AND ELECTROLYTES

A large amount of water and electrolytes, partly dietary, but mainly from intestinal secretions, are absorbed coupled with monosaccharides, amino acids and bicarbonate in the upper jejunum. Some water and electrolytes are absorbed in the ileum and right side of the colon, where active sodium transport occurs but this is not coupled to solute absorption. Intestinal secretion also takes place and abnormalities of this mechanism cause secretory diarrhoea.

Functions

In the body, water is the fluid in which all life processes occur.

Functions in body:
  i. It carries nutrients to the tissues and carries waste products away from the tissues.
  ii. Participates in metabolic reactions.

iii. Serves as the solvent for minerals, vitamins, amino acids, glucose, and many other small molecules so that they can participate in metabolic activities.

iv. Acts as a lubricant and cushion around joints and inside the eyes, the spinal cord, and in pregnancy, the amniotic sac surrounding the foetus in the womb.

v. It is a regulator of normal body temperature (evaporation of sweat from the skin removes excess heat from the body).

Water Balance

Water balance is the balance between water intake and output (losses). The hypothalamus is a brain centre that controls activities such as maintenance of water balance, regulation of body temperature, and control of appetite.

Every cell contains fluid of the exact composition that is best for that cell (intracellular fluid) and is bathed externally in another such fluid (interstitial fluid). Interstitial fluid is the largest component of extracellular fluid. Water imbalance can be devastating, the body quickly responds by adjusting both water intake and excretion as needed. Consequently, the entire system of cells and fluids remain in a delicate, but controlled state of homeostasis.

Water intake: It is normally influenced by thirst and satiety, apparently in response to changes sensed by the mouth, hypothalamus and nerves.

Body gains water in the following ways:

i. By drinking water and beverage,
ii. Water in the food,
iii. Water produced during metabolism.

Water intoxication: It results when water intake in excess of the body's ability to excrete water. Ensuing increased intracellular fluid volume is accompanied by osmolar dilution. This leads to hyponatremia. If left untreated, water intoxication can be fatal.

Water output: It primarily occurs through kidneys as urine and through the GI tract in the faeces (sensible or measurable water loss). But, insensible or non-measurable losses also occur through air expired from the lungs, through the skin in the form of insensible perspiration and as sweat; the level of these losses depends on factors such as body surface area, climate, activity, state of health and dietary intake.

Water Imbalance

Water imbalance usually occurs with people who are critically ill or given inappropriate nutritional or hydration support.

Dehydration results from
• Inadequate fluid intake
• Excessive loss of fluid

- From GI tract due to persistent vomiting or chronic diarrhoea.
- From lungs and skin due to hyperventilation or climatic conditions.
- Excessive urine production due to diabetes insipidus or other conditions.

Overhydration results from
Overhydration is much rarer and usually occurs only in people with impairment in cardiac, hepatic or renal function.

- It is most likely to result from renal failure when ingested water cannot be excreted.

- Fluid retention also occurs following serious injury due to increase in ADH and aldosterone production and fall in urinary output and this is an important aspect of critical care.

Adequate and proper intake of water may help in avoiding the consequences. People can judge whether they are consuming enough fluid by the colour of their urine. If it is a pale straw colour, then their fluid intake is probably sufficient; if it is dark yellow, they may need to drink more.

BLOOD VOLUME AND BLOOD PRESSURE

Water maintains the blood volume, which in turn influences blood pressure. The kidneys are central to the regulation of blood volume and blood pressure. Every time the kidneys reabsorb needed substances and water and excrete wastes with some water in the urine. The kidneys meticulously adjust the volume and the concentration of the urine to accommodate changes in the body, including variations in the day's food and beverage intakes. Instructions on whether to retain or release substances or water come from ADH, renin, angiotensin and aldosterone.

- *ADH and water retention:* Whenever blood volume or blood pressure falls too low, or whenever the extracellular fluid becomes too concentrated, the hypothalamus signals the pituitary gland to release antidiuretic hormone (ADH). ADH is a water-conserving hormone that stimulates the kidneys to reabsorb water. Consequently, the more water you need, the less your kidneys excrete. These events also trigger thirst. Drinking water and retaining fluids raise the blood volume and dilute the concentrated fluids, thus helping to restore homeostasis.

- *Renin and sodium retention:* Cells in the kidneys respond to low blood pressure by releasing an enzyme called rennin. Through a complex series of events, rennin causes the kidney to reabsorb sodium. Sodium reabsorption, in turn, is always accompanied by water retention, which helps to restore blood volume and blood pressure.

- *Angiotensin and blood vessel constriction:* In addition to its role in sodium retention, renin converts the blood protein angiotensinogen to its active form—angiotensin. Angiotensin is a powerful vasoconstrictor that narrows the diameters of blood vessels, thereby raising the blood pressure.

- *Aldosterone and sodium retention:* In addition to acting as a vasoconstrictor, angiotensin stimulates the release of the hormone aldosterone from the adrenal glands. Aldosterone signals the kidneys to retain more sodium, and therefore water, because when sodium moves, fluid follows. Again, the effect is that when more water is needed, less is excreted.

Water Requirements

Thirst is usually an adequate signal for the need to consume water, except in infants, athletes, those who are ill, older adults who may have diminished thirst sensation. Individual requirements for additional fluids vary considerably. The minimum intake should be sufficient to replace losses from all sources and provide adequate dilution for the excretion of solutes through the kidney. Infants need more water because of the limited capacity of their kidneys to handle the renal solute load. Lactating woman's need is also high because of milk production.

UNIT II

CLASSIFICATION OF FOOD
B. Classification by nutritive value

8

Cereals and Cereal Products

INTRODUCTION

Cereals or grains are the seeds of grasses and include the many species of wheat, rice, maize or corn, jowar, barley, ragi, bajra, rye and oats. Cereal products contain flours, breads, meals and pasta, etc. Cereals are the staple diet of the world. Cereals are easy to produce, store, low cost and nutritionally beneficial, hence the usage too high worldwide. From the nutritional point of view, these foods from the base of the food guide pyramid should be 6–11 servings per day.

COMPOSITION AND NUTRITIVE VALUE

The chemical constituents of cereals are carbohydrates, proteins, lipids, minerals and water together with small quantities of vitamins, enzymes and other substances.

Energy

Cereals are the main sources of energy, contributing 70–80% of the requirement. 100 gm gives more than 340 kcal of energy.

Carbohydrate

Carbohydrate is the major constituents comprising about 80% of the dry matter of the cereals. The carbohydrate are the customarily considered in two parts—the crude fibre which is the portion of carbohydrate insoluble in dilute acids and alkalis under prescribed conditions and 'soluble carbohydrate' which are the remainder left after accounting for crude fibre, proteins, fat and mineral matter. The fibre constituents are cellulose, hemicellulose and pentose of the soluble carbohydrates, starch is the most important carbohydrate in all cereals. Free sugars present include simple sugars, such as glucose and galactose and oligosaccharides like sucrose, maltose and raffinose. Of all the cereals, whole wheat, ragi and bajra contain high amount of fibre. Rice contains less fibre. Removal of the husk of rice and oats during processing increases the protein content of the product; dehusked rice is still comparatively low in protein content, but dehusked oats equal or exceed wheat in protein content.

Protein

- The protein content of the different cereals varies.
- Rice contains less amount of protein compared to other cereals. The protein content of the different varieties of the same cereal also varies.
- Proteins are found in all the tissues of the cereal grains, the higher concentration occurring in the embryo, scutellum and aleurone layers than in the starchy endosperm, pericarp and testa. Within the endosperm the concentration of protein increases from the centre to the periphery.
- The types of proteins present in cereal are albumins, globulins, prolamines (gliadins) and glutelins. The proportions of these proteins differ in different cereals. The gliadins and glutelins are known as 'gluten' proteins; they form when flour kneaded with water. The gluten has elasticity and flow properties which are used for baking of bread and other products.
- The amino acid composition of the proteins in the cereal grains vary. They are generally low in the content of lysine. The biological value of the proteins in germ and aleurone is higher than that of the endosperm proteins; the lysine content in the former protein is 2–2.5 times greater than the proteins of the later tissues.

Lipids

Lipids are present to the extent of 1–2 per cent in wheat, rice, rye and barley, 3 per cent in maize and 4–6 per cent in oats. More lipids are present in germ and bran than in other parts of the grain. For example, wheat germ contains 6–11 per cent lipids, the bran 3–5 per cent and the endosperm 0.8–1.5 per cent. Similarly, the lipid content of maize germ is 35 per cent and the bran contains 1 per cent lipid. The lipids are mostly the triglycerides of palmitic, oleic and linoleic acids. Cereals also contain the phospholipid, lecithin.

The lipids in milled cereal products undergo two types of deterioration: hydrolysis due to the action of the enzyme lipase present in the grain and oxidation by the action of the enzyme lipoxygenase or nonenzymatically in the presence of oxygen. These changes give rise to unpleasant flavours. When the germ is separated from the endosperm as in the milling of cereals, the keeping quality of the milled products is improved.

Minerals

The husks of the cereals are rich in minerals about 95 per cent of the minerals being the phosphates and sulphates of potassium, magnesium and calcium. A considerable part of phosphorus in cereals is present in the form of phytin, the calcium, and magnesium salt of phytic acid. Phosphorus and calcium present in phytin are not available for absorption. Copper, zinc, manganese and iron are some other minerals present in very small quantities.

Vitamins

B-group vitamins are present in all cereals in the same extent, except niacin, which is more in wheat, rice, barley and sorghum. The distribution of the vitamins in different grains and in different parts of the same grain is not uniform. Oils from cereal grains are rich in vitamin E.

Enzymes

Cereal grains contain many enzymes and of these the amylases, proteases, lipases and oxidoreductases are of importance from the point of view of cereal technology. Ungerminated wheat, barley and rye have β-amylase activity but exhibit no α-amylase activity. Upon germination, β-amylase activity increases and α-amylase activity slowly appears. The proteases are relatively more in the germ. The lipases of cereals are responsible for the fatty acids appearing during the storage of cereals and their products.

SPECIFIC CEREALS AND THEIR PRODUCTS

Wheat

It belongs to the genus triticum and there are over 30,000 species and varieties. Approximately 90% of wheat consumption in India is in the form of chapathi. More than 1.5 million tonnes of wheat are used in the production of bakery products. Products are discussed below.

Wheat Products

Whole Wheat Flour

It contains the finely ground bran, germ and endosperm of the whole kernel. Whole wheat products have a distinctive flavours and coarser texture than those made from white flour because of the higher fat content of the germ, whole wheat flour is more difficult to keep and sometimes becomes rancid in storage under poor conditions. Iron fortified wheat flour has been successfully used to prevent iron deficiency anaemia in some western countries.

Maida

The bran and germ are separated in making white flour or maida. Maida bakes more uniformly into a loaf of a greater volume and it is more bland in taste and more easily digested. It can be stored in an air-tight container in a refrigerator.

Semolina

It is coarsely ground endosperm and its chemical compositions are similar to that of white flour. It is used in the manufacture of macaroni products. It is roasted before storing to save it from insects and worms.

MACARONI PRODUCTS

These products are also called pasta or alimentary pastes. These products include macaroni, spaghetti, vermicelli and noodles. The main ingredient in the macaroni products is a special durum flour of high gluten content. Durum wheat is used because of its yellow amber colour, nutty flavour and also because they hold their shape and firm texture when cooked. Usually not less than 5.5% by weight of egg solids are added to noodles. Disodium phosphate is added to cook macaroni faster, sometime they also enrich with B vitamins.

Different kinds of wheat are used for different purposes. For cakes and breads soft wheat, for macaroni hard wheat are used. In India, Punjab wheat is used for making chapathi and samba wheat is used for rava (upma) purpose. Maida is used making sweets and snacks.

MALTED WHEAT

The process of malted consists of the following steps:
1. Good quality grain is steeped in cold water for 36 hours in warm climate with two or three changes of water.
2. The steeped grain is spread on wire mesh trays of 2–3" thickness which are kept in a stand. The germination is allowed to proceed for 3 days in a warm climate. During germination amylases and proteases are formed.
3. Germinated grain is allowed to slow dry during which the amylases act on starch, hydrolyzing them. The drying should be at a low temperature to conserve as much of the enzyme activity as possible. During drying, the water soluble carbohydrate and nitrogen (peptones and peptides) increased. The characteristic malt flavour is developed. The malt is dried to a moisture content of about 13%. Amylase Rich Foods (ARF) are germinated cereal flours which can instantly liquefy or reduce the dietary bulk of any viscous multi-mix gruel provided cereal flour is the main ingredient.

Glutamic Acid

It is derived from wheat. A familiar compound of glutamic acid is "mono sodium glutamate", a salt-like product generally available and used to bring out the flavour of other foods or seasonings.

Wheat Bran

It increases the stool weight by increasing the water holding capacity of the bran. Wheat bran prevents constipation and may lower the risk of colon cancer.

Triticale

It is a hybrid cereal from a cross between wheat (Triticum) and rye (Secale). The hybrid cereal has the productivity and disease resistance of wheat with the vigour and hardiness of rye. The protein of triticale has higher lysine content than that of wheat protein. The grains have 14–18 per cent protein as against 12–15 per cent in wheat. Chapatis are acceptable up to a 50 per cent level of incorporation of triticale flour.

Rice

Rice is staple diet for more than half of the world's population. It is principally consumed in Asia. In India, several types of dishes are prepared from rice flavoured with spices and other ingredients. Other rice preparations include parched rice, puffed rice, and fermented preparations like "idli" and "dosa". By-products of rice, such as bran, rice polishing and paddy straw are used for feeding livestock.

RICE PRODUCTS

Rice Flour

This is made from second heads in pulverizing machines. Rice flour 9–13 per cent moisture content, contains 5–9 per cent of protein, 0.4–1.0 per cent of fat and yields 0.4–0.7 per cent ash. It is used in refrigerated biscuit manufacture to prevent sticking, in baby foods as a thickener, and in waffle and pancake mixes as water absorbent, in preparation of vermicelli, papad, sandige (curls) and in many other preparations.

Parched Rice

About 4–5 per cent of the total supplies of rice in India are converted into the rice products—parched rice, parched paddy and rice flakes. Parboiled rice is preferred in making parched rice. Parched rice is a crisp product with a greyish to brilliant white colour and is sold either salted or unsalted.

Parched Paddy (Puffed Rice)

Sun dried paddy is filled in earthen jars and is moistened with hot water. After 2–3 min the water is decanted and the jars are then kept in an inverted position for 8–10 hours. Next the paddy is exposed to the sun for a short time and then parched in hot sand. During parching the grains swell and burst into a soft white product. The parched grains are sieved to remove sand and winnowed to separate the husk.

Flaked Rice

Flaked rice is made from parboiled rice. Flaked rice is thin and papery. It can be stored without deterioration for several months. The vitamin content is equal to that of parboiled rice and many preparations are made out of it by adding suitable flavouring and sweetening agents.

Rice Starch

Rice starch granules are quite small and are embedded in a protein matrix. To separate them from protein, broken rice is steeped for 24 hours in

5 times its weight of 0.3 per cent caustic soda treated granules are washed, dried and grounded into flour. The flour is then mixed with about ten times its weight of caustic soda solution. This removes the gluten. After 24 hours, the starch that settles down is removed, washed and dried.

Rice starch is used as food, especially in puddings, ice creams, pies and custard powder. Its principal use is in laundry as a stiffening agent. Rice starch also finds use in cosmetics, in face and dusting powders, as a thickener, in calico printing, in finishing textiles and for making dextrins, glucose and adhesives.

Rice Bran

The bran is the most nutritious by-product of rice milling and is used almost exclusively as a feedstuff. It is generally contaminated with husk, which lowers its nutritive value. Rice bran contains about 12 per cent protein and 15 per cent fat. Once separated from grain, the fat of rice undergoes oxidation by peroxidation and by peroxidase, which reduces the nutritive value of bran and causes digestive disturbances.

Rice Bran Oil

It is obtained by the extraction of rice bran with solvents. Bran oil is also obtained in the solvent extraction milling of rice. The oil contains a high percentage of unsaturated fatty acids, yet it is quite stable because of the presence of natural antioxidants. When refined, bleached and deodourized, it is used for salad dressing and as cooking oil. Bran after solvent extraction has a higher percentage of protein than the original material. With its low fat content, it keeps well. It is a more palatable feed than the undefatted bran.

Millets

These are hardy plants capable of growing in areas where there is low rainfall and poor irrigation facilities. Apart from maize and sorghum, the major millet crops of India are pearl millet called bajra and finger millet known as ragi.

Maize or Corn

In India, maize is consumed in the form of boiled or roasted as popcorn. In some countries, it is converted into food products by grinding, alkali processing, boiling, cooking and fermentation. Maize contains around 11% of protein. Maize protein is deficient in amino acid like tryptophan and lysine. It is rich in carotene and has appreciable amount of folic acid and thiamine. According to a study conducted at National Institute of Nutrition, Hyderabad, 17–56% of aflatoxin can be reduced in maize by cooking.

There are many varieties of maize. The principal varieties are flint corn, dent corn, sweet corn, popcorn, flour corn and waxy corn. The classification is based on the nature and distribution of starch in the endosperm.

- Flint corn has very hard kernels due to thick layer of hard starch and protein just under the bran layer. In India, mostly flint and semi-flint varieties are grown.
- Dent corn has hard starch at sides, while the major part of the endosperm contains soft starch. At maturity a typical dent-like depression appears at the crown.
- Sweet corn has a large proportion of carbohydrates of the kernel as dextrin and sugar in the unripe kernels which are tender. When matured and dried, the kernels are hard and have a wrinkled surface.
- Popcorn, major part of the endosperm, comprises hard starch on all sides, with a very small core of soft starch. When the corn is popped, the endosperm expands with the formation of a fluffy white irregular mass. The thick outer layers of the corn remain attached to the puffed endosperm in an unexpanded form.
- Flour corn grains are large and soft and the endosperm is very friable. These characteristics permit easy grinding of the grain into flour.
- Waxy corn contains a high proportion of amylopectin. It is of industrial importance.

Sorghum (Jowar)

Jowar or sorghum millet is grown in Maharashtra, Karnataka, Madhya Pradesh, Andhra Pradesh, Gujarat, Uttar Pradesh and Tamil Nadu. Jowar is rich in carbohydrate, B-complex vitamins and dietary fibre. It is poor in vitamin A. It is used as roti or bhakri. From the blend of wheat flour and sorghum flour, baked products like muffins, bread and cakes can be produced. The sugar content of some sorghum stems is high (sweet sorghum) and these are used for making syrup. Sorghum grain is used as a source of starch in the fermentation industry for producing industrial alcohol and solvents.

Sorghum starches are interchangeably used with corn starch in most industrial applications. Sorghum oil after refining is used for salads and general cooking. Kernel residues containing bran and gluten are processed as cattle feed. Sorghum malt is used in the preparation of infant foods and malt extracts produced from sorghum are employed in the pharmaceutical industry.

Ragi

Ragi which is also known as finger millet constitutes a little over 25% of the food grains grown in India. The major proteins of ragi are prolamines and glutelins and they appear to be adequate in all the essential amino acids. It is rich in calcium and fibre. It is also rich in phytate and tannin and hence interferes with mineral availability. It contains B-vitamins but is poor in B_2. Nutritionally it is almost as good as or better than wheat or other cereals. It is converted into flour and a variety of preparations such as mudde, chapathi, dosa, porridge, etc. are prepared. Malted grains are used as a nourishing food for infants.

Bajras

Bajra is also known as pearl millet. It has the same quantity of protein as wheat. The protein contains a high proportion of prolamine, followed by globulin and albumins. Among the amino acids tryptophan content is high and lysine content average to low. Bajra is rich in iron, calcium, thiamin, riboflavin and niacin.

It is dehusked and cooked in the same way as rice flour is made into bhakre. The grain is sometimes eaten after it is parched; the product being similar to popcorn. The grain is also suitable for the preparation of malt.

9   Pulses and Products

Pulses are edible fruits or pod bearing plants belonging to the family of the leguminous. Split pulses are known as dhals. The major pulses which find important place in our dietaries are red gram dhal. Some are used as whole grams. Cow pea, rajmah and dry peas also belong to leguminous family. Legumes not only have dietary values but also play an important role in maintaining or even important soil fertility through their ability to fix atmospheric nitrogen.

NUTRITIVE VALUE OF PULSES

Proteins

Pulse proteins are chiefly globulins but albumins are also present in a few species. Their nutritional importance depends not only on the quantity of protein but also on its quality which in turn depends upon the amino acids composition. Pulse proteins are deficient in sulphur-containing amino acids, particularly in methionine, and in tryptophan. All the pulses contain sufficient amount of leucine and phenylalanine. There are a number of factors which reduce the nutritional value of pulse proteins. Some proteins form complexed with carbohydrates and some with phytin and polyphenols contribute to their low digestibility. Pea and cow pea have high biological value of proteins among pulses.

Carbohydrates

Pulses contain about 55–60 per cent of total carbohydrates including starch, soluble sugars, fibre and unavailable carbohydrates. The unavailable sugars in pulses include substantial levels of oligosaccharides of the raffinose family of sugars (raffinose, stachyose and verbiscose), which are notoriously known for the flatulence production in man and animals. These sugars escape digestion, when they are ingested, due to the lack of α-galactosidase activity in the mammalian mucosa.

Consequently, the oligosaccharides are not absorbed into the blood and are digested by the microflora of the lower intestinal tract resulting in the production of large amount of carbon dioxide and hydrogen and a small amount of methane. Some of the methods used in processing pulses are germination, soaking, cooking and autoclaving which reduce considerable amount of oligosaccharides. Fermentation also reduces oligosaccharides has been observed during the fermentation of black gram and rice.

Lipids

Most pulses contain high amount of polyunsaturated acids. These undergo oxidative rancidity during storage resulting in a number of undesirable changes, such as loss of protein solubility, off-flavour development, and loss of nutritive quality.

Minerals

Pulses contain calcium, magnesium, zinc, iron, potassium and phosphorus. In many pulses 80 per cent of phosphorus is present as phytate phosphorus. Phytin complexes with proteins and minerals and renders them biologically unavailable to human beings and animals. Processing methods, such as cooking, soaking, germination, etc. can reduce or eliminate appreciable amount of phytin.

Vitamins

Pulses are excellent source of B complex vitamins particularly thiamine, folic acid and pantothenic acid. Like cereals they do not contain any vitamin A or C but germinated legumes contain good amount of vitamin C and fresh pulses like peas may have a considerable amount of vitamin A.

PULSES AS SOURCES OF PROTEIN

Pulses are important source of protein in vegetarian diet. They give about 20–25% protein, that is double the amount of protein compared to cereals. Proteins of pulses are of low quality since they are deficient in methionine and red gram is deficient in tryptophan also. However, pulses are rich in lysine. Hence they can supplement cereal protein. A mixture of cereals and pulses is superior to that of the either one.

The most effective combination to achieve maximum supplementary effect is 5 parts of cereals protein and one part of pulse protein. In terms of grains, 8 parts of cereals and 1 part of pulse. This combination gives a quality equivalent to animal proteins.

ANTINUTRITIONAL FACTORS IN SOME PULSES

Most raw legume products contain some antinutritional factors. These are chemical substances which, although non-toxic, generate adverse physiological responses in animals consuming these legumes and, in many cases, interfere with the utilization of nutrients in these products. Antinutritional factors which have been identified in soybean include protease inhibitors, haemogglutinins (lectins), goitrogens, antivitamins and phytates. Other includes saponins, oestrogens, flatulence factors, allergens and lysinoalanine. In addition of those mentioned above, other antinutritional factors have been identified in other legumes. These include cyanogens, favism factors, lathyrism factors, amylase inhibitors, tannins, aflatoxin and presser amines. Although only a few legume seeds may contain all these antinutritionals, many contain a few of them. A study by Walker shows that haemogglutinins, aflatoxin, cyanogens, favism factors and lathyrism factors pose the greatest threat to the health and well-being of humans and animals. Some antinutritional factors are health labile, including the protease inhibitors, haemagglutinins, goitrogens, antivitamins and phytates, and since human consume only legume seeds after cooking, it would appear that they do not constitute any major health hazard as long as the legume seeds or legume products are properly cooked.

TOXIC CONSTITUENTS OF ANTINUTRITIONAL FACTORS

Different types of pulses have different types of antinutritional factors:

1. *Peanuts:* Raw peanuts have very low concentrations of most of the antinutritional factors found in raw soybean. Antinutritional factors which have been isolated, purified and identified are lectins and trypsin inhibitors. A goitrogenic factor has also been isolated and identified in the testa of the peanut and some saponin like compounds which are bitter tasting have been identified in germ. Peanut skin has also been reported to possess trypsin-inhibitors and growth-retarding principles. In warm wet climates, grains are easily infected with toxigenic microorganisms. The best known toxic compounds of peanut are the aflatoxin, metabolic by-products of the moulds—*Aspergillus flavus* and *Aspergillus parasiticus.* There are 4 distinct types of aflatoxin—B_1, B_2, G_1, and G_2. Of these 4, aflatoxin B_1 is the most toxic and best known because it is a very potent hepatocarcinogen. Aflatoxin B1 is reported to be mitogenic, causing chemical modifications of the DNA, inhibiting RNA synthesis and interfering with protein synthesis.

2. *Chick pea:* This chemical composition is found to be very similar with very low contents of trypsin inhibitors and undetectable levels of haemagglutinins. Other antinutritional factors identified include oligosaccharides (flatulence factor) polyphenols, phytic acid, α-amylase inhibitors and saponins. Polyphenols are more abundant in cultivars with dark seed coats than in those which are pale. Dehulling can very effectively reduce levels of polyphenols.

3. *Soybean:* Raw soybean contains various antinutritional factors including antiproteolytic agents which, to some extent, interfere with the utilization of the protein of soy. Liener, lists the heat-labile antinutritional factors in soybean: Protease inhibitors, haemagglutinins, goitrogens, antivitamins and phytates. The heat-stables are: Saponins, oestrogens, flatulence factors, allergens and lysinoalanine.

4. *Mung bean or green gram:* It contains antinutritional factors including protease inhibitors, haemagglutinins, cyanogens, phytic acid, oligosaccharides and saponins.

5. *Cow pea:* The cow pea contain trypsin inhibitors, lectins (haemagglutinins), polyphenols.
6. *Moth Bean:* Moth bean seeds contain antinutritional factors such as trypsin inhibitors, polyphenols, phytic acid, saponins, oxalis acid and amylase inhibitor.
7. *Lentil:* Lentil seeds contain relatively low levels of antinutritional factors. These factors include trypsin inhibitor, haemagglutinins, polyphenols, phytic acid, flatulence factors, α-amylase inhibitor, cyanogens and saponins (Table 9.1).

Table 9.1: Utilization problems of legumes and cereals and possible causes

	Problems	*Causes*
Legumes	• Incomplete protein	• Limiting amount of methionine and cysteins
	• Incomplete availability of amino acids	
	• Low protein digestibility	• Nature of protein, protease inhibitors
	• Antinutritional factors	• Protease inhibitors, haemoagglutin, goitrogens, etc.
	• Flatulence	• Oligosacchariders, dietary fibre, lipoxygenase.
Cereals	• Low protein content incomplete protein	• Limiting amount of lysine, and in some cereals tryptophan, threonine.

Sprouted Pulses

Pulses are good in protein, CHO, vitamin B and fair in mineral content. But vitamin C is not present in them. On sprouting this deficiency can be rectified. To sprout, cleaned pulse is soaked for 24 hours and then it is spread on a muslin cloth, sprinkling water occasionally on it. After 24 hours tiny sprouts appear on the surface. These sprouts are very rich in vitamin C and carotene. Sprouted pulses are very tender and cooking is not necessary. They can be used as raw salad by sprinkling lime juice and salt or as raitas by adding curd and salt to it.

Vitamin C Content of Sprouted Legumes (Table 9.2)

Table 9.2: Vitamin C in sprouted legumes

Period of germination	*Vitamin C*
Dry legumes	Trace
After 24 hours germination	7–12 mg/100 g
After 48 hours germination	11–18 mg/100 g
After 7 hours germination	13–20 mg/100 g

Germinated Pulses as Functional Food

Recent studies revealed that legumes on germination are not only the potential source of linoleic and alfa linolenic acid but also long chain polyunsaturated fatty acid like eicosapentaenoic acid and decosahexaenoic acid. The high ratio of n-3 to n-6 on germination can help to attain the recommended ratio of fatty acids and thus keep the degenerative diseases at bay.

10 Vegetables and Fruits

VEGETABLES

Vegetables are the edible plant or part of a plant other than a sweet fruit or seed. This typically means the leaf, stem, or root of a plant. More than 40 kinds of vegetables belonging to different groups, namely solanaceous, cucurbitaceous, leguminous, cruciferous (cole crops), root crops and leafy vegetables are grown in India in tropical, sub-tropical and temperate regions. Important vegetable crops grown in the country are onion, brinjal, cabbage, cauliflower, okra and peas.

Though Indian population is most vegetarian the intake of vegetable has too low in daily diet, people do not eat vegetable or eat less in quantity because they are expensive, need more preparation time, or due to ignorance of the importance of vegetables. Sometimes unavailability in a particular place or season results in less consumption of vegetables. As they are perishable, the consumption would be limited if storage facilities are not available.

Human body needs foods regularly for strength and to become healthy. Most of our foods should be vegetables and fruits. Vegetables contain terrific colours, flavours and many powerful and important nutrients such as vitamins, minerals, fibre, and that help reduce the risk of many diseases.

Composition of Vegetables

Vegetables differ in their chemical composition. They are called protective foods as they are rich in minerals and vitamins. Vegetables contain pigments, organic acids, flavour compounds, enzymes.

Pigments

Plant pigments include a variety of different kinds of molecules. They are water soluble and fat soluble. Pigments also serve to attract pollinators. These are subject to change with ripening and processing of the raw vegetables or fruits. The four pigments found in plants are: Chlorophyll, the green pigment; carotenoids, a yellow, red, or orange pigment; and the two flavonoids: Anthocyanin, the red, blue, or purple pigmet, and anthoxanthin, the white pigment.

Fat Soluble Pigments

Chlorophyll: Chlorophyll is the primary pigment in plants; it is a porphyrin that absorbs yellow and blue wavelengths of light while reflecting green. It is the presence and relative abundance of chlorophyll that gives plants their green colour. All land plants and green algae possess two forms of this pigment—chlorophyll-a and chlorophyll-b. Chlorophyll-a is present in the florets of blue green broccoli and chlorophyll-b is present in stalks. This pigment is present in green leafy vegetables, capsicum, beans, peas, and chillies. All chlorophylls serve as the primary means plants use to intercept light in order to fuel photosynthesis.

Chlorophyll is structurally a porphyrin ring containing magnesium at the centre of a ring of four pyrrole groups. If the magnesium in chlorophyll is displaced from its central position on the porphyrin ring, an irreversible pigment change occurs. A number of factors including prolonged storage, the heat of cooking, changes in hydrogen ion concentration (pH), and the presence of the minerals, zinc and copper, may cause an off-green, unwanted pigment colour changes.

Carotenoids: Carotenoids are tetraterpenoid organic pigments that are naturally occurring in the chloroplasts and chromoplasts of plants. There are over 600 known carotenoids; they are split into two classes, xanthophylls (which contain oxygen) and carotenes (which are purely hydrocarbons, and contain no oxygen). Carotenoids in general absorb blue light. They serve two key roles in plants and algae—they absorb light energy for use in photosynthesis, and they protect chlorophyll from photo damage. People consuming diets rich in carotenoids from natural foods, such as fruits and vegetables, are healthier and have lower mortality from a number of chronic illnesses. Carotenoids belong to the category of tetraterpenoids (i.e. they contain 40 carbon atoms).

The unoxygenated (oxygen free) carotenoids such as α-carotene, β-carotene and lycopene (present in tomatoes) are known as *carotenes*. Carotenes typically contain only carbon and hydrogen. They contain conjugated double bonds (i.e. double bonds alternating with single bonds), which are responsible for the colour. The greater the number of conjugated double bonds, the deeper will be the colour. For example, β-carotene is orange in colour and contains a six-membered ring at each end of the chain. α-carotene has one less conjugated double bond so it is paler in colour. Lycopene, found in tomatoes and watermelon, has the deepest red colour because it has two openings at each end of the chain and, thus has two more double bonds than β-carotene (Figs 10.1 and 10.2).

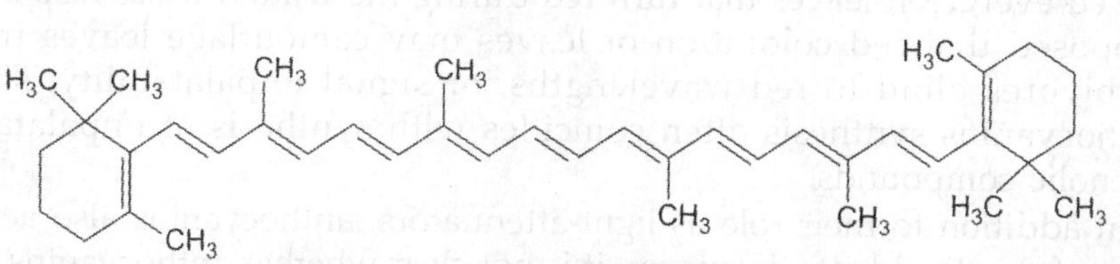

Fig. 10.1: β-carotene

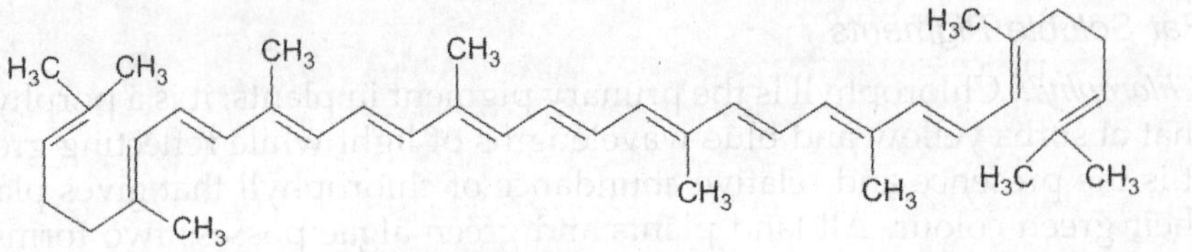

Fig. 10.2: Lycopene

There are hundreds of types of carotenes. The most well-known carotene is the β-carotene, cleaved by an enzyme in the intestinal mucosa to yield vitamin A. In all, 40 or more carotenoids are known to be precursors of vitamin A.

Carotenoids with molecules containing oxygen, such as lutein and zeaxanthin, are known as *xanthophylls*. Xanthophylls are the yellow-orange. coloured derivatives of carotenes containing carbon, hydrogen, and oxygen. Xanthophylls are found in the leaves of most plants, where they act to modulate light energy (Table 10.1).

Table 10.1: Carotenoid pigments in food

Food	Pigments
Yellow corn	Cryptoxanthin
Tomatoes	Lycopene, β-carotene
Red capsicum	Cryptoxanthin, capsorubin, β-carotene, neoxanthin, capxanthin
Green capsicum	Lutein, β-carotene, violaxanthin, neoxanthin
Carrots	β-carotene, α-carotene, γ-carotene, lycopene, xanthophylls.

Water Soluble Pigments

Water soluble pigments are anthocyanins and anthoxanthins.

Anthocyanins: Anthocyanins occur in all tissues of higher plants, including leaves, stems, roots, flowers, and fruits. Cherries, red apples, various berries blue and red grapes, pomegranates, and currants achieve their colour appeal because of predominance of anthocyanins. The red colour in the skin of radishes and sweet potatoes and the leaves of red cabbage is due to anthocyanins too. In photosynthetic tissues (such as leaves and sometimes stems), anthocyanins have been shown to act as a "sunscreen", protecting cells from high-light damage by absorbing blue-green and UV light, thereby protecting the tissues from photo inhibition, or high-light stress. This has been shown to occur in red juvenile leaves, autumn leaves, and broad-leaved evergreen leaves that turn red during the winter. It has also been proposed that red coloration of leaves may camouflage leaves from herbivores blind to red wavelengths, or signal unpalatability, since anthocyanins synthesis often coincides with synthesis of unpalatable phenolic compounds.

In addition to their role as light-attenuators, anthocyanins also act as powerful antioxidants. However, it is not clear whether anthocyanins can significantly contribute to scavenging of free-radicals produced through metabolic processes in leaves, since they are located in the vacuole, and thus spatially separated from metabolic reactive oxygen species. Some studies have shown that hydrogen peroxide produced in other organelles can be neutralized by vacuolar anthocyanins. Most frequent in nature are the glycosides of cyanidin, delphinidin, malvidin, pelargonidin, peonidin and petunidin. Roughly 2% of all hydrocarbons fixated in photosynthesis are converted into flavonoids and their derivatives such as the anthocyanins.

Metals, such as iron from non-stainless-steel preparation tools, change the natural purplish pigment to a blue-green colour. Therefore, food products containing the anthocyanin pigment are often canned in enamel-lined metal cans to prevent the product acid from interacting with the can metal and causing undesirable colour changes.

Anthoxanthins: Anthoxanthins are water-soluble pigments, is also a flavonoid which range in colour from white or colourless to a creamy to yellow, often on petals of flowers. These pigments are generally whiter in an acid medium and yellowed in an alkaline medium. They are water soluble and occur in the vacuoles of plant cells. Anthoxanthins classification represents flavone, flavonol, flavanone, and flavanol pigments, and gives colour to apples, cauliflower, onions, potatoes, turnips and spinach or other leafy vegetables. In green leafy vegetables the colour is masked by chlorophyll. They are very susceptible to colour changes with minerals and metal ions, similar to anthocyanins. As with all flavonoids, they exhibit antioxidant properties, and are important in nutrition, and are sometimes used as food additives. Darkening with iron is particularly prominent in food products. They are considered to have more variety than anthocyanins. Some examples are quercitin. The pigments are frequently found in conjunction with anthocyanin pigments, affecting their colour.

Betalains: The name "betalain" comes from the Latin name of the common beet (*Beta vulgaris*), from which betalains were first extracted. The deep red colour of beets, bougainvillea, amaranth, and many cacti results from the presence of betalain pigments. They are similar to, but not categorized as anthocyanins or anthoxanthins. There are two categories of betalains— betacyanins include the reddish to violet betalain pigments, betaxanthins are those betalain pigments which appear yellow to orange.

Tannins: Tannin is an astringent, bitter plant polyphenolic compound that binds to and precipitates proteins and various other organic compounds including amino acids and alkaloids. The astringency from the tannins causes the dry and puckery feeling in the mouth following the consumption of unripened fruit or red wine. They may be responsible for the unwanted brown discoloration of fruits and vegetables, as well as for the desirable changes that provide tea leaves with their characteristic colour. They range in colour from pale-yellow to light brown. Tannins contain antioxidant properties in it.

Flavour compounds: The flavour of vegetables is determined by taste and odour—active compounds. Taste is perceived on the tongue and odour in the olfactory system. Sugars, acids, salts and compounds that contribute to bitterness, e.g. isocoumarins and polyacetylenes in carrots and related vegetables and sesquiterpene lactones in chicory and lettuce, and to astringency such as phenolic acids, flavonoids, alkaloids, tannins are important to the taste of fruits and vegetables.

The characteristic flavours of onions and garlic are principally made up from a combination of sulphur containing aroma compounds. These volatiles are not present in the whole, raw vegetables but are formed by the action of allinase enzymes on odourless, non-volatile, sulphur containing precursors when the vegetable tissue is injured. Onions and garlic have been traditionally cooked with meat for centuries in order to enhance and modify flavour. Brussel sprouts, cabbage, cauliflower, broccoli, turnip are cruciferace family which contain prominent sulphur compounds. Some of the sulphur compounds, including allyl sulphides may increase carcinogen excretion from the body.

Organic acids: Vegetable contains number of organic acids, metabolic products of the cells. Formic, succinic, citric, acetic, malic, fumaric, tartaric, propoionic, butyric and benzoic acids are present in fruits and vegetables. Organic acids are used by the living plants in their synthetic processes. In the ripening of some fruits some of the acids are progressively utilized in the formation of ethers and carbohydrates. Others are combined to form salts of potassium, sodium, calcium, magnesium, etc. They have a very pleasing flavour and are relished by everyone. Vegetables contain a greater variety of organic acids, yet maintain a less acidic pH level than fruits.

Enzymes: Enzymes are formed in plant cells. They function as catalysts in chemical reactions. They are composed of proteins and destroyed by heat and chemicals that coagulate them. There are two types of enzymes that are normally present in plant substances—hydrolytic enzymes and oxido reductases.

Enzymes bring ripening of tomatoes and bananas. If this enzymatic reaction continues, the vegetable or fruit gets spoilt. They also bring browning in potato, brinjal, and plantain. The enzyme pectinesterase is found in all plants, and many plant pathogens. The enzyme is especially abundant in tomato. In tomato, the enzyme has been detected in fruit,. leaves and roots. In particular, the fruit contains very high levels of the enzyme, leading to the theory that it has an important role in fruit ripening and softening. Green leafy vegetables such as lettuce, spinach, and others are a great source of enzymes. These enzymes are full of antioxidants and will decrease stress in the body.

When bruised or cut during preparation, discoloration of some fruits or vegetables may occur due to the enzymes exposure to the atmosphere, they are subject to undesirable browning. This is referred to as enzymatic oxidative browning. This occurs when a substrate such as the phenolic compound in fruits, oxygen, and an enzyme (phenol oxidase, phenolase, or polyphenolase) are present. One effective control of browning is to avoid contact between the substrate and oxygen. For example, food may be covered by syrup to block oxygen, or it may be covered with a film wrap that limits oxygen permeability.

Nutritive Value of Vegetables

Nutritionally vegetables are classified into 3 groups:
- Green leafy vegetables
- Roots and tubers
- Other vegetables (Table 10.2)

Table 10.2: Classification of vegetables nutritionally

Groups	Example
Green leafy vegetables	Agathi, amaranth, beet greens, brussels sprouts, cabbage, cauliflower greens, carrot leaves, colocasia leaves, coriander leaves, drumstick leaves, fenugreek leaves, gogu, mayalu, spinach
Roots and tubers	Beet root, carrot, colocasia, onion, potato, radish, sweet potato, tapioca, yam
Other vegetables	Bitter gourd, bottle gourd, brinjal, broad beans, cauliflower, cluster beans, cucumber, drumstick, capsicum, ladies finger, raw mango, plantain green

Green leafy vegetables: Leaves are the manufacturing organs of the plant where the life giving process of photosynthesis takes place. In the cells, photosynthesis transforms elements into carbohydrates which are carried to other parts of the plant. Green leafy vegetables deliver a bonanza of vitamins, minerals, and phytonutrients.

They are a rich source of minerals (including iron, calcium, potassium, and magnesium) and vitamins, including vitamins K, C, E, and many of the B vitamins. They also provide a variety of phytonutrients including β-carotene, lutein and zeaxanthin, which protect our cells from damage and our eyes from age-related problems, among many other effects.

- Greens have a very little carbohydrate in them, and the carbs that are there are packed in layers of fibre, which make them very slow to digest. That is why, in general, greens have a very little impact on blood glucose.
- Greens are very good source of folic acid.
- Spinach has a high nutritional value and is extremely rich in antioxidants. It is a rich source of vitamin A (and especially high in lutein), vitamin C, vitamin E, vitamin K, folate, betaine, iron, vitamin B_2, vitamin B_6, folic

acid, niacin, minerals and omega-3 fatty acids. But its high content of oxalate makes the calcium unavailable in diets. Recently, opioid peptides called rubiscolins have also been found in spinach.

- Coriander contains vitamin A, vitamin C and iron.
- Fenugreek is good appetizer and got more medicinal values (see chap. spices).
- Drumstick leaves and flowers are used as vegetables. The leaves are rich in vitamins A and C.
- Lettuce leaves are rich in vitamin A and calcium.

11   Nuts and Oilseeds

Nuts and oilseeds are one of the important sources of plant protein in our diets. Some of the commonly used nuts and oilseeds in India are groundnut, coconut, fresh cashew nuts, gingelly seeds, mustard seeds, almonds, walnut, pistachios, etc.

Both nuts and oilseeds are highly compact foods, containing a high amount of fat and protein. Only moderate quantities of carbohydrate are present. Nutritive composition of nuts and oilseeds is similar; both possess + 40 g% fat, + 15 g% protein, and + 20 g% of carbohydrate and yield + 600 kcal energy per 100 g. Almonds and walnuts have a higher fat content (+ 60 g%) yielding greater energy. Nuts and oilseeds are rich in calcium (+ 400 mg%) and iron (+ 4 mg%). Additionally nuts possess a fair amount of fibre. Nutritive value of selected nuts is given in the following (Table 11.1).

Table 11.1: Nutritive value of selected nuts per 100 g

Nutrient	Almond	Cashew nut	Coconut	Groundnut	Walnut
Protein (g)	20.8	21.2	4.5	25.3	15.6
Fat (g)	58.9	46.9	41.6	40.1	64.5
Carbohydrate (g)	10.5	22.3	13.0	26.1	11.0
Mineral (g)	2.9	2.4	1.0	2.4	1.8
Thiamine (mg)	0.24	0.63	0.05	0.90	0.45
Riboflavin (mg)	0.57	0.19	0.10	0.13	0.40
Niacin (mg)	4.4	1.2	0.8	19.9	1.0
Energy (kcal)	655	596	444	567	687

Recommendation of Storage

Common Storage

1. Dry nuts at 100°F (38°C) to a total moisture content of 7 to 8% for in shell nuts or 3–1/2 or 4–1/2% of shelled nuts.
2. Use properly sealed plastic bags or glass jars.

Refrigerated Storage

1. After drying, nuts can be stored at 32–35°F (0–2°C) for 2 years if packaged in sealed plastic or glass containers. If the relative humidity is maintained at 60–65%, the nuts are stored away from odour-producing substances.
2. After storage allow nuts to warm up in unopened containers to room temperature to avoid drawing of moisture which could cause mold and rancidity.

Freezer Storage

1. Dried nuts can be successfully stored at 2° F (–28°C) or lower for 2 years, with or without plastic containers. There is a little danger of odour pickup and it is not necessary to control humidity.
2. After storage, allow nuts to warm up in unopened plastic bags or in well-ventilated areas if plastic bags are not used, to prevent mold or rancidity.

Almond (*Prunus amygdalus*)

Almonds are extremely nourishing and have long been valued as a muscle and body building substances. They are rich in fat, carbohydrates and protein and their calcium content is particularly valuable for building children's teeth and bone. The chief almond protein is globulin but its biological value is low.

Almonds have large calorie content; being 575.0 per 100 g. Almond is incredibly rich in minerals such as manganese, magnesium, copper, phosphorus, iron, zinc and potassium. However, selenium is also present in good amount. These small nuts are a powerhouse of vitamin E, riboflavin, thiamin, niacin and folate. Good amount of vitamin B_6 and pantothenic acid are also present.

Regular intake of almonds helps the formation of new blood cells and haemoglobin and plays a major role in ensuring the smooth functioning of the brain, nerves, bones, heart and liver.

Almond can be safely eaten by diabetics, obese persons and invalids. Mixing almond cake with wheat flour is a way of increasing the nutritive value of flour.

Almond oil is used in confectionery, pharmaceutical and cosmetic preparations. Almond milk is taken as refreshing drink.

Almonds are of two types—sweet almond and bitter almond. Sweet almond is used domestically, whereas the bitter almond is used only to extract almond oil. Bitter almond is not used like sweet almond since they yield 4–9 mg of hydrogen cyanide per almond which results in death.

Cashew Nut (*Anacardium occidentale*)

Cashew is a highly nutritious and concentrated form of food, providing a substantial amount of energy and consists mostly of glycerides of oleic acid (73.8%) and linoleic acids (7.7%). The cashew nut kernel has a pleasant taste and flavour and can be eaten raw, fried and sometimes salted or sweetened with sugar. It also contributes as an important source of invisible fat in the diet, being widely used in a variety of ways. The nut contains an acrid compound which is a powerful vesicant that is abrasive to the skin. The cashew shell contains 25% of this reddish brown oil, industrially known as Cashew Nut Shell Liquid (CNSL) which is a by-product of the roasting process. Wide differences in the protein content ranging from 13.13 to 25.03% have been reported from various regions of India.

The vitamin content of cashew nut kernels indicates 0.5 to 1.4 mg per 100 g of thiamin, 3.65 mg per 100 g of niacin, and 0.58 mg per 100 g of riboflavin, a good proportion of vitamin E and traces of other vitamins like pyridoxine, vitamin D are present in cashew.

The high magnesium content of cashew nuts also takes the credit for its healthy heart qualities. In their raw form, cashews contain 82.5 mg of magnesium per ounce, or 21% of the daily recommended value of the heart healthy mineral, which also protects against high blood pressure, muscle spasms, migraine headaches, tension, soreness and fatigue. Magnesium also works with calcium to support healthy muscles and bones in the human body.

Cashews provide the body with a good source of copper. Copper plays a role in a wide range of physiological processes including iron utilization, elimination of free radicals, development of bone and connective tissue, production of the skin and hair pigment called melanin. Copper, which is an essential component of the enzyme *superoxide dismutase*, is vital in energy production and antioxidant defense, producing greater flexibility in blood vessels, bones and joints.

Coconut (*Cocos nucifera*)

The coconut contains less protein than other nuts. However, it has very high saturated fatty acid content. Most of the saturated fatty acids are medium chain triglycerides, which are supposed to assimilate well. Lauric acid is the chief contributor, with more than 40% of the share, followed by capric acid, caprylic acid, myristic acid and palmitic. Dried coconut meat, or copra, is rich in oil. In fact, more than 90% of the fatty acids in coconuts are classified as saturated; remarkably, coconut oil is more highly saturated than the fat in butter or red meat.

The high level of saturation in oil results in resists the oil turning rancid, making coconut oil ideal for commercial baking. However, saturated fats tend to raise blood cholesterol levels, hence it is restricted to people who have elevated blood pressure, cholesterol level or any other cardiovascular risk factors. Fatty acid in coconut is easy to digest, and a half cup of coconut meat has about 1 mg of iron and a fair amount of fibre. It is a good source of vitamins E and K. Coconut milk, the sweet white fluid which is extracted from the nut is served as a beverage or used as a marinade. It contains virtually no fat.

Groundnut or Peanut (*Arachis hypogaea*)

Groundnut is the seed of the legume plant. It is nutritious and is eaten raw or roasted or cooked with food. Peanuts are rich in linoleic acid. They provide higher proportion of pantothenic acid. Under certain conditions, substances in peanuts can combine with iodine and act as a blocker so that it cannot reach the blood.

Excessive consumption of groundnuts produces high acidity in the body, spermatorrhoea and premature ejaculation. Eating raw groundnuts in excess causes hyperacidity of the stomach, indigestion and heartburn.

Groundnut is rich in minerals such as manganese, copper, potassium, phosphorus and magnesium. It has good amount of calcium and sodium with small amount of iron, zinc, tryptophan and selenium.

The vitamin content of groundnut is rich in niacin and choline. It has good amount of pantothenic acid and vitamin E and small amount of thiamin, vitamin B_6, folate and betaine. It is also a good antioxidant.

Peanut is a legume used throughout the world for a variety of purposes including production of oil, butter, chocolates, cookies, etc. Peanuts are also eaten raw, roasted or added in various delicacies.

Peanuts may be contaminated with the mold *Aspergillus flavus* which produces a carcinogenic substance called aflatoxin. Aflatoxin is a very powerful and dangerous known carcinogen that may cause liver cirrhosis and cancer. Roasting enhances the taste, antioxidants levels like p-coumaric acid and helps remove toxic aflatoxin.

Walnut (*Juglans regia*)

Walnut is oil-rich food, which is a great source of all important omega-3 fatty acids. As in the cases of nuts, walnut also is a high calorie food. It contains 618 calories for every 100 g. Walnut contains excellent levels of folate. Though walnut is rich in oil, it is low in cholesterol.

Walnut is an excellent source of manganese and copper. They also contain very good levels of magnesium and phosphorous. Good levels of zinc, iron, calcium and selenium can also be found in walnut. They also contain traces of iodine. Walnuts are low in sodium.

Walnuts contain excellent levels of vitamin B_6, thiamin (B_1) and pantothenic acid. They also contain very good levels of vitamin E, niacin (B_3) and riboflavin (B_2). Walnut oil is greenish, yellow or almost colourless with a pleasant odour and a nutty flavour. It is rich in unsaturated fatty acids. Roasting reduces antioxidant quality.

Regular consumption of walnuts helps in lowering cholesterol levels, controlling high blood sugars, and improving cardiovascular functions. It is good for various heart problems. The reason for these benefits of walnuts is that they contain unsaturated fats and little cholesterol, significant amount of omega-3 and antioxidant properties.

Pistachios (*Pistacia Vera*)

Nutrient density, or Index of Nutritional Quality (INQ), is a measurement of a food's nutrient composition compared to its calorie contribution. A food can be considered nutritious if four nutrients have INQs of 1 or more, or if two nutrients have INQs of 2 or higher.

Pistachios are "super nutrient dense" because they are dense in eight nutrients: thiamin, vitamin B_6, copper, and manganese; and INQs ranging from 1 to 1.7 for potassium, fibre, phosphorus and magnesium. It is also a good source of calcium and zinc.

Super nutrient dense, pistachios are a superior snack choice. Low on the glycemic index and naturally cholesterol free, pistachios offer good heart health benefits, plenty of antioxidants and good fat.

Pistachios help your heart:

* Most of the fat in pistachios—almost 90% —is "good" or unsaturated fat, which can lower blood cholesterol along with heart disease.
* Of all snack nuts, pistachios offer the highest level of phytosterols, and are a powerful source of fibre, both of which reduce the absorption of cholesterol from the diet.
* Pistachios provide potassium. An inadequate intake of potassium is characterized by increased blood pressure and may increase the risk of cardiovascular disease and stroke.
* Pistachios offer the second highest amount of polyphenols among nuts. Polyphenols are antioxidants with potential heart health benefits.
* Pistachios contain a significant amount of the antioxidant lutein, about 13 times the amount as the next highest nut, hazelnuts.
* Intakes of lutein are associated with a reduced risk of age-related macular degeneration, the leading cause of irreversible blindness. Macular degeneration is a breakdown of the central portion of the retina and the principal cause of blindness among people ages 65 and older.

Conclusion

Nuts such as cashew nuts and almonds are used in various dishes to enhance the flavour, appearance and texture. Since many of the nuts are quite expensive when compared to cereals and pulses, they are used in small quantities, as garnish or to supplement the nutritive value of cereal and legumes. In some instances consumption of excessive quantities of groundnuts has led to giddiness and vomiting. This is perhaps due to the high amount of fat which is not easily digested. Nuts as such are used to enhance the protein quality of the diet. For more notes on oil seeds, refer to chapter "Fats and Oills".

12

Flesh Foods

MEAT

Much evidence from many civilizations has verified that the meat of wild and domesticated animals has played a significant role in human nutrition since ancient times. In addition to the skeletal muscle of warm-blooded animals, which in a strict sense is "meat", other parts are also used: Fat tissue, some internal organs and blood. Definitions of the term meat can vary greatly, corresponding to the intended purpose. From the aspect of food legislation, for instance, the term meat includes all the parts of warm-blooded animals, in fresh or processed form, which is suitable for human consumption.

Composition of Meat

Muscle of meat is composed of 75% of water, 20% of protein and 5% of fat, carbohydrates and minerals. The composition of meat varies with its sources, season of the year and pH of the meat. Protein comprises about four-fifths of the solid material. True fat, fat-like substances called phospholipids, inorganic substances and vitamins are present.

Veal is the meat from cattle slaughtered three to fourteen weeks after birth. Calf is from fourteen to fifty-two weeks old animal. Beef is from cattle over one year old. A heifer is female cattle that have never borne a calf. Red meat is the meat from mammals, white meat is the meat from poultry, seafood is referred to fish, prawn, etc. and game is from non-domesticated animals.

Meat has skeletal or muscular cuts and organ cuts. Skeletal or muscular cuts have muscle, tissue, connective tissue, bone fats and nerve tissues. Muscle tissue and connective tissue supply the qualities of meat in cookery. Muscle structure is made up of bundles of muscle fibres called fascicule. Connective tissues are scattered throughout the muscles where they play a connecting and supporting role. White fibrous and yellow elastic fibres with proteins like collagen and elastin are present in all muscle. Collagen contributes strength and elastin supplies elastic quality to meat. Collagen reacts with water in hydrolysis to produce gelatin and brings about a tenderizing effect to the meat. But no sack change is brought in elastin and if elastin is more in muscle fibres, meat will be hard even after cooking. This can be remedied by chopping or grinding the elastin fibres. Muscle haemoglobin is present in a small amount.

Water: Water is the major constitute of meat and the greatest percentage is found in lean meat and young animals. Water exists in muscle fibres and to a lesser degree in connective tissue. It is released from the protein structure in a number of ways. For example, water loss occurs as the muscle coagulates during cooking, as muscle fibres are broken (due to chemical, enzymatic, or mechanical tenderization) by salting, and if the pH changes. Inversely, water may be added to meat such as cured ham.

Protein: Meat is made up of high biological value or complete proteins, containing all of the essential amino acids in amounts and proportions that can be used in synthesizing body proteins. The three primary types of proteins in meats are myofibril, stromal proteins, and sarcoplasmic proteins as described in the following.

- *Myofibril protein*: Muscle bundles are groups of myofibrils composed of several protein molecules including actin and myosin which may form an overlap complex called actomyosin. These are soluble in concentrated salt solutions.
- *Stromal proteins* (connective tissue proteins): The watery connective tissue contains fibrils of stromal proteins: collagen, elastin, and reticulin. They are insoluble.
- *Sarcoplasmic proteins*: Sarcoplasmic proteins are a third general classification of meat proteins. They include the pigments and enzymes. For example, the haemoglobin pigment stores oxygen in the red blood cells bringing it to tissues, including the muscles, while myoglobin stores oxygen in the muscle where it is needed for metabolism. They are soluble in water or dilute salt solutions.

Fat: Fat may be a major component of meat, although veal contains only a small amount of fat. The fat content of meat varies from 5 to 40% with the type, breed, feed and age of the animal. Fats in meats are distributed between fascicule. Fat is laid as a protective layer around the organs. The fat deposited with the muscle structure is known as marbling. Marbling is desirable with some meats (like beef) because the amount of fat and consequently the water-holding capacity of the meat greatly influence juiciness.

Fat varies in its degree of saturation. For example, subcutaneous fats are generally more saturated than fat around glandular organs. Saturated fat promotes less oxidation, and therefore, less rancidity. In the animal, fat contributes to the survival of the living animal at low environmental temperatures.

In the diet fat allows the fat soluble vitamins A, D, E, K, to be carried. Moreover, fats contain some essential fatty acids that are precursor materials used in the synthesis of phospholipids for every cell membrane.

Cholesterol, a sterol, presents in the cell membranes of all animal tissues. Typically, lean meats have lower cholesterol content than higher-fat meats. An exception to this is veal, which is low in fat, yet high in cholesterol. The cholesterol content of meat is about 75 mg for 100 g. The lean portion of meat contains greater proportions of phospholipids (0.5–1.0%), and these are located in the membranes of the cell.

Carbohydrates: Carbohydrates are found only in very small quantities in meat. Two carbohydrates found in meat are glycogen and glucose. Carbohydrates are plentiful in plant tissue but are negligible in animal tissue. Approximately half of the small percentage of carbohydrates in animals is stored in the liver as glycogen. The other half exists throughout the body as glucose, especially in muscles and in blood. A small amount is found in other glands and organs of an animal.

Muscle cells of living animals contain glycogen which is otherwise known as animal starch. But immediately after the animal is dead, glycogen is converted into lactic acid. Hence if an animal is exercised or not fed prior to slaughter, low stores of glycogen appear in the liver and muscles.

Vitamins and minerals: The vitamin content of different meats varies. The B-complex vitamins—thiamine, riboflavin, and niacin occur in significant amounts in all meats. The meat of hog origin is rich in thiamine; liver is rich in vitamins A, D, E, and K. The minerals, iron (in haeme and myoglobin pigments), zinc and phosphorus are present in meat. Iron-containing substances and B vitamins are more in organ meats.

Postmortem Changes in Meat

A period of time normally elapses between the slaughter of an animal and the consumption of the meat. In practical terms, the carcass cools down and becomes stiffer or 'sets', the surface dries and the fat becomes firmer. The time period for stiffening is species-specific, and it is known as *rigor mortis*.

The major function of muscles is to contract, the energy for contraction and also for maintaining the functional integrity comes in the form of the ATP. A major role of the enzyme systems in the sarcoplasm and mitochondria is to ensure an adequate supply of ATP to the contractile elements. ATP is also needed to fuel the calcium pump of the sarcoplasmic reticulum. In living muscles, the fuels for producing this ATP are either free fatty acids or glucose from the blood, or glycogen, which is stored directly within the muscle fibres. In the fed animal, the circulating levels of free fatty acids are low and glucose is mostly used. In the fasting state free fatty acids derived from the breakdown of the triglyceride stores in the fat depots of the body are metabolized.

At the death of the animal, the supply of oxygen (and glucose and free fatty acids) to the muscle ceases, when the blood circulatory system fails. Any subsequent metabolism must be anaerobic and ATP can only be regenerated through breakdown of glycogen by glycolysis. As glycogen is broken down, lactic acid accumulates. Because this is not removed by the blood system, the muscle gradually acidifies. The reaction continues until glycogen stores are depleted or until a pH of 5.5 is reached. At this pH, the enzymes that are responsible for glycolysis are denatured and so the reaction stops. If glycogen is in short supply, glycolysis may stop due to depletion of glycogen before the pH drops as low as 5.5.

When glycolysis stops, the ATP supply is quickly depleted. Lack of ATP prevents calcium ions from being pumped out of the sarcoplasm, and so the active site on the actin molecules of the thin myofilaments is available to bind with the myosin of the thick filaments. Actin and myosin unite forming actomyosin cross-links. This cross-links formation is irreversible, as there is no available ATP. (In a live animal, actomyosin cross-links are formed and broken down repeatedly, as part of contraction, but the cycle requires ATP).

The formation of these irreversible actomyosin cross-links causes the muscle to become rigid. This is rigor mortis and correlated with the depletion of ATP in the muscle.

Ageing of Meat

If the meat is held cold for some time after it has gone into rigor mortis, the muscle again becomes soft and pliable with improved flavour and juiciness (resolution of rigor). Some changes take place during this period known as ageing or ripening. During ageing there is progressive tenderization of meat owning to denaturation of muscle protein and mild hydrolysis of denature proteins by the intracellular proteolytic enzymes, the cathepsins. The enzyme slowly breaks down the connective tissue between muscle fibres as well as the muscle fibres themselves.

Tenderizing the Meat

The muscle does not become extensible again in the way it was pre-rigor. This would only occur if the actin and myosin molecules that formed actomyosin at rigor subsequently dissociated, which does not happen. The thick and thin filaments remain locked together by the myosin cross-bridges and tenderization is not caused by the filaments regaining the ability to slide over one another. Instead, the structure of the myofibrils begins to break down.

The myofibrils become more easily fragmented by controlled homogenization of the muscle in aqueous solutions, and this can be monitored by the measurement of the 'myofibrillar fragmentation index'. In this, the degree of fragmentation is estimated from the opalescence of suspensions of myofibrils of equal protein content. Suspensions that are more opalescent indicate smaller particles, reflecting a greater fragmentation of the myofibrils. When longer times of ageing of the muscles after death of the animal, the myofibrillar fragmentation index increases and the meat becomes tenderer when it is cooked.

The use of enzymes like wrapping of meat in papaya leaves before cooking results in tenderization by the action of the enzyme papain in it. Other enzymes are bromelin from pineapple, ficin from fig, trypsin from pancreas and fungal enzymes. The use of low levels of salts and increasing or decreasing the pH of meat increase the tenderness.

Curing of Meat

The prime object of ageing or ripening and use of tenderizers is to increase the tenderness of meat. The curing meat has additional objectives. Curing brings about the modification of meat that effect preservation, flavour, colour and tenderness due to added curing agents. The ingredients used for curing are common salt, sodium nitrate or nitrite, sugar and spices. Cured meat can be dried or smoked.

POULTRY

Poultry meat is defined as meat from chicken, turkey, duck, goose, guinea fowl, and pigeon. Poultry is the most consumed meat in the world. One of the main reasons poultry meat consumption has increased in the last decade is the nutritional value of the meat. Poultry meat is economical, quick and easy to prepare and has a number of desirable nutritional and organoleptic properties.

Composition of Poultry Meat

Meat from poultry contains several important classes of nutrients, is low in calories, and is a source of both saturated and unsaturated fatty acids. The fat contains essential fatty acids and the proteins are a good source of essential amino acids. The fat in poultry meat is located in the skin and is therefore easily removable compared to other meats, enabling consumers to adopt a more low-fat type of meat in their diets. Along with this low-fat aspect, the fat in poultry meat is lower in saturated fatty acids and higher in unsaturated fatty acids. This fat deposition can vary among species and is diet-dependent. Therefore, poultry meat can easily be incorporated into a well-balanced diet to improve health. The meat fibres are tender, easy to chew or grind, easy to digest and the flavour is mild and blends with seasonings and other foods.

Moisture Content

The edible portion of chicken broilers contains about 71% moisture. Carcasses from young birds have a higher proportion of moisture to tissue than old ones.

Calories

Poultry meat is low in calories in relation to other nutrients present. By eating poultry meat as the source of proteins in a diet it is possible to reduce caloric intake, but at the same time help keep other nutrient requirements in proper balance.

Proteins

Poultry meat is not only a good source of protein but it also contains more proteins than red meats. Poultry meat contains high quality protein. It is easy to digest and contains all the essential amino acids presently known to be required in human diet.

Fat

The fat content of poultry carcasses varies according to the age, sex, and species of poultry. The part of the carcass from which the fat is taken also influences the fat content considerably. Cooked turkey skin contains 33.8% fat, whereas the breast meat contains only 6.7 to 8.3%. Unlike red meats, most fat in poultry meat is found under the skin rather than distributed throughout the tissues.

There is increasing evidence that not only the amount of fat in a diet but also the type of fat is important. One measure of the degree of saturation or unsaturation is the iodine number. Low iodine values indicate saturated fats, high ones unsaturated. Poultry meats contain a higher proportion of unsaturated fatty acids than the fats from red meats, but less than fats or oils of vegetable origin. Poultry meats also contain less cholesterol, a fatty alcohol present in the arteries and veins of individuals suffering with atherosclerosis, than other foods of animal origin.

Vitamins

Poultry meat is a good source of niacin, moderately good source of riboflavin, thiamin, and ascorbic acid. Chicken is also rich in folate, choline, betaine, calcium, iron, and vitamin C. Chicken liver is rich in vitamin A.

Minerals

Poultry meat contains sodium, potassium, calcium, iron, phosphorous, sulphur, chlorine and iodine.

FISH

Fish are classified into salt water and fresh water varieties. Their flavour depends on the water in which they were grown. Fish are also classified on the basis of their fat content—lean being less than 2% fat and fat being more than 5% fat. Common species of edible fish include catfish, trout, cod, halibut, haddock, pollock, salmon, tuna, mackerel, herring, shad, and eel. The fish are vertebrates.

Shellfish include the mollusks and the crustaceans. Mollusks are soft-bodied and partially or wholly enclosed in a hard shell composed of minerals. Oysters, clams, abalone, scallops, and mussels are examples of mollusks. Crustaceans are covered in a crust-like shell and have segmented bodies (like insects). Common crustaceans used for food include the lobster, crab, shrimp, prawns, and crayfish. Although fish contains complete proteins and can be an alternative for meat in the diet, fish consumption per capita is far lower than of meat.

Composition

- Fish are easily digestible, good source of protein, important minerals and vitamins.
- Fish contains high quality protein with all the essential amino acids like red meat and poultry.
- It is also low in fat and most of the fat it has is unsaturated. Some fish are relatively high in fat such as salmon, mackerel, and catfish. However, the fat is primarily unsaturated.
- The cholesterol content of most fish is similar to red meat and poultry. Some shellfish contain more cholesterol than red meat. Because the fat is mainly polyunsaturated.
- Fish is also a good source of B vitamins—B_6, B_{12}, biotin, and niacin. Vitamins D and A are found mainly in fish liver oils, but some high fat fish are rich in vitamin A.
- Fish is a good source of minerals especially iodine, phosphorous, potassium, and zinc. Canned fish with edible bones, such as salmons or sardines, are good sources of calcium.
- Oysters are good sources of iron and copper. Salt water fish and shell fish are excellent sources of calcium.

Spoilage

Fish spoil quicker than other meats because bacteria on the skin and in the digestive tract attack all the tissues once the fish is killed and these bacteria are often adapted to cold temperatures. Fish struggle when they are caught, and they convert all their glycogen to lactic acid before death. Associated with the fat of fish are phospholipids containing trimethylamine. Bacteria and enzymes from the fish split the trimethylamine from the phospholipids, producing the characteristic fishy odour. Fresh fish held at 61°F (16°C) remains good for only a day or less. At 52°F (0°C) finfish may remain good for 14 to 28 days depending on the species.

Selection

1. The skin looks bright and shiny. The skin on stale fish may show sign of wrinkling and shrinking away from flesh.
2. The eyes of the freshly caught fish will be convex, the pupil black and the cornea translucent. The eyes should be bright, clear and bulging and not sunken.
3. The gills of freshly caught fish are bright red, but as the blood in them oxidises they rapidly turn brownish and any mucus on them turns opaque.
4. If fish is spilt along the backbone and lifted, the bone should stick firmly to the flesh. If the bone separates easily, the fish is stale.

5. The surface should be free of dirt and slime.
6. The flesh should be firm to touch with no traces of browning or drying around the edges.
7. A fish having odour indicates deterioration due to oxidation of polyunsaturated fat and bacterial growth. Rancidity is revealed by yellowish spots on the surface. Rancidity can be recognized by sour taste, uncharacteristic of fresh fish.
8. Prawns should be fresh and firm, strong colour, and with no unpleasant smell.
9. Scallops should be pinkish white or pale yellow, feel firm, and should give off clear liquid.
10. Clams, cockles, oysters and mussels with tightly closed and heavy for their size, should be selected and their shells should not be cracked.

Grading

Grading determines the quality level. Only products have an established grade standard can be graded. Industry uses the grade standards to buy and sell products. Consumers rely on grading as a guide to purchase products of high quality. Grade A mark indicates that the product is of high quality. It is uniform in size, practically free of blemishes and defects, in excellent condition, and has good flavour and odour.

To determine the grade of processed fish, each fish scored for the following factors:

- Appearance: The overall general appearance of the fish, including consistency of flesh, odour, eyes, gills, and skin.
- Discoloration: This refers to any colour not characteristic to the species.
- Surface defects: These include the presence of fins; ragged, torn, or loose fins; brulses; and damaged portions of fish muscle.
- Cutting and trimming defects: These include body cavity cuts, improper wahing, improper deheading and evis-creation defects.
- Improper boning: for boned styles (fillet) only, this refers to the presence of an unspecified bone or piece of bone.

After inspecting each fish, the number of defects is totaled. Grade A is given when the maximum number of minor defects is three or less and no major defects. Grade B is given to fish with up to five minor defects and one major defect. Grade A fish must also possess good flavour and odour for the species, and grade B must possess reasonably good flavour and odour for the species.

Products: Fresh or frozen fish can be marketed as whole or round, dressed or pan-dressed, fillets, drawn fish, steaks, sticks, or nuggets.

Preservation: Fish are preserved by drying, salting, curing, or smoking. Some progress is being made on the use of irradiation. Refrigeration, freezing, and canning remain the best methods for preserving the quality of fish.

13

Eggs

The eggs of many species of bird have been consumed from prehistoric times, but hen eggs are the largely consumed eggs and the discussion that follows is regarding hen eggs. Eggs are a natural biological structure which protects the development of chick embryos. Eggs are multifunctional foods. World Health Organization considers eggs as the reference protein worldwide.

PHYSICAL STRUCTURE AND COMPOSITION

A fully formed egg, which includes the shell, egg white and yolk, weighs about 57 g. **The shell** of the egg contributes 8–11% of its weight. The dry egg shell contains an organic matrix which composed of 94% calcium carbonate and the remaining percentage contributes to magnesium carbonate, calcium phosphate and protein polysaccharide complex. This organic matrix forms the protective covering for the inner content of the egg, along with the two membranes. Two thin shell membranes are inside of the shell, one is attached to the shell and the other is not attached but moves with the egg contents. The two membranes are loosely attached to one place, usually at the broad end of the egg. These thin membranes help to protect the quality of the egg. Air cell develops as the two membranes separate at the large end of the egg. Shell naturally contains 7,000–17,000 porous for a potentially developing chick inside. Shell is a semi-permeable membrane, which allows air and moisture to pass through its pores. The shell also has a thin outermost coating called *cuticle or bloom* that helps keep out bacteria and dust. A simple wash can remove the shell's outer cuticle lining or open its pores resulting in diminished shelf life. Once this outside protection is removed, microorganisms from the outside can travel to the inside contents and contaminate the egg. Colour of the shell doesn't contribute to nutritive value or quality of the egg.

The egg white is also known as albumen comprises three concentric layers of white: Two thick whites separated by outer and inner thin whites. Egg protein is a "complete protein" since it contains the essential amino acids in a well-balanced proportion. The major protein present in egg white is ovalbumin, and the other proteins present in egg white are conalbumin, ovomucid, and globulins. The protein, avidin, which binds vitamin biotin in raw egg, is denatured by cooking. Vitamins in the egg white are riboflavin (which imparts a greenish tint to the white), niacin, and biotin. Minerals in the egg white are magnesium and potassium.

The yolk carries a germ spot which, under a suitable condition, develops into a chick. The yolk is enclosed in a sac called the "vitelline membrane". Immediately beyond this is another membranous layer known as the chalaziferous layer. Two twisted opaque ropes-like extensions of the chalaziferous layer called chalazae hold the yolk in the centre of the egg. Like little anchors, they attach the yolk's casing to the membrane lining the eggshell. The more prominent they are, the fresher the egg. All the eggs cholesterol and fat are present in the yolk. Egg yolk contains all three lipids—triglycerides, phospholipids, and sterols. The primary phospholipid is phosphatidyl choline, or lecithin, the best known sterol is cholesterol. Protein present in yolk is primarily vitelline that is present in a lipoprotein complex as lipovitellin and lipovitellinin. It also contains phosphorus-containing phosvitin and sulphur-containing livetin. The colour of the yolk differs from dark to pale yolk depending on the hen's feed. The yellow pigment may be carotene, xanthophylls, or lycopene.

The physical structure inside the shell changes as the egg ages. The content inside the shell shrinks and the air cell enlarges due to water loss. The vitelline membrane and the surrounding thick white become thinner, the chalazae cord appears less prominent, this makes the yolk flatten and it doesn't stay in the center of the egg as in the fresh ones. CO_2 loss leads to higher pH (from 7.6 to 9.7) which allows bacterial growth (Fig. 13.1).

EGG QUALITY

The abundance nutritional advantages of the egg can be utilized only when the egg is in good quality. Hence it is very essential to take steps to check and maintain the quality of the egg. Quality of egg is determined considering both external and internal factors. External factors are size and shape of the egg and condition of the shell. Internal factors are size of the air cell and condition of the albumen, yolk and the germ spot.

The size of the egg is indicated by the weight of the egg. The weight of the egg varies from 40–70 g. Several factors influence the size of the egg; major factor is the age of the hen, an older hen produces a larger egg. Secondary factors are the breed and weight of the hen. The size does not reflect the quality of the egg. There is no grading of eggs depending upon its size. Though the shell is not an edible portion, it protects the edible portion of the egg. The strength, porosity, texture, and cleanliness determine the quality of the shell. Soft-shelled eggs generally occur when an egg is prematurely laid and insufficient time in the uterus prevents the deposit of the shell. Thin-shelled eggs may be caused by dietary deficiencies, heredity, or disease. Glassy-shelled eggs are less porous and will not hatch but retain their quality. If the porosity of the egg shell is high, then CO_2

Vitelline (yolk) membrane
• Holds yolk contents

Shell membrane
• Two membranes — inner and outer shell membranes surround the albumen
• Provide protective barrier against bacterial penetration
• Air cell forms between these two membranes

Air cell
• Pocket of air formed at the large end of egg
• Caused by contraction of the contents during cooling after laying
• Increases in size as egg ages

Shell
• Outer covering of egg, composed largely of calcium carbonate
• May be white or brown depending on bread of chicken
• Colour does not effect egg quality, cooking characteristics, nutritive value or shell thickness

Thin albumen (liquid)
• Nearest to the shell
• Spreads around thick white of high-quality egg

Thick albumen (dense)
• Major source of egg riboflavin and protein
• Stands higher and spreads less in higher-grade eggs
• Thin and becomes indistinguishable from thin white in lower-grade eggs

Chalazae
• Twisted, cordlike strands of egg white
• Anchor yolk in centre of egg
• Prominent chalazae indicated freshness

Yolk
• Yellow portion of egg
• Colour varies with feed of the hen, but doesn't indicate nutritive content
• Major source of egg vitamins, minerals, and fat

Albumen layers
Outer liquid
Dense (albuminous sac)
Inner liquid

Vitelline membrane
White yolk
Germ
Membranes
Egg membrane
Shell membrane
Air cell
Chalaza
Cuticle
Chalaza
Yellow yolk
Egg shell

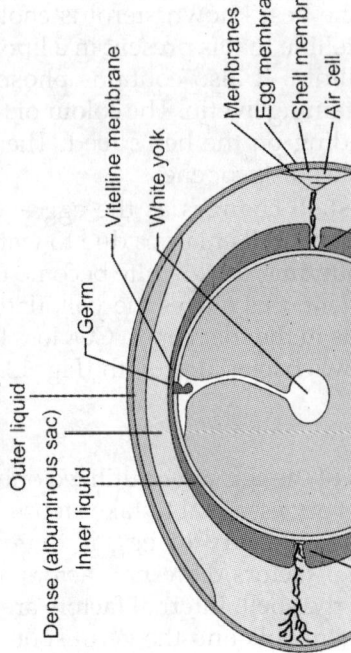

Fig. 13.1: Physical structure and composition of egg

and moisture losses occur while O_2 enters the shell and this leads to deterioration in the quality of egg on storage. The high porous shell is graded low than a shell with fine pores (Fig. 13.2).

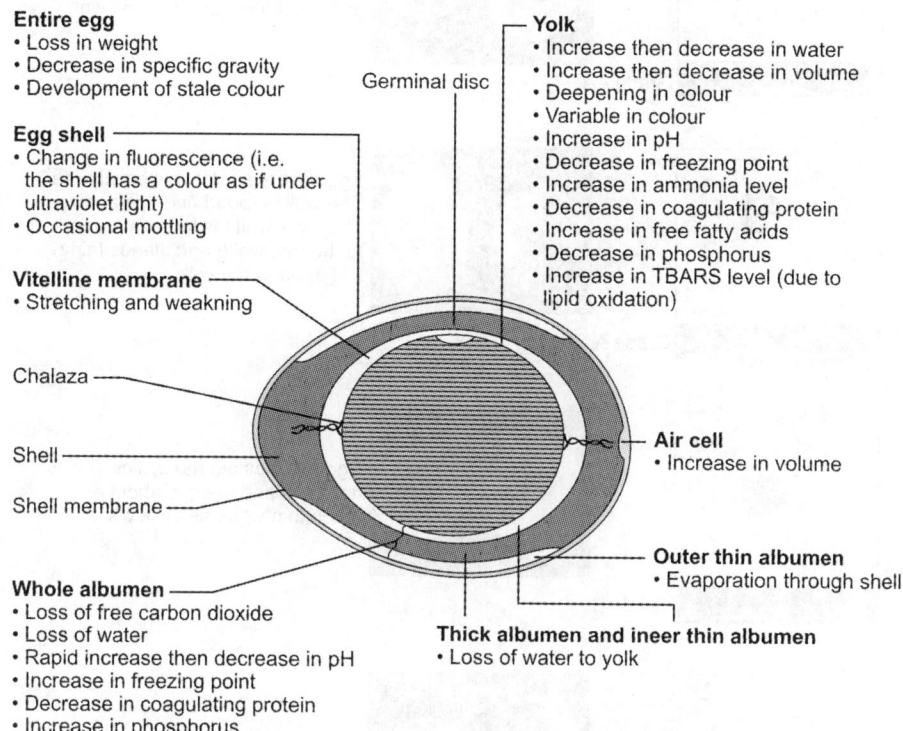

Entire egg
• Loss in weight
• Decrease in specific gravity
• Development of stale colour

Egg shell
• Change in fluorescence (i.e. the shell has a colour as if under ultraviolet light)
• Occasional mottling

Vitelline membrane
• Stretching and weakning

Germinal disc

Chalaza

Shell

Shell membrane

Whole albumen
• Loss of free carbon dioxide
• Loss of water
• Rapid increase then decrease in pH
• Increase in freezing point
• Decrease in coagulating protein
• Increase in phosphorus

Yolk
• Increase then decrease in water
• Increase then decrease in volume
• Deepening in colour
• Variable in colour
• Increase in pH
• Decrease in freezing point
• Increase in ammonia level
• Decrease in coagulating protein
• Increase in free fatty acids
• Decrease in phosphorus
• Increase in TBARS level (due to lipid oxidation)

Air cell
• Increase in volume

Outer thin albumen
• Evaporation through shell

Thick albumen and ineer thin albumen
• Loss of water to yolk

Fig. 13.2: Summary of changes in quality as the egg ages

When it comes to internal factor the condition of air cell or also known as air sac, is examined to evaluate the quality of egg. Initially there is no air cell when an egg is laid. Later an air cell is formed between two shell membranes at the large blunt end of the egg, and it enlarges during storage. When storage continues in warm, dry atmosphere, there will be increase in loss of moisture and the size of air cell increases. Through candling method the size of air cell inside the shell can be examined for its quality evaluation. An acceptable air cell size for different grades are: 1/18 inch for Grade AA, 3/16 inch for Grade A, and 3/8 inch for Grade B quality eggs. As the moisture loss increases, the egg content shrink and the inner membrane pulls away from the outer membrane and this ultimately increases the size of air cell, thinners the white and the yolk enlargers and becomes less viscous (Fig. 13.3).

EVALUATION OF EGG QUALITY

Candling is the most common and best available method to evaluate the quality of the egg. Candling is done either by hand (where egg content is

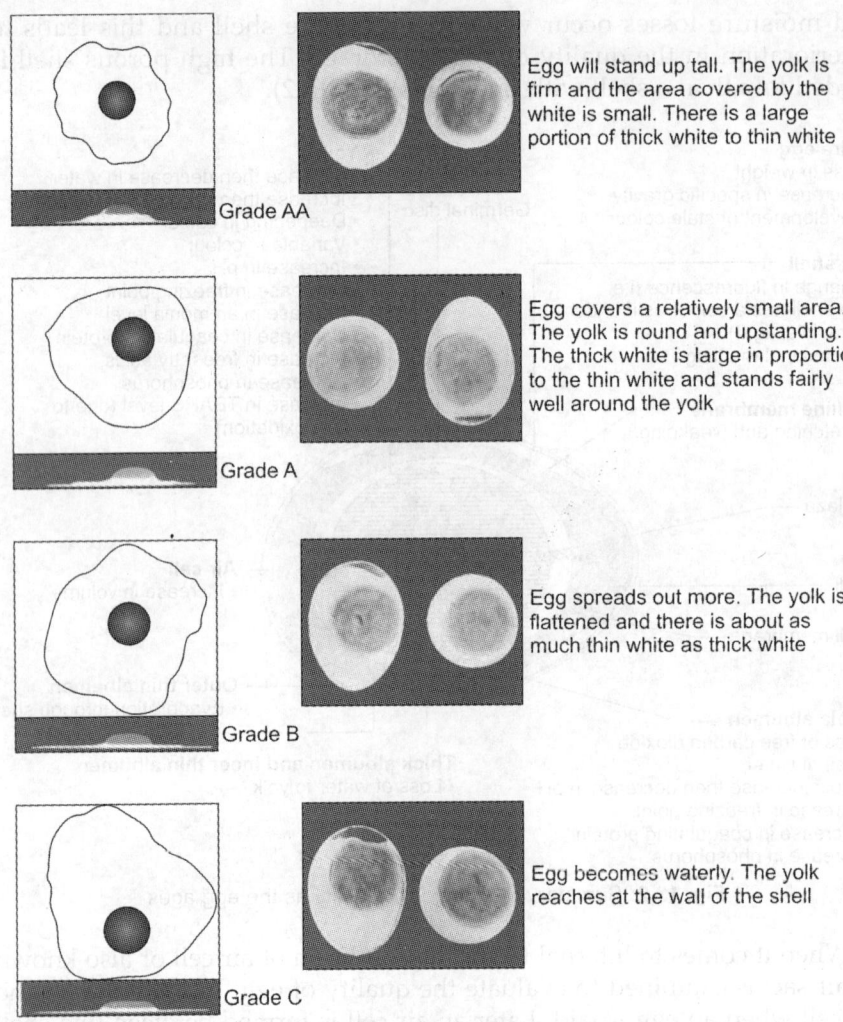

Egg will stand up tall. The yolk is firm and the area covered by the white is small. There is a large portion of thick white to thin white

Grade AA

Egg covers a relatively small area. The yolk is round and upstanding. The thick white is large in proportion to the thin white and stands fairly well around the yolk

Grade A

Egg spreads out more. The yolk is flattened and there is about as much thin white as thick white

Grade B

Egg becomes waterly. The yolk reaches at the wall of the shell

Grade C

Fig. 13.3: Grades of egg

seen when held up to a candle while being rapidly rotated) or mass scanning (commercial eggs may be scanned in mass, with bright lights under trays of eggs). Candling helps to examine the cracks in the shell and without breaking the content, the size of the air cell, the firmness of albumin, the position and mobility of yolk and the possible presence of foreign substances such as blood spots, moulds and developing embryo can also be examined.

Domestically, the quality of the egg can be determined by dropping the egg in the water. Fresh eggs or the eggs which are of good quality fall at once to the bottom, the eggs which are a few days old floats midway and the eggs with deterioration in quality will float on the surface of the water. The egg floating in water is due to an increase in the size of the air cell, loss in weight due to dehydration.

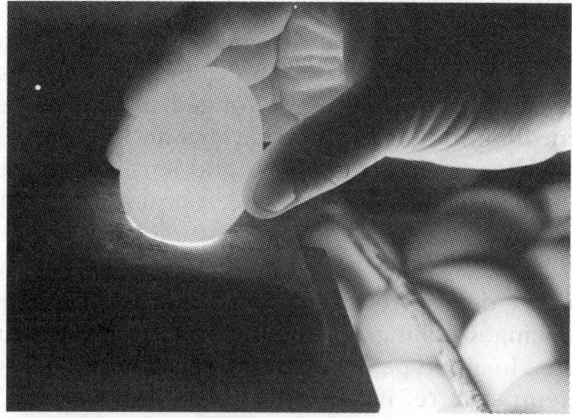

(a) Candling done by hand

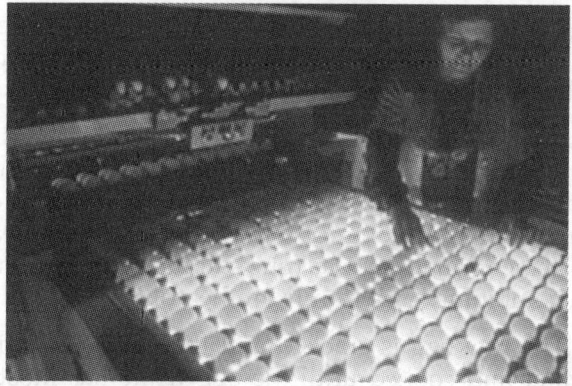

(b) Candling by mass screening

Egg has to be bought and stored carefully since it is easily deteriorate. Egg should be bought which is crack free. It should be refrigerated at 4–7°C, if stored in room temperature it reduces the quality of eggs within a week.

Heat Effect on Egg Proteins

When a protein molecule retains the peptide linkages between amino acids, yet unfolds, *denaturation* occurs by producing irreversible changes in the specific folding and the shape that a protein assumes in space. Denaturation occurs due to heat, mechanical actions like beating or whipping, or due to an acidic pH. The helical chains with intramolecular bonds uncoil and align in a parallel fashion, forming intermolecular bonds, and the protein chains shrink. In this process, the egg changes in appearance from translucent to opaque.

Coagulation represents the process that occurs when denatured protein molecules from either the white or yolk form a solid mass. Various proteins coagulate at different temperatures and also by other factors such as beating, pH, use of sugar and salt. By heat egg white proteins begin to coagulate at 52°C and is completed at 65°C. Egg yolk begins to coagulate at 65°C and is completed at 70°C. Prolonged or intense heating causes *Curdling*. In curdling, the precipitate shrinks and becomes tough which brings negative changes like water loss and shrinkage. Beating changes the helical protein structure. Acid pH, sugar and salt help in coagulation.

Changes While Cooking

Eggs, nutritionally dense product, undergo various changes in different methods of cooking. Cooking is done to produce tender, edible and high quality products. In any type of cooking eggs as to be cooked only at low to moderate temperature, if cooked at high temperature, it results in toughening of the proteins. Some of the examples of changes while egg cooking is as follows:

Soft-cooked eggs: Eggs are placed in sufficient boiling water (eggs should be fully covered with water). Eggs are left in simmering temperature for 3–5 min. This will make the white firm but tender and yolk as a thick liquid.

Hard-cooked eggs: The same method is used as in soft-cooked eggs but the time of cooking here is increased to 15–20 min. By this, white becomes an opaque tender gel and the yolk is completely coagulated. Green discolouration occurs if cooking for a long time and high heat. The green colour is due to the formation of ferrous sulphide from sulphur in the egg white protein combining with iron from the yolk.

Poached eggs: The raw egg is cracked and then gently slid into a pan of simmering water and cooked until the egg white has mostly solidified, but the yolk remains semi-liquid and covered by a thick coating of white. Fresh eggs will yield the best results. When the egg white is completely coagulated, it should be removed from water immediately. Addition of vinegar or salt will increase the quality of the end product.

Fried eggs: Frying eggs in a measurable amount of fat and basting the top of the egg with fat to increase the cooking speed. The egg may be turned over and a lid placed on the pan so that the steam may speed the cooking of the upper surface. In fried egg the white should be uniformly coagulated, tender, thick and compact. The yolk should be unbroken and covered with a layer of coagulated white.

Scrambled eggs: Raw eggs are whisked to blend the egg white and yolk into a homogeneous liquid. Liquids such as stock, cream, butter, milk, water, or oil may be added during the whisking to create a softer texture. The amount of liquid added is typically about 1tbsp per egg. Salt, pepper, or other seasonings can be added to taste. The mix is then heated slowly and the egg is scraped, as it coagulates. This will create small and soft curds which are moist, tender and fluffy. Overcooking will make the product shrunken, tough and dry. If any liquid is seeping from the eggs, this is a sign of undercooking. For best result double boiler can be used.

French omelet: Raw egg is blended thoroughly and poured on a greased pan. It is cooked with its lid covered until it is coagulated. Flavoring agent can be added while blending the raw egg.

Custards: Custards are cooked with slow rate of heating. If proper temperature is not maintained, it results in undesirable curdling where the protein structure shrinks and releases water. There are two types of custards, soft or stirred custards and baked custards. Soft custards are soft and creamy and does not form gel. If overheated or heated too quickly, the mixture curdles and whey separates. For better control of temperature and rate of cooking double boiler is suggested. Baked custards are firm, yet tender and forms gel. If overheated, it becomes porous filled with watery serum. To control heat and prevent the mixture from burning baking in water bath is recommended.

Egg White Foams

As liquid egg white is whisked, the mechanical action causes its proteins to unfold and form a network, trapping air in tiny pockets. The colour changes from translucent to brilliant white. Foam holds its shape as protein coagulates around air cells. Thus, foams are used in various food applications. If the foam is left to stand, it will eventually collapse back into a liquid. But the physical change caused by whisking denatures the protein, depriving it of elasticity and become stiff and brittle.

Factors affecting volume and stability of egg white foams:
- *Over-beaten egg whites* will lose its elasticity and not able to expand.
- *Thin blades or fine wired beater* is the best choice for making fine foams.
- *Older eggs* and *cold eggs* will not give high volume and stable foams and do not work as a leavening agent. Hence fresh eggs and eggs at room temperature are preferred because of lowered surface tension at the room temperature.
- By adding cream of tartar or lemon juice (acid) to the alkaline egg white the pH is lowered. If acid is added at the beginning of beating, it gives greater stability but less volume hence, acid should be added when egg reaches the foamy stage while whipping it.
- Addition of *water* to the egg white will increase the volume but decrease the stability of the foam.
- Presence of *fat* in the form of oil, cream or the yolk itself will hinder the foam formation.
- When *salt* is added, it results in very less foam with no peaks and the foam formation is also very slow.
- In addition of *sugar* it takes double the time in foam formation and the finished foam looks glossy and shine, which is preferred in various food products for its finished texture.

- Soft and hard meringues, soufflés, foam cakes are the few examples of food products created by using egg white foams.

Nutritive Value of Eggs

Eggs are a complete protein, with a high biological value of 100 which means all the absorbed protein is retained by the body. Egg whites are given the highest protein-digestibility-corrected amino acid score (PDCAAS) of 1.0, which corrects the amino acid composition with its digestibility. Egg 12–14% of protein contains all essential amino acids in a balanced form. Eggs constitute 10–12% of lipids, they contain essential fatty acids—linoleic and arachidonic fatty acids. The interactions between lipids and proteins result in the formation of lipoproteins (low and high density), which represent the main constituents of yolk. Cholesterol is the sterol found in egg yolk. It results partly from hen feed and partly from synthesis in the liver during the elaboration of lipoproteins. Egg yolk contains 250 mg of cholesterol, whereas the normal man RDA is 300 mg of cholesterol per day, hence it has to be restricted by some individuals. Egg is an excellent source of vitamin A, good source of vitamin D and vitamin B, and poor source of vitamin C. Minerals in eggs are iron, phosphorus, zinc, iodine, potassium, and sulphur. Most of the calcium in an egg is found in the shell as calcium carbonate. Levels of most nutrients in the eggs are influenced by age, breed, season and diet of the hen.

Functions of Eggs

Eggs are multifunctional product.

- Eggs are viscous and have coagulating property hence this can help to bind the ingredients together in food preparation. Therefore, eggs are used as a *binding agent,* e.g. cutlet, French or Bombay toast, banana fritters.
- Egg whites are used as *clarifying agent*, when protein in egg coagulates, they trap the loose particles in liquid and clarify it and hence used to clarify broth and soups.
- Egg yolks act as an *emulsifying agent.* Yolk itself is an emulsion. Egg yolks contain phospholipid emulsifiers, including lecithin. Emulsifier allows mixing two immiscible liquids, such as oil-in-water to mix. This emulsion is used in the preparation of salad dressing, mayonnaise, various baked products such as cheese soufflés, cream puffs, shortened cakes, etc.
- Eggs as *foaming agent and leavening agent.* Egg white when beaten forms foam which is six to eight times in volume than the unbeaten eggs. Egg white foams are used in making meringues, soufflés, fluffy omelets, foam cakes, etc. Egg yolk also foams but the volume change is much less than that of the egg white. Egg yolk foam is used in sponge cake preparation.
- Eggs as a *thickening* property and these are made use in different food preparations. The protein in the egg coagulates on heating and this

increases the viscosity of the entire food preparation, e.g. custards, soups, puddings and cream pie fillings.

- Eggs work on *inhibition of crystal formation*. Egg white minimizes the crystallization of sugars in icings and candies. In candy it helps to ensure creamy smoothness as well as whiteness in such confections as divinity fudge and fondant. As the hot syrup is added to the beaten egg white, the albumen forms thin films around the tiny sugar crystals and prevents them from clustering together, which results in a grainy and crumbly candy.
- Eggs also add colour, flavour and nutritional value to the food.
- The other nonfood uses of eggs are:
  - The principal nonfood use of egg is that it reproduces the species.
  - Industrial egg albumen is used in finishing certain types of leather, particularly glazed, coloured stock.
  - Inedible eggs are utilized also in animal feedstuffs and plant fertilizers.
  - To improve the glossy sheen of the fur coat eggs are fed to animals.
  - Eggs are used in production of vaccines in chick embryos.

14   Milk and Milk Products

Milk is a white liquid produced by the mammary glands of mammals. It provides the primary source of nutrition for young mammals before they are able to digest other types of food. The exact components of raw milk vary by species, but it contains significant amount of saturated fat, protein and calcium as well as vitamin C. Milk is as ancient as mankind itself, as it is the substance created to feed the mammalian infant. All species of mammals, from man to whales, produce milk for this purpose. Many centuries ago, perhaps as early as 6000–8000 BC, ancient man learned to domesticate species of animals for the provision of milk to be consumed by them. These included cows, buffaloes, sheep, goats, and camels, all of which are still used in various parts of the world for the production of milk for human consumption.

Composition of Milk

Milk is often described as a colloidal suspension, containing emulsified globules of fat, a heterogeneous family of major and minor proteins, the carbohydrate lactose, minerals, vitamins and enzymes. While the classes of constituents are similar for milk from most species, there are considerable inter-species differences, both qualitatively and quantitatively.

The composition and properties of fresh cow's milk shows considerable variability. The main factors from which such variability arises are: (a) genetic factors (breed and individual), (b) stage of lactation, (c) health status of the cow and (d) environmental factors (e.g. feed climate or method of milking).

Milk Fat

Milk fat is excreted in the form of small droplets which, in cow's milk, range from 1 to 18 μm in diameter with a mean size of about 3 μm. The mean size appears to be related to the fat content of the milk and the higher the fat content, the bigger is the average size of the individual fat globules. Globule membrane comprises largely proteins and phospholipids and provides stabilization for the hydrophobic fat particles in the aqueous environment of the milk serum.

Fat content in milk may vary greatly in calories. It contains fat-soluble vitamins, and it contains the pigments carotene and xanthophyll. Fat contains lipids such as cholesterol and the phospholipids, but it is primarily triglyceride (95%) with saturated, polyunsaturated, and monounsaturated fatty acid components that have varying melting points and susceptibility to oxidation. The fatty acid chains vary from 4 to 22 carbons in length and contain many short-chain fatty acids such as the saturated butyric acid and caproic, caprylic, and capric acids.

The milk fat globule membrane is, however, a delicate structure and can easily be ruptured by either physical or thermal shock. The lypolytic enzymes present in great excess in raw milk. Lypolytic action leads to the hydrolysis of milk fat and the liberation of free fatty acids, resulting in development of unacceptable rancid flavour and odour. For these reasons raw milk must be carefully handled during all stages of transport and storage. Milk fat will absorb volatile odour very readily. Because of this property, butter, milk and cream should not be stored near the source of volatile odours which might contribute to the off-flavour of these products.

Milk Proteins

Protein represents 3–4% of the composition of milk and components may be fractioned out of milk by ultracentrifugation. Milk protein is a heterogeneous mixture which can be separated based on solubility at specific values of pH and in presence of salt solutions. The proteins in milk fall into two distinct types, whey proteins and caseins.

Caseins: Casein is the primary protein of milk, comprising approximately 80% of the milk protein. The largest structures in the fluid portion of the milk are casein protein micelles: Aggregates of several thousand protein molecules, bonded with the help of nanometer-scale particles of calcium phosphate. There are four different types of casein proteins, and collectively they make up around 80% of the protein in milk, by weight. Most of the casein proteins are bound into the micelles. The casein proteins distinctively subdivided into 4 main classes—the alpha$_{s1}$, alpha$_{s2}$, beta, gamma and kappa caseins. Alpha$_{s1}$-casein and alpha$_{s2}$-casein are two fractions which are difficult to separate from each other. All four fractions are phosphoproteins containing phosphate groups esterified to the amino acid serine. They are modest of size and do not possess an organized structure. Because of this property, they cannot be denatured by heating.

The alpha and beta caseins contain several phosphate groups, and as a result they are "calcium-sensitive," and may be coagulated by addition of calcium. First, they account for the calcium sensitivity of milk protein. When calcium added to casein solutions, the casein promptly coagulates as intermolecular calcium bridges are formed. The reaction is the key to cheese making and to the formation of acidic gels such as yogurt.

The gamma caseins are the result of post-secretary hydrolysis of beta casein. In good quality milk from cows in mid-lactation, gamma casein should constitute a very low proportion of the total casein fraction in milk certainly less than 5%. Casein is a glycoprotein; glutamic acid is predominant one in this. Other amino acids such as proline, aspartic, leucine, lysine and valine are also present at relatively higher levels in casein. Kappa casein contrasts with other caseins as it has one serine ester group and contains a charged carbohydrate. Carbohydrates present in casein are galactose, glucose, mannose, and glucosamine. Rennin, an enzyme secreted by the young calves, brings about the coagulation of milk. The coagulation is due to the change in physicochemical status of casein.

Whey proteins: In contrast to the casein, the whey proteins are typical globular proteins which may be denatured on heating at temperature above 65°C. The major components are beta lactoglobulin and alpha lactalbumin, and the water-soluble nutrients, such as riboflavin. The major whey proteins contain sulphur amino acid which, on heating, may participate in sulphydryl exchange reactions leading to inter- and intra-molecular cross-linking.

Whey are used to make ricotta cheese and also used in beverages, frozen dairy desserts, and in baked products. In a dried form it is used as an emulsifier and as a fortifier to provide extra protein to foods. Whey is concentrated by ultrafiltration to yield whey protein concentrates. Whey protein concentrates are frequently added to yogurt, and dried for use in items such as coffee whitener, whipped toppings, fruit beverages, and chocolate drinks. On future, purification yields whey protein isolates, they are used in infant formulas.

Milk Sugar (Lactose)

Lactose is a milk sugar, by weight most abundant of the milk solids. Its concentration in milk is related to yield and may range from 4.2 to 5.0%. Lactose is a disaccharide which on hydrolysis gives glucose and galactose. Lactose has only about one-sixth the sweetness of sucrose and one-third of its solubility in water. Lactose is a reducing sugar and, in some circumstances, reacts freely with free amino groups in protein and thus develops a brown colour (Maillard reaction). The Maillard reaction is characterized by browning but, in the earlier stages of the reaction, there is a loss of nutritive value as the essential amino acid, lysine reacts with reducing sugar. On fermentation of lactose to lactic acid by the intestinal microorganisms, it promotes absorption of minerals. The acid fermentation is also needed for the curd, cheese and butter making.

Vitamins and Minerals

Milk contains both water-soluble and fat-soluble vitamins. Both depend on the feed consumed. Under water-soluble vitamins, milk is a good source of thiamin, riboflavin and vitamin B_{12}. Milk contains small amount of niacin, pantothenic acid, vitamin B_6, vitamin C, and folate and is not considered a major source of these vitamins in the diet. Milk is rich in B vitamin riboflavin, a greenish fluorescent coloured vitamin. It acts as a photosynthesizer and is readily destroyed upon exposure to sunlight. Under fat-soluble vitamins, milk contains vitamins A, D, E, and K. The content level of fat soluble vitamins in dairy products depends on the fat content of the product. Reduced fat (2% fat), low fat (1% fat), and skim milk must be fortified with vitamin A to be nutritionally equivalent to whole milk. Fortification of all milk with vitamin D is voluntary. Milk contains small amounts of vitamins E and K and is not considered a major source of these vitamins in the diet.

Minerals (ash) such as calcium and phosphorous are the major minerals found in milk. Calcium is combined with the protein casein as calcium caseinate, and with phosphorus as calcium phosphate and as calcium citrate. Milk also contains almost all other minerals such as sodium, potassium, magnesium, iron, sulphur and chloride. In addition to these, milk contains many trace elements such as copper, zinc, aluminium, molybdenum, iodine, etc., depending upon the feed of the animal.

Enzymes

More than 25 enzymes found in milk. It originates from the mammary glands, or may be released by contaminating bacteria.

These enzymes may be grouped into following categories:

Lipases — Lipases are fat splitting enzymes

Proteases — Proteases are protein decomposing enzymes

Amylases — Amylases are starch hydrolyzing enzymes

Catalases — Catalases are hydrogen peroxide decomposing enzymes

Phosphatases — Phosphatases decompose phosphoric acid

Lactases — Lactases hydrolyze lactose into lactic acid

Peroxidases — They cause oxidation, responsible for peroxidase test.

Xanthine oxidase: An enzyme associated with the cell membrane and on the inner surface of the milk fat globule membranes. It is a conjugated protein complexed with FAD, iron, and molybdenum. The enzyme degradation of FAD (Flavin Adenine Dinucleotide) gives FMN (Flavin Adenine Mononucleotide) and riboflavin. The riboflavin content of milk may thus be due to xanthine oxidase.

Lactoperoxidase: It is one of the most heat-stable enzymes found in milk. Lactoperoxidase, when combined with hydrogen peroxide and thiocyanate, has antibacterial properties. It is suggested that the presence of lactoperoxidase in raw milk inhibits the disease causing microorganisms (pathogens) present in milk. However, since there is no hydrogen peroxide or thiocyanate present in fresh milk, these compounds would have to be added to milk in order to achieve the antibacterial benefits.

Lysozyme is another enzyme that has some antibacterial activities, although the amount of lysozyme present in milk is very small.

Lipase: Lipases are enzymes that degrade fats. The major lipase in milk is lipoprotein lipase. It is associated with the casein micelle. Agitation during processing may bring the lipase into contact with the milk fat resulting in fat degradation and off-flavours. Pasteurization will inactivate the lipase in milk and increase shelf life.

Proteases: These are enzymes that degrade proteins. The major protease in milk is plasmin. Some proteases are inactivated by heat and some are not. Protein degradation can be undesirable and result in bitter off-flavours, or it may provide a desirable texture to cheese during ripening. Proteases are important in cheese manufacture.

Alkaline phosphatase enzymes are able to split specific phosphoric acid esters into phosphoric acid and the related alcohols. Unlike most milk enzymes, it has a pH and temperature optima differing from physiological values; pH of 9.8. The enzyme is destroyed by minimum pasteurization temperatures; therefore, a phosphatase test can be done to ensure proper pasteurization.

Properties of Milk

- The white colour (apolescence) of milk is due to reflection of light by the fat globules and the colloidal protein, calcium caseinate and phosphate. The bluish colour of separated milk or whey is due to another pigment known as riboflavin (vitamin B_{12}) or lactochrome.
- Milk average pH value is 6.7. On titrating it with an alkali, it is found to contain 0.1to 0.17% acidity. This acidity is not due to lactic acid (developed) but due to phosphates of milk proteins citrates and carbon dioxide present in milk (natural).
- The sweet taste of lactose is balanced against the salty taste of chloride in milk.
- The specific gravity of freshly drawn milk is lower than specific gravity obtained after an hour or later.
- The rise in specific gravity is regular, more rapid at low temperature than at higher ones and amounts on an average to 0.001. This attributed to: (i) change in the specific gravity of fat due to partial cooling and solidification, (ii) hydration of the proteins, (iii) loss of carbon dioxide, and (iv) presence of air bubbles.
- The specific gravity ranges from 1.025 to 1.032 at 60°F or 15.5°C.
- Milk has lower freezing point than water due to the presence of lactose and slats in aqueous phase; it freezes at − 0.55°C to − 0.56°C.
- Average milk boils at 212.3°F (100.17°C). As specific gravity boiling point affects by the same factor, the specific heat of milk at 15°C is 0.938.

MILK PRODUCTS

Milk is used in both fermented and non-fermented forms.

NON-FERMENTED MILK PRODUCTS

Whey Protein Concentrates

• The milk is first coagulated by application of either rennet or acid. Whey is passed through the membranes called ultra filtration technology to concentrate protein to various levels between 20 and 80%.

• Removing the water results in Whey Protein Concentrate (WPC) Powder. WPC is the most efficient protein for the human body. Research has shown that, of all protein sources, WPC is digested and absorbed better than any other protein.

• WPC has no flavours and no sweeteners — it is merely 100% pure whey, of which more than 80% is the quality protein. Flavours and/or sweeteners can be added on our own choice (such as vanilla, cloves, ginger root, cyclamate sweeteners, etc.).

Typical Nutrition Information for Whey Protein Concentrate

Serving size: 1 oz.	—	28.4 g
Protein (dry basis)	—	23.0 g (81%)
Total carbohydrates	—	2.0 g
Sugars (as lactose)	—	2.0 g
Total fat	—	2.0 g
Saturated fat	—	1.2 g
Cholesterol	—	65 mg
Energy	—	110 calories (kcal)
Energy from fat	—	18 calories (kcal)
Potassium	—	160 mg
Sodium	—	55 mg
Calcium	—	110 mg
Vitamin A	—	200 I.U.

Specialty Milks

This includes lactose-reduced milk (e.g. Pauls zymil and zerolac are the two products which is currently getting popular in India), calcium-fortified (e.g. Amul Calci+), as well as flavoured milks, and shakes. One of the most useful products, lactose-reduced milk, is available in both nonfat and low-fat compositions as well as in many flavoured versions. The lactose is reduced by 70 to 100%, making it possible for lactose-intolerant individuals. Lactose reduction is accomplished by subjecting the appropriate milk to the action of the enzyme lactase in a refrigerated tank for approximately 24 hours. The enzyme breaks down the lactose to more readily digestible glucose and galactose. The reaction is halted when the lactose is consumed or when the milk is heat-treated. The resulting beverage is sweeter than regular milk but acceptable for most uses.

Condensed Milk

Whole, low-fat, and skim milk, as well as whey and other dairy liquids, can be efficiently concentrated by the removal of water, using heat under vacuum. Since reducing atmospheric pressure lowers the temperature at which liquids boil, the water in milk is evaporated without imparting a cooked flavour. Water can also be removed by ultra filtration and reverse osmosis, but this membrane technology is more expensive. Usually about 60% of the water is removed, which reduces storage space and shipping costs. Whole milk, when concentrated, usually contains 7.5% milk fat and 25.5% total milk solids. Skim milk can be condensed to approximately 20 to 40% solids.

Evaporated Milk

Condensed milk is often sold in refrigerated tank-truck loads to manufacturers of candy, bakery goods, ice cream, cheese, and other foods. When preserved by heat in individual cans, it is usually called "evaporated milk." In this process the concentrated milk is homogenized, fortified with vitamin D, and sealed in a can. A stabilizer, such as disodium phosphate, is also added to keep the product from separating during processing and storage. The sealed can is then sterilized at 118°C (244°F) for 15 minutes, cooled, and labeled. Evaporated milk keeps indefinitely, although staling and browning may occur after a year.

Ultra-High Temperature (UHT) Processing Milk

UHT processing (sterile, aseptic) is done at 280–302°F (138–150°C) for 2–6 seconds. With this treatment, milk is sterilized by reaching temperatures beyond the normal pasteurization temperature. Packaging is also done under sterile conditions, which are aseptically sealed and does not allow microorganisms to enter. Thus, it is aseptically packaged, and the milk does not require refrigeration until it is opened.

Sweetened Condensed Milk

It is also made by removing the water (as in evaporated milk) and adding sugar. The final product contains about 8.5% milk fat and at least 28% total milk solids. Sugar is added in sufficient amount to prevent bacterial action and subsequent spoilage. Usually, at least 60% sugar in the water phase is required to provide sufficient osmotic pressure for prevention of bacterial growth.

Khoa

A concentration of milk to one-fifth volume is normal in the production of khoa. Khoa is used as the base for a wide variety of Indian sweets. Khoa is made from both cow and buffalo milk. Kzhoa is normally white or pale yellow. Khoa is made by simmering milk in an iron karahi (open pan) for several hours, over a medium fire. Milk is cautiously stirred in a circular motion with a scraper to avoid scorching. When the viscocity increases, the rate of stirring also increases to maintain a uniform consistency. The gradual vaporization of its water content leaves coagulated solids in milk, which is khoa. The ideal temperature to avoid scorching is 175–180°F (about 80°C). There is decrease in vitamin A and some water-soluble vitamins of milk in khoa formation.

Skimmed Milk

Whole milk fat content is reduced to 0.5–2% by centrifugation. By removing fat from the milk not only taste or flavour is reduced but also fat-soluble vitamins such as vitamins A and D are decreased. Skimmed milk powder should be fortified with vitamins A, D and pyridoxine, to make high nutritive value food. It is useful for the treatment of malnutrition, the nephrotic syndrome and the cirrhosis of liver. It is also used for low calorie diets.

Toned Milk

Toned milk is prepared by mixing equal parts of fresh buffalo milk (rich in fats) and reconstituted skimmed milk powder. The fat, protein, carbohydrate, vitamin and mineral contents — and thus the nutritive value — are the same as fresh cow's milk. Toned milk is a useful source of proteins for malnourished children and pregnant women.

Double Toned Milk

This is prepared by admixture of cows or buffalos milk or both with fresh skimmed milk or by admixture with skim milk reconstituted from skim milk powder or by partial removal or addition of milk to skim milk. It should be pasteurized and show negative phophotase test. It contains only 1.5% fat and S.N.F. not less than 9%.

Recombined Milk

Recombined milk is a homogenized product prepared from milk fat, non-fat milk solids and water. It should be pasteurized and show a negative phophotase test. Its fat content should be less than 3% and S.N.F. 8.5%.

Sterilized Milk

Standardized cow's or buffalo's milk is sterilized in bottles by heating continuously to a temperature of 115°C for 15 minutes to ensure destruction of all microorganisms and preservation at room temperature for not less than 85 days from the date of manufacture. Sterilized milk shall be sold only in the container in which milk was sterilized.

Malai (Clotted cream)

After milk is boiled and allowed to cool, a thick layer of fat and coagulated proteins collects at the surface and can be skimmed off; by repeating the process twice, most of the fat is removed. Buffalo's milk, being rich in fat, produces better malai. Good malai supplies 43 kcal (181 kJ) per tablespoon.

Ice Cream

The essential ingredients in ice cream are milk, cream, sugar, flavouring, and stabilizer. Cheaper ingredients such as dry whey, corn syrup, and artificial flavourings may be substituted to create a lower-cost product.

The first step in ice cream making is formulating a suitable mix. The mix is composed of a combination of dairy ingredients, such as fresh milk and cream, frozen cream, condensed or dried skim, buttermilk, dairy whey, or whey protein concentrate. Sugars may include sucrose, corn syrup, honey, and other syrups. Stabilizers and emulsifiers are added in small amount to help prevent formation of ice crystals, particularly during temperature fluctuations in storage. The ice cream mix is pasteurized at no less than 79°C (175°F) for 25 seconds. The heated mix is typically homogenized in order to assure a smoother body and texture. Homogenizing also prevents churning (i.e. separating out of fat granules) of the mix in the freezer and increases the viscosity. (Since smaller fat globules have more surface area, the associated milk protein can hydrate more water and produce a more viscous fluid.)

After homogenization, the hot mix is quickly cooled to 4.4°C (40°F). The mix must age at this temperature for at least four hours to allow the fat to solidify and fat globules to clump. This aging process results in quicker freezing and a smoother product. The next step, freezing the mix, is accomplished by one of two methods: Continuous freezing, which uses a steady flow mix, or batch freezing, which makes a single quantity at a time. For both methods, the objective is to freeze the product partially and, at the same time, incorporate air. The freezing process is carried out in a cylindrical barrel that is cooled by a refrigerant. The barrel is equipped with stainless steel blades, called dasher blades, which scrape the frozen mixture from the sides of the freezing cylinder and incorporate or whip air into the product. The amount of air incorporated during freezing is controlled by a pump or the dasher speed. Depending on individual conditions, freezing can be instantaneous in the continuous freezer or require approximately 10 minutes in the batch freezer.

Ice cream and other frozen desserts require no preservatives and have long shelf lives if they are kept below −23°C (−10°F) and are protected from temperature fluctuations. Airtight packaging materials have made it possible to consider frozen storage of six months or longer without loss of flavour or body and texture. When ice cream is finally dipped, composition and overrun will determine ideal scooping temperature. This can vary from "16° to "9°C (3° to 15°F), with lower temperatures resulting in less dipping loss but more effort on the part of the server.

Ice cream can also be freeze-dried by the removal of 99% of the water. Freeze-drying eliminates the need for refrigeration and provides a high-energy food for hikers and campers and a "filling" centre for candy and other confections.

Dry Milk

It is a manufactured dairy product made by evaporating milk to dryness. One purpose of drying milk is to preserve it; milk powder has a far longer shelf life than liquid milk and does not need to be refrigerated, due to its low moisture content. Another purpose is to reduce its bulk for economy of transportation.

Milk first passes into the evaporator where about one-third of its water is removed. The evaporator has a partial vacuum put on it, lowering the boiling point to about 135°F. This is important for two reasons. First, it makes it possible for the water in the milk to be evaporated at a low enough temperature that won't damage the milk. And second, it reduces costs a substantial amount. Fresh, raw milk contains about 12% solids if the butterfat is included. During the evaporation process, water in the milk is removed until the solids increase to 50%.

During the evaporation process the milk is pasteurized. The pasteurization process reduces the bacteria content without heating the milk to the point that it is damaged. In a creamery, the milk is ran through small tubes where it is heated up to the desired temperature of 175°F for just 20 seconds, then it is immediately force-cooled to prevent the milk from getting damaged.

Separating the milk: From evaporator the milk runs through the separator which removes the cream or butterfat. The butterfat is placed in a separate storage tank to be used later. The skimmed milk now moves to the tanks where standardizing takes place.

Standardizing the milk: After the milk has been separated, it is then standardized which means the different components of the milk are mixed automatically until we have a consistent product. Every batch must be exactly the same. During the standardization process, even some of the vitamins in the milk are checked to ensure that they meet our standards.

The remaining evaporated, condensed milk is turned into powdered milk. Depending on needs, standardize this milk with butterfat levels ranging from less than 1% all the way up to 30% fat. Most of the milk powders make, however, either non-fat milk or whole milk powder which contains 0% to 28.5% butterfat after it has been reconstituted. But there is a huge difference in the taste. After the condensed milk has been standardized, its next is the drying.

Whole milk powder can be stored only for six months because of the propensity of fat to oxidize. A more acceptable flavour is developed when the milk is reconstituted and chilled several hours before consumption. 1–1/3 cups of dried milk powder is needed to yield 1 quart of fluid milk.

FERMENTED MILK PRODUCTS
Butter

Butter is one of the most highly concentrated forms of fluid milk, produced through churning of pasteurized cream. Churning involves agitation that breaks fat globule membranes so the emulsion breaks, fat coalesces, and water (buttermilk) escapes. Twenty litres of whole milk are needed to produce one kilogram of butter. The original 20/80 oil-in-water emulsion of milk becomes a 20/80 water-in-oil emulsion. It may have a yellow colour due to the fat-soluble animal pigment, carotene.

Commercial butter is 80–82% milk fat, 16–17% water, and 1–2% milk solids other than fat (sometimes referred to as curd). It may contain salt, added directly to the butter in concentrations of 1 to 2%. Unsalted butter is often referred to as "sweet" butter. This should not be confused with "sweet cream" butter, which may or may not be salted. Reduced-fat, or "light," butter usually contains about 40% milk fat. The cream was often sour and needed to be neutralized (with sodium hydroxide) before churning.

Butter is produced when the cream emulsion in unhomogenized milk is destabilized by agitation, or churning. Breaking the emulsion produces butterfat granules of the size of rice grains. The granules mat together and separate from the water phase or serum, which is known as buttermilk. The butterfat is then washed with clean water and "worked" (kneaded) until more buttermilk separates and is removed. Ultimately, only about 16% of the water and milk solids present in the original milk remains trapped in the butter.

The churning process can take 40 to 60 minutes to complete in a traditional churn, but butter is more commonly made by high-speed continuous "churns" in factories. Although the basic principle is the same, in the continuous churn cream is pumped into a cylinder and mixed by high-speed blades, forming butter granules in seconds. The butter granules are forced through perforated plates while the buttermilk is drained from the system. A salt solution may be added if salted butter is desired. The butter is then worked in a twin screw extruder and emerges ready to be packaged.

Cheese

Cheese is a concentrated form of milk that contains casein, various percentages of fat, primarily saturated fat, mineral salts, and a small portion of milk serum (whey proteins, lactose, and water-soluble vitamins). The cheese-making process consists of removing a major part of the water contained in fresh fluid milk while retaining most of the solids. Since storage life increases as water content decreases, cheese making can also be considered a form of food preservation through the process of milk fermentation. The fermentation of milk into finished cheese requires several essential steps: Preparing and inoculating the milk with lactic acid producing bacteria, curdling the milk, cutting the curd, shrinking the curd (by cooking), draining or dipping the whey, salting, pressing and ripening. These steps begin with four basic ingredients: Milk, microorganisms, rennet and salt.

Inoculation and Curdling

Milk for cheese making must be of the highest quality. Because the natural microflora present in milk frequently include undesirable types called psychrophiles, good farm sanitation and pasteurization or partial heat treatment are important to the cheese-making process. In addition, the milk must be free of substances that may inhibit the growth of acid-forming bacteria (e.g. antibiotics and sanitizing agents). Milk is often pasteurized to destroy pathogenic microorganisms and to eliminate spoilage and defects induced by bacteria. However, since pasteurization destroys the natural enzymes found in milk, cheese produced from pasteurized milk ripens less rapidly and less extensively than most cheese made from raw or lightly heat-treated milk.

During pasteurization, the milk may be passed through a standardizing separator to adjust the fat-to-protein ratio of the milk. In some cases the cheese yield is improved by concentrating protein in a process known as ultra filtration. The milk is then inoculated with fermenting microorganisms and rennet, which promote curdling.

The fermenting microorganisms carry out the anaerobic conversion of lactose to lactic acid. The type of organisms used depends on the variety of cheese and on the production process. Rennet is an enzymatic preparation that is usually obtained from the fourth stomach of calves. It contains a number of proteolytic (protein-degrading) enzymes, including rennin and pepsin. Some cheeses, such as cottage cheese and cream cheese, are produced by acid coagulation alone. In the presence of lactic acid, rennet, or both, the milk protein casein clumps together and precipitates out of solution; this is the process known as curdling, or coagulation. Coagulated casein assumes a solid or gel-like structure (the curd), which traps most of the fat, bacteria, calcium, phosphate, and other particulates. The remaining liquid (the whey) contains water, proteins resistant to acidic and enzymatic denaturation (e.g. antibodies), carbohydrates (lactose), and minerals.

Lactic acid produced by the starter culture organisms has several functions. It promotes curd formation by rennet (the activity of rennet requires an acidic pH), causes the curd to shrink, enhances whey drainage (syneresis), and helps prevent the growth of undesirable microorganisms during cheese making and ripening. In addition, acid affects the elasticity of the finished curd and promotes fusion of the curd into a solid mass. Enzymes released by the bacterial cells also influence flavour development during ripening.

Salt is usually added to the curd. In addition to enhancing flavour, it helps to withdraw the whey from the curd and inhibits the growth of undesirable microorganisms.

Cutting and Shrinking

After the curd is formed, it is cut with fine wire "knives" into small cubes approximately one centimeter (one-half inch) square. The curd is then gently heated, causing it to shrink. The degree of shrinkage determines the moisture content and the final consistency of the cheese. Whey is removed by draining or dipping. The whey may be further processed to make whey cheeses (e.g. ricotta) or beverages, or it may be dried in order to preserve it as a food ingredient.

Ripening

Most cheese is ripened for varying amounts of time in order to bring about the chemical changes necessary for transforming fresh curd into a distinctive aged cheese. These changes are catalyzed by enzymes from three main sources: Rennet or other enzyme preparations of animal or vegetable origin added during coagulation, microorganisms that grow within the cheese or on its surface, and the cheese milk itself. The ripening time may be as short as one month, as for Brie, or a year or more, as in the case of sharp cheddar.

The ripening of cheese is influenced by the interaction of bacteria, enzymes, and physical conditions in the curing room. The speed of the reactions is determined by temperature and humidity conditions in the room as well as by the moisture content of the cheese. In most cheeses lactose continues to be fermented to lactic acid and lactates, or it is hydrolyzed to form other sugars. As a result, aged cheeses such as emmentaler and cheddar have no residual lactose.

In a similar manner, proteins and lipids (fats) are broken down during ripening. The degree of protein decomposition, or proteolysis, affects both the flavour, and the consistency of the final cheese.

Not all cheeses are ripened. Cottage, cream, ricotta and most mozzarella cheeses are ready for sale as soon as they are made. All these cheeses have sweet, delicate flavours and often are combined with other foods.

Curd

Curd has a better nutritive value than milk. Though there is no increase in the fat or protein content of milk during fermentation, the digestibility is better when compared to ordinary milk. Calcium and phosphorus content of curds are more easily assimilated. Curds contain more B vitamins than milk.

Milk is fermented by lactobacillus and streptococci bacteria which convert the lactic acid which is responsible for the sour taste of curd. The preparation of curd is the way of preserving the milk. During curd formation, the lactose of milk is converted into lactic acid and there is break down of protein into non-protein nitrogen.

Yogurt

The production process used to make yogurt is similar to buttermilk and sour cream, but the incubation temperature and the types of bacteria are different. The milk cuddled by a specific type of lactic acid bacillus called *Lactobacillus bulgaricus* and *Streptococcus thermophilus* and held at 40–42°C for several hours. Microorganisms in yogurt exist in a "friendly" form, known as probiotic flora. Such probiotic yogurt is able to survive destruction during gastrointestinal passage and offer health benefits such as immune stimulation, and positive balance to the GI microflora.

Lassi (Butter Milk)

When curd is churned with water and fat is removed, the residual acid buttermilk is called lassi. Curd and lassi can be prepared from whole or skimmed milk. It is consumed as beverage.

Ghee

The composition of cow and buffalo ghee is similar: 99.5% fat, mostly saturated. Ghee from cow milk is distinctly yellow. Buffalo and goat milk have no colour since they impart a little carotene to their milk. Ghee contains some fat-soluble vitamins. Vitamin D content varies with the exposure of cattle to the sunshine. Ghee contains practically no calcium, phosphorus, iron, vitamin B, or vitamin C. It contains only small quantity of essential fatty acids. Ghee contains cholesterol oxide (which is not found in butter), which is suspected to produce thickening of arteries (Atherosclerosis) leading to heart disease. Its keeping quality is high since the moisture content in ghee is low.

15

Fats and Oils

Fats and oils have been used in food preparations for many centuries. It is the most concentrated kind of energy that we consume. In spite of its high concentration, fat is used because it added richness of flavour, texture, aroma, palatability and colour to the food preparation. Oils and fats of animal and vegetable origin and many products developed from them are consumed by man. We consume fat in both visible form and invisible forms. Invisible fats are not apparent in their appearance but they are present in food in a few percentages, e.g. avocados (16%), egg-yolk (31%), almonds (58%).

Fats and oils are triglycerides, the major component of lipids. Lipids also include the phospholipids and sterols. In common usage, fats that have a relatively high melting point and are solid at room temperature. It contributes 9 kilocalories in one gram. Fats can be solid or liquid at room temperature. For example, cooking oil is a type of liquid fat. Butter is a solid fat. Some fats come from animals, others come from plants. Fat from plants is called vegetable fat. Examples of vegetable fats are margarine and vegetable oil. Examples of animal fats are butter, cream and lard.

The different types of fats are saturated, unsaturated and trans fats. Trans fats are created in the food industry by treating other types of fats and giving them a different structure. This happens when oil is hardened to make margarine, for example. Many restaurants also use trans fats for deep-frying food. Trans fats are the most unhealthy fats to eat and can cause disease. Fats are usually not soluble in water, but they can be dissolved in other organic solvents. Fats are trimesters of fatty acids and glycerol.

FUNCTIONS OF FAT

Nutritionally,

- It is a concentrated source of energy providing 9 kcal/g. Excess intake of fat gets stored in the fat cells (adipocytes) within fat tissue (adipose), whose main function is to store fat. When this storage is increased, it leads to obesity.

- Only source for fat soluble vitamins (A, D, E, K) to get carried and stored in body.
- It helps in biosynthesis of several long chain fatty acids.
- Two polyunsaturated fatty acids are essential—linoleic and linolenic acids are components of membranes of living cells.
- Fats depositing under the skin (subcutaneous fat) act as an insulator to the body.
- Deposited fat also surrounds around the vital organs like kidney, heart, etc., this helps in guarding the heart from physical shock.

In addition to their nutritional function, oils and fats add or modify flavour, aerate (leaven) batters and dough, contribute flakiness and tenderness, emulsify, transfer heat, and provide satiety. During the baking process, fat performs a multitude of chemical functions, such as tenderizing, leavening, aiding in moisture retention, and creating a flaky or crumbly texture. The products range from breads and layered doughs to cakes, biscuits (cookies), and biscuit fillings, pie-crusts, short pastry, and puff pastry. The fats used to produce this wide range of baked goods vary in their properties and particularly in their melting behaviour and plasticity.

COMPOSITION OF DIETARY FATS AND OILS

Polyunsaturated fats are liquid at room temperature and found primarily in plants. Safflower oil is 76% polyunsaturated, sunflower oil is 71%, soybean oil is 54%, and corn oil is 57% ("partially hydrogenated" oils are hydrogenated to have a greater degree of saturation).

Monounsaturated fats are liquid at room temperature and found chiefly in plants. Olive oil is 75% monounsaturated, high-oleic safflower oil is 80% (versus 76% polyunsaturated safflower oil), and canola (rapeseed oil) is 61% monounsaturated. These fats are associated with a decrease in serum cholesterol and a decreased risk of coronary heart disease.

Saturated fats are solid at room temperature and found primarily in animals, although it is found in some tropical oils. These fats are implicated in a greater rise in serum cholesterol than in dietary cholesterol.

Animal Fats

Oils and fats are essential ingredients of foods. Several animal and vegetable fats are used in food preparations. The animal fats used are butter and lard.

Butter

Butter is produced by churning cream until the fats separate from the liquid (buttermilk) and the butter is in a semi-solid state. It is used widely because of its sensory properties and the perception of added value and naturalness. The raw material for butter is milk fat, usually in the form of cream, which is separated from the milk to contain about 30–35% fat. The cream is pasteurized at a somewhat higher temperature than for pasteurizing milk since the high fat content has a slight protective effect on bacteria. Butter, with yellow colour, solid consistency, and about 80% fat content, is valued for its sweet flavour, pleasant aroma, and ability to contribute great tenderness to baked products.

It is popular for specialty breads, cookies, and pastries and is rolled into doughs from which flaky and tender pastries, such as Danish pastry and puff-paste products, are made. Because of its high cost, it is used, alone or in shortening mixtures, mainly in higher priced baked goods. It is fairly perishable, requiring storage at low temperature, and is not easily creamed (blended with sugar), producing cakes with lower volume and coarser grain than those made with more easily creamed shortenings.

Lard

Lard obtained from the fatty tissue of hogs (pigs) has solid consistency, white colour, about 98% fat content, and mild, pleasing flavour and odour considered desirable in breads, crackers, cookies (sweet biscuits), and pie-crusts. It has 43% saturated fatty acids. It lacks natural antioxidants and is therefore less stable than equally saturated vegetable oils that have been partially hydrogenated.

Lard is pig fat in both its rendered and unrendered forms. Lard was commonly used in many cuisines as a cooking fat or shortening, or as a spread similar to butter. Its use in contemporary cuisine has diminished because of its saturated-fat content. The culinary qualities of lard vary somewhat depending on the part of the pig from which the fat was taken and how the lard was processed. Lard is still commonly used to manufacture soap. Lard can be obtained from any part of the pig as long as there is a high concentration of fatty tissue

Lard may be rendered by either of the two processes: Wet or dry. In wet rendering, pig fat is boiled in water or steamed at a high temperature and the lard, which is insoluble in water, is skimmed off of the surface of the mixture, or it is separated in an industrial centrifuge. In dry rendering, the fat is exposed to high heat in a pan or oven without the presence of water. The two processes yield somewhat differing products. Wet-rendered lard has a more neutral flavour, a lighter colour, and a high smoke point. Dry-rendered lard is somewhat more browned in colour and flavour and has relatively lower smoke point.

Margarine

Margarines are emulsions containing about 80% fat, from either animal or vegetable sources, plus water, salt, emulsifiers, and sometimes milk solids. They are white to yellow in colour, with neutral or butter like flavour and solid consistency. Margarine has a high melting point, produces tender products, and is especially popular for use in puff pastes.

The basic method of making margarine today consists of emulsifying a blend of purified vegetable oils with cultured skimmed milk, chilling the mixture to solidify it and working it to improve the texture. Vegetable and animal fats are similar compounds with different melting points. Those fats that are liquid at room temperature are generally known as oils. The melting points are determined by the presence of double bonds of unsaturated acyl groups on fatty acids; the higher the number of double bonds, the lower the melting point.

Vegetable Oils

Vegetable oils, obtained from such oil-bearing seeds as corn (maize), cottonseed, peanuts, mustard, sesame, rice bran, palm nuts (coconuts), and soybeans, are 100% fat and remain liquid at fairly low temperatures. They are processed to achieve neutral to yellow colour and to eliminate odour or produce mild odour. Oils are used mainly in rolls, breads, and other fairly hard baked goods and in chiffon and other cakes in which their liquid consistency is useful.

Groundnut oil is a clear amber coloured liquid extensively used in cooking, as salad oil, making vanaspathi, peanut butter and also in making margarine. The major proteins of groundnut are arachin and conarachine but lack in lysine and methionine. It contains 40% of fat which is twice the amount of soybeans. They are rich in niacin. After the extraction of oil from groundnut, the residues are used as fodder or purified and used as supplementary mix.

Soybean oil considered as nutritionally best when compared to other oils due to its high polyunsaturated fatty acid (n-6 and n-3) composition next only to sunflower oil. It is used in vanaspathi, salad oil, mayonnaise, sandwich spreads, baby food, cake mixes and non-dairy creamers. It has 40% of protein and 20% fat. Soybean yields all essential amino acids except methionine and cystine. It is rich in lecithin and linolenic acids. The other products of soybean are soybean milk, okara, tofu, tempeh, natto, soya sauce, miso, etc. Soybean oil is the only (other than canola oil) major edible oil that contains a significant amount of linolenic acid (approx. 8%). However, the ratio of linoleate-to-linolenate in soybean oil is nearly 7:1.

Coconut oil is extracted from the dried white fleshy part of the coconut called "copra". It is the highest saturated fat vegetable oil (over 91%), oleic and linoleic acids are present to the extent of about remaining 9%. It is very stable against oxidation, and, to a lesser degree stable against hydrolysis. Coconut oil is used in cookery and in manufacturing of soaps, vanaspathi, margarine, pharmaceutical preparation, etc. after extraction of oil the cakes are used as cattle feed.

Sunflower seeds are 22% protein and contain 50% oil. For every 100 g, sunflower seeds contain 30 g of unsaturated fats and 30 mg of essential linoleic acid. Its oil is an excellent source of vitamin E than any other oil. It is rich in linoleic acid. It is a very good source of thiamin as well as of manganese, magnesium, copper, tryptophan, selenium, phosphorus, vitamin B_5 (pantothenic acid) and folate.

Mustard oil has a strong sinus-irritating aroma, a hot nutty taste, and is often used for cooking in many parts of India. The oil makes up about 30%

of the mustard seeds. It can be produced from black mustard (*Brassica nigra*), brown Indian mustard (*Brassica juncea*), and white mustard (*Brassica hirta*). It contains the pungent allyl isothiocyanate and has about 60% monounsaturated fatty acids of which 42% erucic acid and 12% oleic acid, it has 21% polyunsaturates of which 6% is the omega-3 alpha-linolenic acid and 15% is the omega-6 linoleic acid and it has 12% saturated fats.

Sesame or gingelly oil or till oil has low level of saturated fat. The components of the fats include 43% oleic acid and 43% linoleic acid, 9% palmitic acid and 4% stearic fatty acids. It contains high levels of anti-oxidants, which preserve its chemical composition. It has a long shelf life and resists becoming rancid. Storing the oil in a dark glass bottle will preserve it for longer periods.

Sesame seeds contain sesamol (3, 4-methylene-dioxyphenol), sesaminol, furyl-methanthiol, guajacol (2-methoxyphenol), phenylethanthiol and furaneol, vinylguacol and decadienal. Sesamol and sesaminol are phenolic antioxidants. Together, these compounds help stave off harmful free radicals from the body. They are very good sources of B-complex vitamins such as niacin, folic acid, thiamin (vitamin B_1), pyridoxine (vitamin B_6) and riboflavin. 100 g of sesame contains 97 mcg of folic acid, about 25% of recommended daily intake. Folic acid is essential for DNA synthesis. Essential minerals such as calcium, iron, manganese, zinc, magnesium, selenium and copper are especially concentrated in sesame seeds.

Rice bran oil is the product obtained from outer husk of the rice. It contains gamma-oryzanol which increases HDL (good) cholesterol and lowers LDL (bad) cholesterol and triglycerides. It has the ideal ratio of saturated, monounsaturated and polyunsaturated fatty acids and is the closest to WHO recommendation. Food fried in rice bran oil absorbs 15% less oil. It contains squalene which improves the health of the skin. It has natural antioxidants. It has 4 hydroxy 3 methoxy cinnamic acid which stimulates hormonal secretion and rejuvenates health. Tocopherol in it helps in nervous system and tocotrienol has anti-thrombotic and anti-cancer properties.

It does not require hydrogenation for stability and has a high percentage of fatty acids (oleic 46%, linoleic 36%, and linolenic 1%). It has a pleasant, nutty aroma and taste that complements the flavour of many foods, and its excellent cooking characteristics [It is notable for its very high smoke point of 490 °F (254 °C) (high flash point and low smoke)] make it ideal for frying and stir-frying applications. Many gourmet Asian restaurants have switched to rice bran oil for these reasons.

Canola oil is characterized by a very low level of saturated fatty acids (< 7% of total fatty acids), a relatively high level of monounsaturated fatty acids (oleic acid 58%) and an intermediate level of polyunsaturated fatty acids (32%), with a good balance between the omega-6 and omega-3 fatty acids. It contains only 7% saturated fatty acids. The most abundant fatty acid in nature is the monounsaturated fatty acid (MUFA), oleic acid. It is present in virtually all fats and oils and in some, such as olive oil and canola oil. Oleic acid makes up 58% of the total fatty acids in canola oil. Among the common vegetable oils, canola oil is second only to olive oil in oleic acid content. It contains appreciably higher levels of PUFA than palm oil or olive oil but lower levels of PUFA than corn oil, cottonseed oil, safflower oil, soybean oil and sunflower oil. Canola oil contains an appreciable amount (11%) of linolenic acid. Hence, there is a very favourable balance (approx. 2:1) between linoleic acid (omega-6 PUFA) and linolenic acid (omega-3 PUFA).

Canola oil may contain a natural toxin erucic acid and glycosinolates. Erucic acid is an omega-9 fatty acid which occurs in brassica family of plants such as rapeseed, mustard, etc. Unrefined rapeseed oil contains up to 45% erucic acid. It is always recommended to consume refined oil to avoid toxin.

Flax oil or linseed oil has 55% plant-based omega-3 but is uncommon as a table or cooking oil. Although flax seeds contain lignans, a class of phytoestrogens considered to have antioxidant and cancer-preventing properties, the extracted linseed oil does not contain the lignans found in flax seed, and therefore does not have the same antioxidant properties. Flax seed oil is easily oxidized, and rapidly becomes rancid, with an unpleasant odour. Regular flaxseed oil contains between 52% and 63% ALA (C18:3 *n*-3). The nutritional properties of flax seed differ majorly with flax seed oil.

Corn oil, corn germ contains about 85% of the total oil of the kernel. The rest is dispersed in endosperm and hull fractions and is generally utilized in feed products. Corn oil is a concentrated source of energy (like any other oil), is very digestible, provides EFA and vitamin E, and is a rich source of PUFA. Animal and human studies show that at least 97% of the oil is digested and absorbed. Corn oil is a rich source of linoleic acid, an essential fatty acid. Refined corn oil contains 99% triglyceride, with proportions of approximately 55% polyunsaturated fatty acid, 30% monounsaturated fatty acid, and 15% saturated fatty acid. Of the saturated fatty acids, 80% are palmitic acid, 14% stearic acid, and 3% arachidic acid. Over 99% of the monounsaturated fatty acids are oleic acid, 98% of the polyunsaturated fatty acids are the omega-6 linoleic acid with the 2% remainder being the omega-3 alpha-linolenic acid.

METHODS OF EXTRACTING EDIBLE OILS FROM SEEDS

There are two methods in practice for oil extraction. The residue remaining behind in the case of most edible oil industries is used as a concentrated source of protein for use in food and feeds.

1. Mechanical extraction of oil

The oil seed is dehulled or shelled to remove the outermost covering. The kernel remaining behind is boiled in water and the oily meat is hydrolyzed by subjecting it to a mechanical process incorporating steam and pressure. During the extraction process the amino acids in the protein and the sugars present combine together to cause the browning reaction. It is desirable to prevent this chemical reaction as far as possible.

2. Solvent extraction of oil

The oil bearing seeds can simply be pressed to extract the oil mechanically. However, a considerable portion of the oil which is intricately bound with the fibres in the plant tissue will remain behind, thus resulting in wastage of valuable oil. In the solvent extraction process, the fat interspersed in the tissue fibres can be dissolved in suitable solvents and flushed out. Separation of the solvent and the dissolved fat is done by distillation thus obtaining the pure fat from oil seed. Benzene, chloroform, hexane and ethyl alcohol are some of the chemicals used as solvents in extracting fat.

In the solvent extraction processing of edible oils, it is important to select a solvent that does not have any harmful effects when consumed. The usual solvent used in the extraction of fat is hexane.

This should not remain in the residue in a considerable amount, because when the oil seed cake is used as supplement in foods, it can have undesirable effects on the body.

Oil seeds are not only used as a source of edible oil but also in the preparation of protein concentrates which find wide application in the food industry.

16 Sugar and Sugar Products

Sugar has been produced in the Indian subcontinent since ancient times. It was not plentiful or cheap in early times, honey was more often used for sweetening in most parts of the world.

Sugars are simple carbohydrates that may be classified as monosaccharide or disaccharides. In food, sugar almost exclusively refers to sucrose, which primarily comes from sugarcane and sugar beet. Other sugars are used in industrial food preparation, but are usually known by more specific names—glucose, fructose or fruit sugar, high fructose corn syrup, etc (Table 16.1).

Table 16.1: Nutritional value per 100 g

Foodstuff	Energy (kcal)	Carbohydrates (g)	Calcium (g)	Phosphorus (mg)	Iron (mg)
Sugarcane	99.4	398	12	1	0.155
Jaggery	95.0	383	80	40	2.64

Sources of Sugar

Sugarcane is the chief source of sugar. Sugarcane contains 12–15% sugars. Raw canes are processed to extract the juice and the extracted juice is centrifuged to create raw sugar with its slightly brown colour. While centrifuged, molasses separate from the crystals and become a by-product of sugar production. The crystals are further refined to yield usable sugar. Roots of the beet are also less frequently used to produce sugar.

Sugar provides only energy to the body. Sugar and sugar-related products generally have low nutrient density—proportionately less protein, minerals and vitamins.

Properties of Sugar

Sensory Properties

Taste: Sweetness is generally the most recognized functional property of sugar.

Flavour: Flavours result when tastes (sweet, sour, bitter, salty) are combined with sense of smell when food is consumed. Through interaction with other ingredients, sugar is an important contributor to flavour. Depending on the food applications, sugar has the unique ability to heighten flavour or depress the perception of other flavours. For example, sugar is added to tomato-based products (e.g. barbeque, spaghetti and chilli sauces) to reduce the acidity of the tomatoes. Sugar itself also provides flavour when it is heated due to caramelization.

Texture: Sugar makes an important contribution to the way we perceive the texture of food. For example, adding sugar to ice-cream provides body and texture which is perceived as smoothness. This addition helps prevent lactose crystallization and thus reduces sugar crystal formation that otherwise causes a sandy, grainy texture that is sometimes associated with frozen dairy products.

Tenderizer: Sugar acts as an important tenderizing agent in foods such as baked products. During the mixing process, sugar competes with other ingredients for water. In bread making, for example, the affinity of sugar to bind to available water will delay the development of gluten, which is essential for maintaining a soft or tender product.

Appearance: Sugar is responsible for the yellow-brown colours that develop in baked foods. Sucrose itself develops colour through caramelization. However, the monosaccharide components of its hydrolysis (glucose and fructose) can also undergo browning reactions (Maillard reaction). For example, the reactivity of glucose upon heating contributes to the subtle orange-red colour in bread crust which is a result of this browning.

Physical Properties

Solubility: Sugar is very soluble in water. Sucrose is more soluble than glucose and less soluble than fructose. The ability to produce solutions of varying sugar concentrations is important in many food applications. A high level of solubility, for example, is essential in beverages to provide sweetness and to increase viscosity to create a desirable 'mouthfeel'.

Freezing point: Sugar is effective in lowering freezing points. Freezing point depression is an important property in ice-creams, frozen desserts and freeze-dried foods to ensure the development of fine crystal structure and product smoothness.

Boiling point: The concentration of sugar in a solution affects the boiling point by raising it. Increasing concentrations of sucrose increase the boiling point. This characteristic is important in candy manufacture as boiling point elevation allows for more sugar to be dissolved in solution, creating a 'supersaturated' and more concentrated solution. It is this specific concentration of the supersaturated sugar syrup, which is achieved at specific boiling points, which inevitably determine the candy's final consistency.

Microbial Properties

Preservation: Sugar plays a role in the preservation of many food products. The addition of sugar to jams and jellies, for example, inhibits microbial growth and subsequent spoilage. Having the ability to readily absorb water (hygroscopicity), sugar withdraws moisture from microorganisms. As a result, microorganisms become dehydrated, and cannot multiply and cause food spoilage.

The interaction between sugar and water controls the level of moisture in baked products. Sugar's high affinity for water helps to slow moisture loss in cakes and biscuits, for example, to prevent drying out and staleness, thereby extending their shelf life.

Fermentation: Sugar is extremely important in the baking and brewing industries. Yeasts use sugars as food to produce ethanol, carbon dioxide and water through the process of fermentation. In baking, sugar increases the effectiveness of yeast by providing an immediate and more utilizable source of nourishment for its growth. This hastens the leavening process, by producing more carbon dioxide which allows the dough to rise at a quicker and more consistent rate.

Chemical Properties

Antioxidant activity: Sucrose has been reported to exhibit antioxidant properties which help to prevent the deterioration of textures and flavours in canned fruits and vegetables. These effects may be partially attributed to sucrose's ability to lower water activity.

In addition, the products of the hydrolysis of sucrose (glucose and fructose) appear to have the ability to block the reactive sites of ions such as copper and iron and, to a lesser extent, cobalt. This characteristic of monosaccharide aids in food preservation by impeding catalytic oxidation reactions.

Furthermore, Maillard reaction products are known to have antioxidant properties in food systems. For this reason, some mixtures of Maillard reaction products have been employed in the food industry as food additives for biscuits, cookies and sausages.

Caramelization: It is a nonenzymatic browning reaction that results from the action of heat on sugars. At high temperatures [338°F(170°C)], it dehydrates and decomposes. The sugar ring (either pyranose or furanose) opens and loss water. The sugar becomes brown; more concentrated, and develops a caramel flavour as it continues to increase in temperature.

Maillard reaction: It results from chemical interactions between sugars and proteins at high heat. It involves the reaction of the carbonyl group of sugar with the amine group of an amino acid and occurs with heat, a high pH, and low moisture. This is responsible for the brown colour in a variety of foods.

Sugar-related Products

Molasses: To make molasses, the sugarcane plant is harvested and stripped of its leaves. Its juice is extracted from the canes, usually by crushing or mashing. The juice is boiled to concentrate it, which promotes the crystallization of the sugar. The result of this first boiling of the sugar crystals is first molasses, which has the highest sugar content because comparatively a little sugar has been extracted from the source. Second molasses is created from a second boiling and sugar extraction, and has a slight bitter tinge to its taste.

The third boiling of the sugar syrup makes blackstrap molasses. The majority of sucrose from the original juice has been crystallized and removed. The calorie content of blackstrap molasses is still mostly from the small remaining sugar content. However, unlike refined sugars, it contains trace amounts of vitamins and significant amounts of several minerals. Blackstrap molasses is a source of calcium, magnesium, potassium, and iron; one tablespoon provides up to 20% of the daily value of each of those nutrients. Blackstrap is used in the manufacture of ethyl alcohol for industry and as an ingredient in cattle feed. Generally molasses is used for edible purposes and in manufacture of confectionery.

Cane syrup: Cane syrup is similar to molasses and is obtained by simply boiling sugarcane juice to a syrup consistency. The term "liquid sugar" is used for commercial products, such as a solution of sucrose and solutions containing varying proportions of invert sugar. They are made from raw sugar and their composition varies from pure sucrose to full invert sugar.

Corn syrup: Corn syrup is prepared by hydrolyzing corn starch with hydrochloric or sulphuric acid with heat and pressure. The syrup is a mixture of glucose, maltose and dextrin. The principal element in composition of the syrup is the sugar and is present to the extent of hydrolysis. Glucose is the principal sugar and is present to the extent of 35%. The dextrin content varies from 30% to 35%. The presence of dextrin makes the syrup inhibit crystallization to be controlled. It may also be prepared by the enzymic hydrolysis of starch.

Artificial Sweeteners

A sugar substitute is a food additive that duplicates the effect of sugar in taste, usually with less food energy. Some sugar substitutes are natural and some are synthetic. Those that are not natural are, in general, called artificial sweeteners.

An ideal sweetener, as sweet as or sweetener than sucrose, has a pleasant taste, with no after taste, is colourless, odourless readily soluble, stable, functional and economically feasible.

It is also nontoxic, does not promote dental cavities and is either metabolized normally or excreted from the body a changed without contributing to any metabolic abnormalities. They reduce the cost and improve the product taste and stability.

Artificial sweeteners are available in many categories, they are as follows.

Low Caloric Sweeteners

The majority of sugar substitutes approved for food use are artificially-synthesized compounds. However, some bulk natural sugar substitutes are known, including sorbitol and xylitol, which are found in berries, fruit, vegetables, and mushrooms. It is not commercially viable to extract these products from fruits and vegetables, so they are produced by catalytic hydrogenation of the appropriate reducing sugar. For example, xylose is converted to xylitol, lactose to lactitol, and glucose to sorbitol.

Polyols

Some non-sugar sweeteners are polyols, also known as "sugar alcohols." Polyols are caloric, chemically reduced carbohydrates that provide sweetness to foods. The sugar alcohols are similar in chemical structure to glucose, but an alcohol group replaces the aldehyde group of glucose. Sorbitol is commercially produced from glucose and contains 2.6 cal/g while mannitol contains 1.6 cal/g. Both of these naturally occurring sugar alcohols provide half the sweetness of sucrose and may be used as humectants because they increase the water-holding capacity of the food.

Sorbitol is also used as a bulking agent. In combination with aspartame and saccharin, it provides the volume, texture, and thick consistency of sugar. Xylitol, isomalt, hydrogenated starch hydrolysate (HSH), and hydrogenated glucose syrup (HGS) are also sugar alcohols.

The body does not metabolize sugar alcohols and, when consumed, these sugars do not require insulin, therefore, diabetic patients may use sugar alcohols sparingly.

Non-caloric Sweeteners

Acesulfame Potassium

It is a calorie-free artificial sweetener, also known as *Acesulfame K*. It is a synthetic derivative of acetoacetic acid that received FDA approval in 1988. It is a white crystalline powder with molecular formula $C_4H_4KNO_4S$. Acesulfame K is 180–200 times sweeter than sucrose (table sugar). Like saccharin, it has a slightly bitter aftertaste, especially at high concentrations. Acesulfame K is often blended with other sweeteners (usually sucralose or aspartame). These blends are reputed to give a more sugar-like taste, whereby each sweetener masks the other's aftertaste, and/or exhibits a synergistic effect by which the blend is sweeter than its components. Acesulfame K is stable under heat, even under moderately acidic or basic conditions, allowing it to be used in baking, or in products that require a long shelf life. In carbonated drinks, it is almost always used in conjunction with another sweetener, such as aspartame or sucralose. It is also used as a sweetener in protein shakes and pharmaceutical products, especially chewable and liquid medications, where it can make the active ingredients more palatable.

Alitame

It is an artificial sweetener developed by Pfizer in the early 1980s and currently marketed in some countries under the brand name **Aclame**. Like aspartame, alitame is an aspartic acid-containing dipeptide. It is about 2000 times sweeter than sucrose. Alitame does not contain phenylalanine, and can therefore be used by people with phenylketonuria.

Aspartame

It is an artificial, non-saccharide sweetener used as a sugar substitute in some foods and beverages. Aspartame is a methyl ester comprising two amino acids—aspartic acid and phenylalanine; thus it should not be consumed by those with genetic disease phenylketonuria because it contains phenylalanine, which is not metabolized. Under strongly acidic or alkaline conditions, aspartame may generate methanol by hydrolysis. Under more severe conditions, the peptide bonds are also hydrolyzed, resulting in the free amino acids is approximately 200 times sweeter than sucrose. Due to this property, even though aspartame produces four kilocalories of energy per gram when metabolized, the quantity of aspartame needed to produce a sweet taste is so small that its caloric contribution is negligible. According to the joint committee of FAO/WHO, allowed daily intake of aspartame is 40 mg/kg body weight.

Cyclamate

It is 30 times sweeter than sugar, making it the least potent of the commercially used artificial sweeteners. Some people find it to have an unpleasant aftertaste, but, in general, less than saccharin or Acesulfame potassium. It is often used synergistically with other artificial sweeteners, especially saccharin; the mixture of 10 parts cyclamate to 1 part saccharin is common and masks the off-tastes of both sweeteners. It is less expensive than most sweeteners, including sucralose, and is stable under heating. Cyclamate is the sodium or calcium salt of cyclamic acid (cyclohexanesulfamic acid), which itself is prepared by the sulfonation of cyclohexylamine.

Controversy developed when, in 1966, a study reported that some intestinal bacteria could desulfonate cyclamate to produce cyclohexylamine, a compound suspected to have some chronic toxicity in animals. Further research resulted in a 1969 study that found the common 10:1 cyclamate:saccharin mixture to increase the incidence of bladder cancer in rats, so it was banned.

Saccharin

In this basic substance, benzoic sulfilimine, has effectively no food energy and is 300–700 times sweeter than sucrose, but has a bitter or metallic aftertaste, especially at high concentrations. It is used to sweeten products such as drinks, candies, biscuits, medicines and toothpaste.

Saccharin is unstable when heated but it does not react chemically with other food ingredients. As such, it stores well. According to the joint committee of FAO/WHO allowed daily intake (ADI) of saccharin is 0–2.5 mg/kg of body weight. Calcium or sodium saccharin, combined with dextrose and an anticaking agent may be used in tabletop sweeteners.

Sucralose

The majority of ingested sucralose is not broken down by the body and therefore it is non-caloric. Sucralose is approximately 600 times as sweet as sucrose, twice as sweet as saccharin. It is stable under heat and over a broad range of pH conditions. Therefore, it can be used in baking or in products that require a longer shelf life. It is a noncaloric trichloro derivative of sucrose [three hydroxyl (hydrogen–oxygen) groups on a sugar molecule are selectively replaced by three atoms chlorine], plus maltodextrin, which gives it bulk.

Natural Sugar Substitutes

Glycyrrhizin: It is the main sweet-tasting compound from liquorice root. It is 30–50 times as sweet as sucrose. Pure glycyrrhizin is odourless.

In chemical terms, glycyrrhizin is a triterpenoid saponin glycoside of glycyrrhizic (or glycyrrhizinic) acid. Upon hydrolysis, the glycoside loses its sweet taste and is converted to the aglycone glycyrrhetinic acid plus two molecules of glucuronic acid. The acid form is not particularly water-soluble, but its ammonium salt is soluble in water at pH greater than 4.5.

Thaumatin: It is a low-calorie sweetener and flavour modifier. The substance, a natural protein, is often used primarily for its flavour-modifying properties and not exclusively as a sweetener.

The thaumatins were first found as a mixture of proteins isolated from the katemfe fruit (*Thaumatococcus daniellii* Bennett) of west Africa. Some of the proteins in the thaumatin family are natural sweeteners roughly 2000 times more potent than sugar. Although very sweet, thaumatin's taste is markedly different from sugars. The sweetness of thaumatin builds very slowly. Perception lasts a long time, leaving a liquorice-like aftertaste at high usage levels. Thaumatin is highly water soluble, stable to heating, and stable under acidic conditions.

17

Spices

A spice is a dried seed, fruit, root, bark, or vegetative substance used in nutritionally insignificant quantities as a food additive for flavour, colour, or as a preservative that kills harmful bacteria or prevents their growth. It may be used to flavour a dish or to hide other flavours. Spices were among the most demanded and expensive products available in Europe in the Middle Ages, the most common being black pepper, cinnamon, cumin, nutmeg, ginger and cloves.

Some spices come in the form of seeds such as aniseed, caraway, celery, coriander, etc. Some are in the form of leaves, e.g. basil leaves, chervil, curry leaves, thyme leaves, mint, parsley, etc. Some are in flowers form, e.g. saffron, some in fruits form, e.g. cardamom, kokam, mace and nutmeg, star anise, tamarind, etc., some in roots form, e.g. galangal, garlic, ginger, onion, stone leek, lovage. Some spices constitute the bark of a plant, e.g. cassia, cinnamon, etc.

Below are the few spices which are commonly used for ages:

Ajowan

Botanical Name: *Trachyspermum ammi*
Syn: Carum Copticum Heirn
Family: Umbelliferae
English Name: Bishop's Weed

Indian names are as follows:
Hindi: Ajowan; Bengali: Jowan or Joan; Gujarati: Yavan; Kashmiri: Jawind; Kannada: Oma; Malayalam: Omum; Marathi: Onva; Oriya: Juani; Urdu: Ajowain; Sanskrit: Ajamoda Yavanika; Tamil: Omum; Telugu: Vamu. Ajowan seeds, are more known as adjuncts used in small quantities for flavouring numerous foods, as anti-oxidants, as preservatives, or in medicine or for the manufacture of essential oils for ultimate use in perfumery, essences and medicines, etc. The physicochemical composition is as follows:

Moisture: 8.9%
Protein: 15.4%

Fat [ether extract]: 18.1%
Crude fibre: 11.9%
Carbohydrates: 38.6%
Mineral matter [total ash]: 7.1%
Calcium: 1.42%
Phosphorus: 0.30%
Iron: 14.6 mg/100 g
Calorific value: 379/100 g

Bishop's weed can be used in a wide variety of food items. It possesses preservative and medicinal properties. In India it is used with pulses, meat and liver. Bishop's seed is rich in calcium and iron and is used to enhance digestion. It is an anthelmintic and antiseptic. Bishop's weed oil is used for treating cholera, stomach pains, diarrhea and indigestion.

Steam distillation of crushed seeds yields 2.5 to 4.0% essential oil which is valued considerably in medicine on account of the presence of thymol therein. Oil of ajowan is much valued in medicine, as it has nearly all the properties ascribed to the ajowan seeds. This was used in surgery as an antiseptic and was also found to be of great value in the treatment of hookworm disease. The aqueous solution of thymol is an excellent mouthwash and thymol is a constituent of many toothpastes. Extracts of seeds in 70% and 40% alcohol are toxic to *Staphylococci* and *E.coli*.

Aniseed

Botanical Name: *Pimpinella anisum*
Family: Umbellifereae
Syn: Nisum vulgare Gaertner

Indian names are as follows:

Hindi: Valaiti Saunf or Aawonf; Bengali: Muhuri; Gujarati: Anisi or Sowa; Kannada: Sompu; Malayalam: Shombu; Marathi: Somp; Oriya: Sop; Punjabi: Valaiti Sounf; Sanskrit: Shetapuspa; Tamil: Chombu; Telugu: Kuppi Sopu.

Aniseed is ground-gray to grayish-brown in colour, 3.2 to 4.8 mm in length, oval in shape and with a short stalk [pedicel] attached. Five longitudinal ridges are available on each pericarp. It has a characteristic agreeable odour and a pleasant aromatic taste.

The chemical composition of aniseed varies with the origin of the fruits; the reported ranges of values are:

Moisture: 9 to 13%
Protein: 18%
Fatty oil: 8 to 23%
Essential oil: 2 to 7%
Sugar: 3.5%
Starch: 5%
N-free extract: 22 to 28%

Crude fibre: 12 to 25%
Ash: 6 to 10%
Choline is also present.

Aniseed, on steam distillation, yields an essential oil, known as 'Oil of Anise', which has now replaced the fruits for medicinal and flavouring purposes. Anise oil is a colourless or pale-yellow liquid having the characteristic odour and taste of the fruit.

The yield of oil generally varies from 1.9 to 3.1%. Higher values up to 6% have been reported from Syrian aniseed. The chief constituent of aniseed oil is anethole, which is present to the extent of 80 to 90% and is mainly responsible for the characteristic flavour of the oil. The oil also contains methyl chavicol, p-methoxyphenyl acetone, and small amount of terpenes and sulfur containing compounds of disagreeable odour.

- Aniseed possesses a sweet, aromatic taste and emits, when crushed, a characteristic agreeable odour and is used for flavouring food, confectionary, bakery products, beverages, anisette and other liquors.
- The fruit is considered mild expectorant and is used as an antiseptic, and for treatment of cholera.
- It is also stimulating, carminative, diuretic and diaphoretic and is used in flatulent colic, in the preparation of asthma powders due to its expectorant properties and also in veterinary medicine.
- It may be used for preparation of gripe water.
- Aniseed is esteemed in medicine for its properties to relieve flatulence.
- It helps to remove catarrhal matter and phlegm from the bronchial tube.
- The seed also induces perspiration and increases the volume and discharge of urine thus helping the body detoxify.
- Alcoholic extract of aniseed possesses fungicidal activity.
- Aniseed can be externally used as an insecticide against small insects such as head lice, mites and vermin.

Caraway

Botanical Name: *Carum carvi*
Family Name: Umbellife

Indian names are as follows:
Hindi: Shia Jira, Siya Zira; Bengali: Sada Jira or Sa-Zira; Kannada: Shime Jeerige; Kashmiri: Gunyun; Malayalam: Shima Jirakam; Marathi: Wilayati Zirah; Punjabi: Zira-siah; Sanskrit: Sushavi; Sindhi: Kalu daru; Tamil: Shimai Shembu; Telugu: Sima Jirakaia.

The caraway plant usually has a fleshy root and a slender branched stem that attains a height of 0.5 to 0.6 m; the compound, pinnate leaves are divided into very narrow segments; the small white flowers are borne in flat compound umbels; the fruit when ripe, splits into narrow, elongated carpels 4 to 6.5 mm long, curved, pointed at the ends, and with five longitudinal ridges on the surface. This spice thrives in temperate climate and prefers moderately light clay soil that is well tilled and rich in humus. The dried fruit or seed is brown in colour, has a pleasant odour, aromatic flavour, warm and somewhat sharp taste. Seeds are hard sharp to the touch. They are free from stalk ends. The seeds, on steam distillation, yield an aromatic essential oil (4 to 6%), which finds greater use in medicines than the seeds as such.

In India, the fruits are collected before ripening. Well-ripened fruits may also be reaped in the early mornings when the plants are bathed in dew; otherwise many seeds fall during harvesting itself. The plants are dried and the fruits threshed out, cleaned and stored in bags. The yield is variable. Caraway seed has the following composition:

Moisture: 4.5%

Protein: 7.6%

Fat: 8.8%

Fibre: 25.2%

Carbohydrates: 50.2%

Total ash: 3.7%

Calcium: 1.0%

Phosphorus: 0.11%

Sodium: 0.02%

Potassium: 1.9%

Iron: 0.09%

Vitamin B_1 (thiamine): 0.38 mg/100 g

Vitamin B_2 (riboflavin): 0.38 mg/100 g

Niacin: 8.1 mg/100 g

Vitamin C (ascorbic acid): 12.0 mg/100 g

Vitamin A: 580 I.U

Calorific value (food energy): 465 per 100 g of spice.

Caraway oil, distilled from fresh seeds, is colourless or pale yellow oil. Carvone content of oil is 45 to 65%. The volatile oil contains a mixture of ketone and carvone; a terpene formerly called carvene but now recognized to be dl-limonene and traces of carvacrol. Pure carvone is prepared by decomposing the crystalline compound of carvone with hydrogen sulfide.

- Caraway is widely used as a spice for culinary purposes and for flavouring bread, biscuits, cakes and cheese.
- Used in the manufacture of 'Kummel'.
- As an ingredient of sausage seasoning and pickling spice.
- It is a mild stomachic and carminative, occasionally used in flatulent colic.
- Carvone isolated from caraway oil is used as anthelmintic in hookworm disease.
- Caraway oil is used chiefly for flavouring purposes and in medicine

as a carminative. It is also used to correct the nauseating and griping effects of medicines.

- Caraway seed oil is used in oral preparations for overcoming an unpleasant odour or taste.
- Decarvonised oil consists of limonene with traces of carvone and it is used for scenting soaps.

Celery Seeds

Botanical Name: *Apium graveolens*
Family: Umbelliferae
Indian names are as follows:
Hindi: Shalari, Ajmud; Bengali: Bandhuri, Chanu; Gujarati:Bodiajmoda; Marathi: Ajmoda; Punjabi: Kernauli; Sanskrit: Ajamoda; Tamil: Ajmada. Celery seed is the dried ripe fruit, usually 60 to 180 cm high, erect, with conspicuously jointed stems bearing well-developed leaves on long expanded petioles. The rigid fruit is small, 1 to 1.5 mm long and 1 mm in diameter, contains a small seed, united or separated, some pericarp with stalk ends, brown in colour and somewhat bitter in taste. The pericarp is intercepted with oil ducts. It is widely used as a spice.
Average composition of the seed is as follows:

Moisture: 5.1%
Protein: 18.1%
Fat (ether extract): 22.8%
Crude fibre: 2.9%
Carbohydrates: 40.9%
Total ash: 10.2%
Calcium: 1.8%
Phosphorus: 0.55%
Iron: 0.45%
Sodium: 0.17%
Potassium: 1.4%
Vitamin B_1 (thiamine): 0.42 mg/100 g
Vitamin B_2 (riboflavin): 0.49 mg/100 g
Niacin: 4.4 mg/100 g
Vitamin C (ascorbic acid): 17.2 mg/100 g
Vitamin A: 650 I.U
Calorific value: 450 calories/100 g

The celery fruit (or seed) yields 2 to 3% of a pale yellow volatile oil with a persistent odour. In trade, this is known as celery seed oil and is much valued both as a fixative and as an ingredient of novel perfume. The principal constituents are: d-limonene (60%), d-selinene (10%), sedanonic acid anhydride (0.5%) and sedanolide (2.5 to 3%). The last two are responsible for aroma of the oil.

Oleoresin of celery seed is prepared by extracting the crushed dried celery seeds with suitable volatile solvents, filtration and desolventisation under vacuum. The oleoresin not only possesses the volatile top note of the essential oil, but also the 'body', i.e. the fixed or non-volatile extractive matter of the celery used. Oleoresin could rightly be considered as 'liquid celery seed', which is easier to handle in the preparation of tinctures and extracts.

- The dried ripe fruits (celery seeds) are used as spice. Leaves and stalks are used as salads in soups and as a pre-dinner appetizer.
- They are used in asthma and for liver diseases.
- This is used as an anti-spasmodic and nerve stimulant.
- It has been successfully employed in rheumatoid arthritis and probably acts as an intestinal antiseptic.
- The root is considered alternative and diuretic and is given in anasarca (massive edema) and colic.

Coriander

Botanical name: *Coriandrum sativum*

Family name: Umbelliferae

Indian names are as follows:

Hindi: Dhania; Bengali: Dhane; Gujarati: Kothmiri, Libdhana; Kannada: Kothambri; Kashmiri: Daaniwal, Kothambalari; Malayalam: Kothumpalari bija; Marathi: Dhana; Oriya: Dhania; Punjabi: Dhania; Sanskrit: Dhanyaka; Tamil: Kothamalli; Telugu: Dhaniyalu.

The composition of coriander seeds varies, depending upon its country of origin and the agro climatic conditions under which grown, harvested, dried and stored. The following typical analysis gives a fair idea of its composition:

Moisture: 6.3%
Protein: 1.3%
Volatile oil: 0.3%
Non-volatile ether extract: 22%
Total ether extract (fat): 19.6%
Crude fibre: 31.5%
Carbohydrates: 24.0%
Total ash: 5.3%
Calcium: 0.08%
Phosphorus: 0.44%
Sodium: 0.02%
Potassium: 1.2%
Vitamin B_1: 0.26 mg/100 g
Vitamin B_2: 0.23 mg/100 g
Niacin: 3.2 mg/100 g
Vitamin C (ascorbic acid): 12.0 mg/100 g
Vitamin A: 175 I.U./100 g

Coriander seed contains volatile oil, fixed oil, tannins, cellulose, pentosans and pigments.

Coriander fresh leaves have the following composition:

Moisture: 87.9%
Protein: 3.3%
Carbohydrates: 6.5%
Total ash: 1.7%
Calcium: 0.14%
Phosphorus: 0.06%
Iron: 0.01%
Vitamin B$_2$: 60 mg/100 g
Niacin: 0.8 mg/100 g
Vitamin C (ascorbic acid): 135 mg/100 g
Vitamin A: 10, 460 I.U./100 g

The aromatic odour and taste of coriander fruits (seeds) is due to an essential oil. The amount of oil varies considerably according to the source of the fruits. The volatile oil is made up of hydrocarbons and oxygenated compounds. The hydrocarbon accounts for about 20% of the essential oil. The major oxygenated compounds present are: d-linalool or coriandrol (45 to 70%). The entire plant and unripe fruit also yield essential oil. The good quality oleoresin can be extracted from coriander seeds.

- All parts of the coriander plant, that is, tender stem, the leaves, flowers and the fruits have a pleasant aromatic odour.
- The coriander leaves also constitute one of the richest sources of vitamins C and A.
- Its use as a condiment in curries and particularly as fresh leaves for garnishing of curries and other dishes, and in chutney, as an appetizer is well known.
- The oleoresin is used for flavouring beverages, pickles, sweets and other delicacies.
- Coriander seeds are considered to be carminative, diuretic, stomachic, antibilious, refrigerant and aphrodisiac.
- Alcoholic extracts as mother tincture of this herb is popular among homeopaths.

Cumin

Botanical name: *Cuminum cyminum*

Family name: Umbelliferae

Indian names are as follows:

Hindi: Jira, Safaid Jeera, Zeera; Bengali: Jeere; Punjabi: Jira, Safaid Jeera; Gujarati: Jeeru; Kannada: Jeerige; Kashmiri: Zyur; Malayalam: Jeerakam; Marathi: Jeregire; Oriya: Jeera; Sanskrit: Jiraka, Jeera; Sindhi: Zero; Tamil: Ziragum; Telugu: Jidakara, Jikaka.

Cumin comprises the dried yellowish to grayish brown seeds of a small slender annual herb of the coriander family. It grows to the height of 30 to 45 cm and produces a stem with many branches bearing long, finely divided, deep green leaves and small flowers, white or rose in colour, borne in umbels. The aromatic seed-like fruit is elongated, oval, approximately 6 mm long and light yellowish brown in colour.

The physicochemical composition of cumin seeds is as follows:

Moisture: 6.2%

Protein: 17.7%

Fat: 23.8%

Crude fibre: 9.1%

Carbohydrates: 35.5%

Total ash: 7.7%

Calcium: 0.9%

Phosphorus: 0.45%

Iron: 0.48%

Sodium: 0.16%

Potassium: 2.1%

Vitamin B_1: 0.73 mg/100 g

Vitamin B_2: 0.38 mg/100g

Niacin: 2.5 mg/100 g

Vitamin C: 17.2 mg/100 g

Vitamin A: 175 I.U./100 g

Calorific value: 460 calories/100 g

The seed yield volatile oil on an average is 3.1%.

The dried fruit is crushed and soon thereafter, it is steam distilled to yield 2.5 to 4.5% of valuable volatile oil, colourless or pale yellow, turning dark on keeping. The chief constituent of the oil is cuminaldehyde (20 to 40%). In addition to volatile oil, the seed also contains about 10% fixed (non-volatile) greenish brown oil with a strong aromatic flavour.

- Cumin seeds are largely used as condiment and form an essential ingredient in all mixed spices and curry powders for flavouring soups, pickles, curries, and for seasoning breads, cakes, etc.
- Aqueous extract of cumin seed is frequently used for removing intestinal worms.
- The seeds have been considered as stimulant, carminative, stomachic, astringent and useful in diarrhea and dyspepsia.
- Cuminaldehyde is used in perfumery.
- The oil cake is used as good cattle fodder.
- The flowers yield sufficient nectar, thus can assure us with tasty honey. Cumin honey is viscous, contains higher quantity of iron and unsaturated sugar. It also has attractive aroma.

Fennel

Botanical name: *Foeniculum vulgare*
Family name: Umbelliferae
Indian names are as follows:
Hindi: Saunf, Sonp; Bengali: Mauri, PanMuhuri; Gujarati:Variari; Kannada: Badi-sopu; Malayalam: Perum-jeerakam; Marathi: Badi-shep; Punjabi: Saunf; Sanskrit: Madhurika; Tamil: Shombei; Telugu: Sopu, Pedda-jilakara.
The plant is a biennial or perennial, aromatic, stout, glabrous herb, 1.5 to 1.8 m high, cultivated in Mediterranean countries, Rumania and India. The seed (or the fruit) is small, oblong, ellipsoidal or cylindrical, 6 to 7 mm long, straight or slightly curved, and of greenish yellow or yellowish brown colour; Mesco carp is 5-ridged; it possesses an agreeable, sweet aroma resembling aniseed.
In India, fennel is classified for trade purposes according to their place of origin. Some of the well-known types are Bombay, Bihar and U.P fennels; seeds from Lucknow are considered to be the best and are priced higher than those from other areas.
The composition of fennel seed is given below:

Moisture: 6.30%
Protein: 9.5%
Fat: 10%
Crude fibre: 18.5%
Carbohydrates: 42.3%
Total ash: 13.4%
Calcium: 1.3%
Phosphorus: 0.48%
Iron: 0.01%
Sodium: 0.09%
Potassium: 1.7%
Vitamin B_1: 9.41 mg/100 g.
Vitamin B_2: 0.36 mg/100 g
Niacin: 6.0 mg/100 g.
Vitamin C (ascorbic acid): 12.0 mg/100 g
Vitamin A: 1040 I.U./100 g
Calorific value: 370 calories/100 g

On steam distillation of crushed fennel seed, 0.7 to 6.0% volatile oil is obtained. The essential oil of fennel seed is a colourless or pale yellow liquid with a characteristic taste and odour. Two types of oil are recognized in commerce — sweet fennel oil from the fruits of var dulce and bitter fennel oil from the fruits of var vulgare. The taste and odour of sweet fennel oil are superior to those of bitter oil. Indian fennel oil contains over 70% anethole and 6% fenchone. It possesses a sweet taste. The main constituent of the oil from the fruits of cultivated Foeniculum vulgare is anethole. Oils of good quality contain 50 to 70% anethole.

The oil of sweet fennel fruits contains anethole, d-phellandrene and d-limonene. The high percentage of anethole (up to 90%) and the absence of fenchone are responsible for its delicate sweet odour and flavour. Oil from wild variety does not have any commercial importance.

Fennel seeds also contain 9.0 to 13% fixed oil. The components of fatty acids of the oil are:

Palmitic: 4%, Oleic: 22%, Linoleic: 14%, Petroselinic: 60%.

- The plant is pleasantly aromatic and is used as a potherb. The leaves are used in fish sauce and for garnishing; leaf stalks are used in salad. They are used for flavouring soups, meat dishes, sauces, liquors, pickles, and bakery products.
- Dried fruits of fennel have a fragrant odour and a pleasant aromatic taste.
- In India and neighbouring countries, they are used as a masticatory or for chewing alone or with betel leaves.
- The leaves have diuretic properties. The roots are regarded as purgative; they have an aromatic odour and taste. The fruits are aromatic, stimulant and carminative.
- They are official in the pharmacopoeias and are considered useful in diseases of the chest, spleen and kidney.
- Fennel has been found to stimulate appetite, and to aid digestion.
- Fennel is one of the safest herb for colic.
- Fennel is also believed to be beneficial for kidney stones, menopausal problems, nausea, obesity and increasing milk yield during breast feeding.

Fenugreek

Botanical name: *Trigonella foenum-graecum*
Family: Leguminosae

Indian names are as follows:

Hindi, Bengali, Gujarati, Marathi, Oriya, Punjabi, Sanskrit, Urdu: Methi; Kannada: Menthya; Malayalam:Ventayan, Uluva; Tamil: Vendayam; Telugu: Menthulu.

The plant is grown as a green leafy vegetable and for its seeds. Both plant and the seeds are considered medicinal.

The robust herb has light green leaves, is 30 to 60 cm tall, and produces slender beaked pods 10 to 15 cm long. Each pod contains 10 to 20 small hard yellowish brown seeds, which are smooth and oblong, about 3 mm long; each is grooved across one corner, giving it a hooked appearance. The composition of seed on an average is given below:

Moisture: 6.3%
Protein: 9.5%
Fat: 10.0%
Fibre: 18.5%
Carbohydrates: 42.3%

Total ash: 13.4%

Calcium: 1.3%

Phosphorus: 0.48%

Iron: 0.011%

Sodium: 0.09%

Potassium: 1.7%

Vitamin B_1: 0.41 mg/100 g

Vitamin B_2: 0.36 mg/100 g

Niacin: 6.0 mg/100 g

Vitamin C: 12.0 mg/100 g

Vitamin A: 1040 I.U./100 g

Calorific value: 370 calories/100 g

Gums: 23.06%

Mucilage: 28.00%.

Fenugreek seed contains many substances such as protein, starch, sugars, mucilage, mineral matters, volatile oil, fixed oil, vitamins and enzymes. Seeds are rich in essential amino acids. Fenugreek leaves and stems are also rich in calcium, iron, vitamin A and vitamin C (ascorbic acid). Although fresh leaves contain only 3 to 5% protein, on dry basis, they are comparable to pulses.

The fixed oil content of the seed is about 7%. The fatty acids consist largely of oleic, linoleic and linolenic. The volatile oil content of fenugreek is less than 0.02%.

- Fenugreek stimulates the digestive process as well as the metabolism in general.
- The seeds are used in colic flatulence, dysentery, dyspepsia with loss of appetite, diarrhea, chronic cough, dropsy, enlargement of liver and spleen, rickets, gout and diabetes.
- The seeds are used as carminative, aphrodisiac; infusion is given to small pox patients as a cooling drink.
- The seeds of fenugreek made in gruel, given to nursing mothers, increase the flow of milk.
- During the early stages of any of the respiratory tract infections such as bronchitis, influenza, sinusitis, catarrh and suspected pneumonia, fenugreek helps to perspire, dispels toxicity and shortens gestation period of fever.
- Fenugreek has a soothing effect on the inflamed stomach and intestines.
- It cleans the stomach, bowls and kidneys.
- It helps healing peptic ulcers by providing coating of mucilaginous matter.
- Fenugreek is used to lower blood sugar levels. An infusion of the fenugreek leaves is used as a gargle for recurrent mouth ulcers.
- When used externally, fenugreek has a soothing effect on the skin.

Mustard

Botanical names: *Brassica nigra*
Family names: Crucifereae
English names: True mustard or black mustard, white mustard, India mustard or brown mustard.

Indian names are as follows:
Hindi, Punjabi and Urdu: Banarasi Rai, Rai, Safed Rai, Kalee Sarson; Bengali: Sarisha; Assamese: Soriha; Gujarati: Rai; Kannada: Sasave; Kashmiri: Aasur, Sorisa; Sanskrit: Asuri, Bimbata; Tamil: Kadugu; Telugu: Avalu; Oriya: Soriso.

In India, mustard is known both as oilseed and spice. Internationally, however, it is more popular as a spice. The seeds yield 23 to 33% of the fixed oil. The volatile oil of mustard is obtained in a yield of 0.7 to 1.2% after the hydrolysis of the glucoside sinigrin, by the enzyme myrosin. For the preparation of volatile oil, the fixed oil is first expressed from the seeds, which are subsequently macerated with tepid warm water for several hours, and steam distilled.

In India seeds of black mustard are used in pickles and curries.
The seeds contain:

Moisture: 6.2%
Fat: 35.5%
Nitrogenous matter: 24.6%
Fibre: 8%
Ash: 5.3%.

The oil content of the seeds is usually 30 to 38%. There are also a number of hybrid mustards introduced and grown in India, which have commercial values for various reasons. Some are known for higher oil yield while some others are known for appropriate pungency for which they are popular as spice or as ground mustard.

Three related species of mustard are grown for their seeds:
White Mustard (*Brassica alba* or *Brassica hirta*) is a round hard seed, beige or straw coloured. Its light outer skin is removed before sale. With its milder flavour and good preservative qualities, this is the one that is most commonly used in pickling.

Black Mustard (*Brassica nigra*) is a round hard seed, varying in colour from dark brown to black, smaller and much more pungent than the white.

Brown Mustard (*Brassica juncea*) is similar in size to the black variety and varies in colour from light to dark brown. It is more pungent than the white, less than the black.

- The oil contained in the mustard seed is edible and it is also used in making pharmaceutical products, soap, leather and wool articles.
- Whole white mustard seed is used in pickling spice and in spice mixtures for cooking meats and seafood. It adds piquancy to sauerkraut and is sometimes used in marinades.

- In India, whole seeds are fried in ghee/oil until the seed pops, producing a milder nutty flavour that is useful as a garnish or seasoning for other dishes.
- Mustard oil is made from B. juncea, providing piquant oil widely used in India in the same way as ghee and other oil.
- Powdered mustard acts as an emulsifier in the preparation of mayonnaise and salad dressings.
- Although the volatile oil of mustard is a powerful irritant capable of blistering skin, in dilution as a liniment or poultice it soothes, creating a warm sensation.
- Over the years mustard has been prescribed for scorpion stings and snake bites, epilepsy, toothache, bruises, stiff neck, rheumatism, colic and respiratory troubles.
- It is a strong emetic (used to induce vomiting) and rubefacient (an irritant) that draw the blood to the surface of the skin to warm and comfort stiff muscles. It is useful in bath water or as a foot bath.

Poppy Seed

Botanical name: *Papaver somniferum*
Family name: Papaveraceae

Indian names are as follows:
Hindi: Kaskash; Bengali: Posta; Gujarati: Khuskhush; Kannada: Khasksi; Malayalam: Kashakasha; Marathi: Khus Khus; Oriya: Posta, Apu manji; Punjabi: Khus Khus; Sanskrit: Khasa; Tamil: Gashagasha; Telugu: Gasagaslu; Urdu: Kashkash Safaid.

The plant's species name, *somniferum*, means 'sleep inducing' and it is this narcotic effect that has provided so much incentive to its cultivation. The gum from the fruit is known as `Opium` that is ill-famed for addiction. Opium, apart from its addiction values, is also considered as medicine. Many of the traditional herbal preparations are manufactured with opium as one of the important ingredient. Poppy seeds of culinary use have none of the alkaloids that comprise the narcotic.

Poppy seeds are like tiny hard grains. The Western type is slate blue; the Indian type, off-white. Both are kidney-shaped. The blue seeds average 1mm in length, while the white seeds are somewhat smaller. They are similar in flavour and texture and their uses are interchangeable. They are widely available in a dried form.

The analysis of seeds from five types of Indian poppy gave the following ranges of values:

Moisture: 4.3 to 5.2%
Protein: 22.3 to 24.4%
Ether extract: 46.5 to 49.1%
Nitrogen free extract: 11.7 to 14.3%
Fibre: 4.8 to 5.8%

Total ash: 5.6 to 6.0%

Calcium: 1.03 to 1.45%

Phosphorus: 0.79 to 0.89%

Iron: 8.5 to 11.1 mg/100 g

It also yields thiamine, riboflavin and nicotinic acid considerably, but carotene is absent. There are also small quantities of minerals such as iodine, manganese, copper, magnesium and zinc. The seeds also contain lecithin (2.80%), oxalic acid (1.62%), pentosans (3.0 to 3.6%), traces of narcotine and an amorphous alkaloid, and the enzymes diastase, lipase and nuclease. The seeds have high protein content, the major component being a globulin, which accounts for 55% of the total nitrogen. The amino acid make up of the globulin is similar to that of the whole seed protein and is as follows (g/11g N):

Arginine: 10.4

Histidine: 2.9

Lysine:1.5

Tyrosine: 4.7

Tryptophan: 2.0

Phenylalanine: 4.1

Cystine: 2.0

Methionine:2.3

Threonine: 4.2

Valine: 7.1

The proteins are deficient in lysine and methionine. At 10% level of intake, they have a biological value of 57.9% and a digestibility coefficient of 81%. Poppy seeds contain up to 50% of edible oil. It has iodine value of 132 to 142 and saponification value of 188 to 196. Raw cold-pressed oil is pale to golden yellow in colour.

The cake or the meal left after extraction of the oil from the seeds is sweet and nutritious and eaten by the poor people as the source of protein. It is readily consumed by cattle and sheep.

Analysis of the cake gave the following values:

Moisture: 10.8%

Crude protein: 36.6%

Nitrogen free extract: 20.7%

Ether extract: 1.6%

Total ash: 2.4%.

The cake may also be used as manure.

- Poppy seed oil is edible without refining; it does not develop rancidity easily.
- It is largely used in soap making.
- Poppy seed oil is widely used for culinary purposes. It is free from narcotic properties.

- On hydrogenation, it yields a product similar to hydrogenated groundnut oil, which is useful for industrial purposes such as manufacture of paints and varnishes.
- The plant itself can be used for manufacture of paper and pulp.
- The culinary uses:
  - In the West, the blue poppy seeds are used principally in confectionery and in baking, they are sprinkled on breads and buns and used in a variety of Western cakes and pastries.
  - Fried in butter, poppy seed is added to noodles or pasta.
  - It is added to flavour vegetables and their accompanying sauces.
  - Its function in curry is partially to thicken the liquid and add texture.
- In medicinal properties:
  - Western poppy syrup is an anodyne and expectorant.
  - Eastern poppy is an anodyne and narcotic.
  - Cough mixtures and syrups are also made from this variety, which is further used as a poultice with chamomile.
  - An infusion of seeds is said to help ear and toothache.

Following are some of the commonly used spices which come under the leaf category:

Basil leaves

Botanical name: *Ocimum basilicum*
Family name: Lamiaceae
General Indian name: Tulsi
Indian names are as follows:

Bengali: Babui Tulsi, Dulal Tulsi; Gujarati: Damaro, Nasabo; Kannada: Kama Kasturi, Sajjagida; Kashmiri: Niazbo; Oriya: Dhala Tulasi; Telugu: Bhutulsi; Punjabi: Furrunz Mushk; Marathi: Marva, Sabza. In all Indian dialects it is commonly known as Krishna Tulsi.

Basil or Tulsi is an erect glabrous herb, 30–90 cm high and very common to India. The leaves of basil have numerous oil glands in which the aromatic volatile oil of the herb is contained. The herb bears cluster of small, white, two-lipped flowers in raceme fashion. The freshly picked bright green leaves turn brownish green when dried and become brittle and curled. American basil, French basil, Egyptian basil and Indian basil are its major types. The odour of sweet basil is aromatic fragrant and sweet. Most of the basil species possess a clove-like scent with an aromatic and somewhat saline taste. However, 'Kilimandscharicum' species gives camphor-like odour and its essential oil tend to crystallize just like camphor.

Dried leaves and tender four-sided stems of this plant are used as spice for flavouring and for recovery of essential oil. The flavour is warm, sweet and somewhat pungent and peculiar. In dried sweet basil leaves the fragrant, fresh-smelling top notes disappear upon drying, a concentration of volatile oils in the cells of the dehydrated leaves gives a pungent clove and allspice bouquet.

Oil of basil is produced by the distillation of the herb. Primary chemical constituents of basil include essential oil (estragole, eugenol, limonene, and linalool), caffeic acid, tannins, beta carotene, and vitamin C. Basil is aromatic, and carminative. The essential oil is also used for flavouring not only food items but also in various dental and oral products.

- Basil helps to expel flatulence, and ease griping pains in the abdomen.
- Basil is antispasmodic, carminative, galactagogue, and stomachic.
- The herb has been used in the preparation of cough medicine, used to expel worms, essential ingredient in a snuff used to ease headache.
- It is also considered as good insecticide and pesticide.
- Basil has also been used for various topical applications— as a poultice or salve for fungal infection, insect bites, acne and ringworm; as a gargle or mouthwash for thrush; as a bath herb; and as eyewash. The essential oil of basil is added to massage oils for sore muscles.

Chervil

Botanical name: *Anthriscus cerefolium Hoffm*
Family name: Umbelliferae
Common Indian name: Baz-Atrila

Chervil flavour is similar to that of mild parsley and aniseed. Chervil is a member of the Carrot family and its leaves highly resemble carrot tops. There are two main varieties of chervil, one plain and one curly. The young green leaves are collected before they lose their pungency and often preserved in vinegar. Chervil's flavour is lost very easily, either by drying the herb, or too much heat. That is why it should be added at the end of cooking or sprinkled on in its fresh, raw state.

- Chervil is a favourite ingredient in French cuisine. It enhances the flavours of other herbs accompanying it in recipes.
- Chervil has been used in the past as a diuretic, expectorant, digestive aid, and skin freshener. It was also thought to relieve symptoms of eczema, gout, kidney stones, and pleurisy.
- It is most widely known as a remedy for high blood pressure.
- Chervil is also a rich source of bioflavonoid.

Curry Leaves

Botanical name: *Murraya koenigii*
Family name: Rutaceae

Indian names are as follows:
Hindi: Curry pata, Gandhel, Barsenga; Assamese: Narsingha, Bisharhari; Bengali: Barsanga, Curry pata; Marathi: Karhinimb, Poospala, Gandla, Jhirang; Gujarati: Goranimb, Mitha nimb, Kadhilimbdo; Kannada:

Karibevu; Malayalam: Kariveppilei; Oriya: Bhursunga patra, Barsan, Basango; Punjabi: Curry patia; Tamil: Karivempu; Telugu: Karepaku. The composition of leaves is as follows:

Moisture: 66.3%

Protein: 6.1%

Fat (ether extract): 1.0%

Carbohydrates: 16.0%

Fibre: 6.4%

Ash (mineral matters): 4.2%

Iron: 3.1 mg/100 g

Calcium: 810 mg/100 g

Phosphorus: 600 mg/100 g

Vitamin A (carotene): 12600 I.U./100 g

Vitamin C (ascorbic acid): 4 mg/100 g

Nicotinic acid: 2.3 mg/100 g

Volatile oil: 0.5 to 0.8%.

The fresh leaf has a spicy, strong piney-lemony aroma, and a slightly tangerine peel-like taste. The leaves are a fair source of vitamin A; they are also a rich source of calcium, but due to the presence of oxalic acid in high concentration (total oxalates 1.35% and soluble oxalates 1.15%), its nutritional availability is affected. Moreover, the presence of oxalates may cause kidney stones.

The free amino acids present in the leaves are asparagines, serine, aspartic acid, glutamic acid, threonine, alanine, proline, tyrosine, tryptophan, histidine, etc.

Fresh leaves, on steam distillation under pressure yield 0.5% to 2.5% volatile oil, mostly monoterpenes. With advancing maturity, there is a gradual decrease in volatile oil and oleoresin (acetone extracted). Curry leaf has a good amount of vitamin A (β-carotene is 12,600 IU/100 g), with calcium (810 mg/100 g), phosphorus (600 mg/100 g), iron (3.1 mg/100 g), vitamin C (4 mg/100 g), and fibre (6.1%). It also has high levels of oxalates (1.35%).

- Used as a natural flavouring agent in various curries, chutneys, vegetables, and beverages.
- The leaves, bark and the root of the plant are used in indigenous medicine as a tonic, stomachic, stimulant and carminative.
- An infusion of the roasted leaves is used to stop vomiting.
- The leaves are used to help blood circulation and menstrual problems. The fresh leaves are taken to cure dysentery.
- It is also recommended for relieving kidney pains.
- Studies have shown that it has a hypoglycemic action.
- It is found to prevent formation of free radicals.
- It prevents rancidity of ghee (or clarified butter).

Mint

Botanical name: *Mentha arvensis Linn*
Family name: Labiatae.

Indian names are as follows:
Hindi, Bengali, Gujarati, Marathi, Punjabi, and Urdu: Pudina; Kashmiri: Pudyanu; Malayalam: Muthina; Tamil and Telugu: Pudina.
The composition of leaves is as follows:

Moisture: 84.9 g
Protein: 4.8 g
Fat: 0.6 g
Carbohydrates: 5.8 g
Fibre: 2.0 g
Ash (mineral matters): 1.9 g
Iron: 15.6 mg/100 g
Calcium: 200 mg/100 g
Phosphorus: 62 mg/100 g
Vitamin A (carotene): 1620 I.U./100 g
Vitamin C (ascorbic acid): 27 mg/100 g

Pudina is known to almost all the Indians, as used in 'chutney' and as an old popular remedy for relieving stomach complaints and cough and cold. Many other branded medicines are now being prepared using Pudina as principal raw material.

By steam distillation and filtration, a golden yellow volatile oil is obtained. Leaves and flowering tops give the highest yield. About 50% of menthol can be separated out in crystalline form on cooling the oil. The remaining (dementholised) oil is used as peppermint oil.

The peppermint oil is stored in coloured bottles, airtight aluminium or galvanized containers in cool dry place. Since it is acidic in nature, it should not be stored in tin containers. Peppermint oil is used for the production of natural menthol.

The natural oil yields on an average 40 to 50% menthol and 50 to 60% dementholised oil, which can be used both in confectionery and medicine in place of imported peppermint oil.

- The oil and the dried plant are antiseptic, carminative, stimulative, stomachic, diaphoretic, antispasmodic, refrigerant and diuretic.
- The menthol in peppermint soothes the lining of the digestive tract that stimulates the production of bile, which is an essential digestive fluid.
- Dementholised oil is employed flavouring in mouthwashes, toothpastes, chewing gum, liquor and pharmaceutical preparations like in medicines for stomach disorders, in ointment or balm for headache, rheumatism and other pains, in cough drops, inhalation, etc.
- Infusion made with mint leaves is useful for cold, flu, hiccups and flatulence.

- Traditionally, peppermint essential oil has been used to treat indigestion, headache, colic, gingivitis, irritable bowel syndrome, spasms and rheumatism. It relaxes muscles and has antiviral and bactericidal qualities.
- Essential oils promote formation of white cells and acts against microbial germs, while being completely harmless to skin tissue.

Parsley

Botanical name: *Petroselinum crispum (curled parsley)*
Petroselinum neapolitanum (Italian parsley)
Petroselinum sativum (Hamburg parsley)
Family name: Apiaceae formerly Umbelliferae

Indian names are as follows:
Hindi: Ajmood; Kannada: Achu mooda; Malayalam: Kothambeluri.

There are three common varieties of this popular, bright green biennial: flat leaf (Italian), curly leaf, and parsnip rooted (Hamburg). This spice is not traditionally popular in India but gaining popularity in recent years. It is a hardy, aromatic biennial umbelliferous herb. Leaves and seeds are used as spice. The colour of the dried herb is green. Its aroma is pleasant and characteristic is fragrant and spicy.

There are two main types of horticultural parsleys: those cultivated for the leaves (var. crispum) and those grown for their turnip-like roots (var. radicosum Danert). Only the former type of parsley is cultivated in India. In the latter case, roots are cut after the fruits are harvested. The seeds are used for the extraction of parsley oil.

Analysis of the green leaves gave the following values:

    Moisture: 68.4%
    Protein: 5.9%
    Fat: 1.0%
    Carbohydrates: 19.7%
    Fibre: 1.8%
    Total ash: 3.2%
    Calcium: 390 mg/100 g
    Phosphorus: 200 mg/100 g
    Iron: 17.9 mg/100 g
    Vitamin A (carotene): 3200 I.U/100 g
    Thiamine: 0.04 mg/100 g
    Nicotinic acid: 0.5 mg/100 g
    Vitamin C (ascorbic acid): 281 mg/100 g
    Riboflavin and biotin are also present.

The oil is recovered by steam distillation and is used mainly for flavouring food products.

The volatile oil includes myristicin, limonene, eugenol, and alpha-thujene and the flavonoids-including apiin, apigenin, crisoeriol and luteolin. The fruit yields about 20% of greenish fatty oil with a peculiar odour and disagreeable sharp flavour. It can be tried for a variety of industrial purposes, such as making of plastics, synthetic rubber, lubricating oil additives and protective coatings. It may be tried as a raw material for manufacture of soap. The oil cake can be used for manufacture of industrial adhesives.

- The roots are used as vegetable in soups. The dried leaves and roots are used in condiments.
- The herb is reported to possess diuretic, carminative, emmenagogue and antipyretic properties.
- The herb has long been used for uterine troubles.
- The juice of fresh leaves is used as an insecticide.
- Parsley root has been used medicinally since ancient times for digestive disorders, bronchitis, and urinary tract problems.
- In the past Hippocrates parsley was used in medicinal recipes for cure-all, general tonics, poison antidotes, anti-rheumatics and formulas to relieve kidney and bladder stones.
- High chlorophyll content in it acts as a great breath freshener.
- An isolated compound, apiol, is now used in medications to treat kidney ailments and kidney stones.
- Parsley is an excellent source of vitamin C and vitamin A and good source of folic acid.
- It is a rich source of antioxidant nutrients.
- The flavonoids—especially luteolin—have been shown to function as antioxidants that combine with highly reactive oxygen-containing molecules (called oxygen radicals) and help prevent oxygen-based damage to cells.

Following are some of the commonly used spices which come under the flower category:

Saffron

Botanical name: *Crocus sativus*

Family name: Iridaceae

Indian names are as follows:

Hindi: Zaffran, Kesar; Bengali: Zaffran; Gujarati: Keshar; Kannada: Kunkuma Kesari; Kashmiri: Kong; Marathi: Kesar, Kesara; Punjabi: Zaffran, Kesar; Sanskrit: Keshara, Kunkuma, Aruna, Asra, Asrika; Tamil: Kungumapu; Telugu: Kunkumapuva; Urdu: Zaffran, Jafranekar.

Saffron is well known all over the world added to various food items for colouring, flavouring and for taste. Saffron is one of the oldest and certainly among the world's most expensive spices since it takes 75,000 blossoms or 225,000 hand-picked stigmas to make a single pound.

The average composition of saffron is as follows:

Moisture: 15.6%
Starch and sugars: 13.00%
Essential oil: 0.6%
Fixed oil: 5.63%
Fibre: 4.48%
Total ash: 4.27%
Nitrogen free extract: 43.64%.

The ash is rich in potassium and phosphorus and contains races of boron. The flower stigma are composed of many essential volatile oils but the most important being **safranal**, which gives saffron its distinct hay-like flavour. Other volatile oils in saffron are 3,5,5-trimethyl-4-hydroxy-1-cyclohexanone-2-ene, cineole, phenethenol, pinene, borneol, geraniol, limonene, p-cymene, linalool, terpinen-4-oil, etc.

This spice has many non-volatile active components; the most important of them is **á-crocin**, a carotenoid compound, which gives the stigmas their characteristic golden yellow colour. It also contains other carotenoids including zeaxanthin, lycopene, á- and â-carotenes. These are important antioxidants that help protect body from oxidant induced stress, cancers, infections and acts as immune modulators.

- Saffron is famous for its extraordinary flavouring and colouring properties.
- Because of its expense, intense flavour, and strong dying properties, a very little saffron is required for culinary purposes.
- It has been recognized of value as an antispasmodic, diaphoretic, carminative, emmenagogue and sedative.
- Saffron is an important ingredient of the Ayurvedic and Unani systems of medicine in India.
- It has been popularly known as stimulant, helping in urinary, digestive and uterine troubles.
- Stigmas in overdoses are narcotic.

Following are some of the commonly used spices which come under the fruit category:

Cardamom

Botanical name: *Elettaria cardamomum Mation*
Family name: Zingiberaceae
Indian names are as follows:
Hindi: Chhoti Elaichi; Bengali: Chhoto Elach; Gujarati: Elaychi; Kannada: Yelakki; Kashmiri: Aa'l Budu aaa'l; Malayalam: Elathari; Marathi: Velchi; Oriya: Aloichi; Sanskrit: Ela; Tamil: Yelakkai; Telugu: Yealak-Kayulu or Elakkayi.

Cardamoms are the dried capsules of a small group of species or plants belonging to the family Zingiberaceae, which contains seeds possessing a pleasant characteristic aroma. Broadly there are two types of cardamoms, such as small or green cardamom and large or black cardamom. Cardamom is popularly known as the 'Queen of Spices'. Indian cardamom tops in quality with its characteristic flavour or aroma.

Cardamoms are the dried fruits (capsules) of a medium-sized herbaceous perennial. The composition of cardamom varies slightly with the variety, region and age of the product. The following data cover the range of variations in Indian cardamom (seeds):

Moisture: 7 to 10% (av. 8.3)

Volatile oil: 5.5 to 10.5% (av.8.3)

Total ash: 3.8 to 6.9% (av. 5.0)

Alkalinity of ash: 0.4 to 2.4% (av. 1.1)

Water soluble ash: 0.4 to 2.4% (av. 2.7)

Acid soluble ash: 0.4 to 1.9% (av.1.1)

Non-volatile ether extract: 2.0 to 4.5% (av.2.9)

Crude fibre: 6.7 to 12.8% (av. 9.2)

Crude protein: 7.0 to 14.0% (av. 10.3)

Starch (by acid hydrolysis): 39.0 to 49.9 (av. 45.4)

Calcium: 0.3%

Phosphorus: 0.21%

Sodium: 0.01%

Potassium: 1.2%

Iron: 0.012%

Vitamin B_1 (thiamine): 0.18 mg/100 g

Vitamin B_2 (riboflavin): 0.23 mg/100 g

Niacin: 2.3 mg/100 g

Vitamin C (ascorbic acid): 12 mg/100 g

Vitamin A: 175 I.U./100 g of seeds

The spicy pods contain many essential volatile oils that include pinene, sabinene, myrcene, phellandrene, limonene, 1, 8-cineole, terpinene, p-cymene, terpinolene, linalool, linalyl acetate, terpinen-4-oil, a-terpineol, a-terpineol acetate, citronellol, nerol, geraniol, methyl eugenol, and trans-nerolidol.

- The therapeutic properties of cardamom oil have found applications in many traditional medicines as antiseptic, antispasmodic, carminative, digestive, diuretic, expectorant, stimulant, stomachic and tonic.
- Cardamom in India is consumed internally, as a masticatory, as a common ingredient of special seasonings and curry powders and flavouring various kinds of foods.
- Cardamoms are used as medicine for scanty urination, diarrhea, dysentery, palpitation of the heart, exhaustion due to over work, depression, etc.
- Infusion of cardamom is gargled to cure pharyngitis and sore throat.
- Cardamom is an excellent source of manganese and iron, good source of minerals such as potassium, calcium, and magnesium.

Nutmeg and Mace

Botanical name: *Myristica fragrans Hout*

Family name: Myristicaceae

Indian names are as follows:

Hindi, Bengali, Gujarati, and Marathi: Jaivitri, Japatri, Jotri, Joitri, Jaiphal, Payapatri; Kannada: Japatre; Kashmiri: Jaabvatur; Malayalam: Jathipatri; Oriya: Joitri; Punjabi: Jaiphal, Jaivatri, Jaipatri; Sanskrit: Jatiphala; Tamil: Jadhipattiri; Telugu: Japatri.

The nutmeg tree is a large evergreen which produces two spices — mace and nutmeg. Nutmeg is the seed kernel inside the fruit and mace is the lacy covering (aril) on the kernel. The mace is skilfully removed, gently pressed flat, dried. On drying, the original scarlet colour of the mace turns rather pale yellowish brown or reddish brown and becomes brittle. The flavour of mace is similar to that of nutmeg but is more refined. Both the spices are used for flavouring besides being used as medicine.

The composition of mace is given below:

Moisture: 5.9%

Protein: 6.5%

Ether extract: 24.4%

Carbohydrates: 47.8%

Fibre: 0.8%

Ash: 1.6%

Calcium: 0.18%

Phosphorus: 0.13%

Iron: 12.6 mg/100 g

Vitamin B_1: 0.37g/100 g

Vitamin B_2: /0.56 mg/100 g

Niacin: 1.2 mg/100 g

Vitamin C: 12 mg/100 g

Vitamin A: 175 I.U/100 g

It contains a volatile oil (4 to 15%), amylodextrin (25%), reducing sugar, pectin, resins and colouring matters. Oil of mace resembles nutmeg oil in odour, flavour and composition and no distinction is made between them in the trade. Like nutmeg oil, mace oil also becomes viscous on storage due to absorption of oxygen. Nutmeg's flavour and fragrance come from oil of myristica, containing myristicin, a poisonous narcotic. Myristicin can cause hallucinations, vomiting, and epileptic symptoms.

- Nutmeg and mace are generally classified as baking spices.
- Both nutmeg and mace are much used for culinary purpose. Nutmeg, in general, tends to be sweeter and more delicate than mace.
- Nutmeg volatile oil is used as a flavorant in liquor, tobacco and dental creams.

- In India, mace and nutmeg are used more as drugs as both are stimulant, carminative, astringent and aphrodisiac and are used in pharmaceutical preparations for dysentery, stomach ache, flatulence, nausea, vomiting, malaria, rheumatism, sciatica and early stages of leprosy.
- It is also an effective medicine for insomnia, irritability and depression.
- It is used beneficially in the treatment of skin diseases such as ringworm and eczema. A nutmeg coarsely powdered is used as external application to relieve any rheumatic pain, neuralgia and sciatica.

Kababchini Fruit

Botanical name: *Pimenta dioica*
Family name: Piperaceae

Indian names are as follows:
Sanskrit: Kankol and Kakkol; All other Indian languages: Kababchini
Kababchini is otherwise known as allspice or Cubeb or tailed pepper.
Allspice takes its name from its aroma, which smells like a combination of spices, especially cinnamon, cloves, ginger and nutmeg. It is well known as a spice in India. It is used for flavouring curries particularly non-vegetarian dishes in India besides in soups and sauces.

- Allspice is a good source of potassium, manganese, iron, niacin and vitamin C.
- The oil is classed as rubefacient, meaning that it irritates the skin and expands the blood vessels, increasing the flow of blood to make the skin feel warmer.
- The tannins in allspice provide a mild anesthetic that, with its warming effect, make it a popular home remedy for arthritis and sore muscles.
- Eugenol present in allspice has local anesthetic and antiseptic properties that are very useful in gum and dental treatment procedures.
- It is widely used as a home remedy for throat infections and also by singers to maintain a clear throat.
- According to modern science it is stimulant, diuretic, and expectorant. It is used for treatment of dysentery, asthma, leucorrhoea, broken voice, cough, and rheumatism.

Star anise

Botanical name: *Illicium verum Hook*
Syn: Illicium anisatum
Family name: Magnoliaceae

Indian names are as follows:
Hindi: Anasphal; Marathi: Badian; Tamil: Anashuppu, Anasipu; Telugu: Anaspuvu.

Star anise fruit has an agreeable, aromatic, sweet taste and a pleasant odour resembling anise. Anethole is the main constituent (85 to 90%) of the volatile oil. The fatty oil can be used as a raw material for soap. After refining it can be consumed as edible oil.

- It is used as a condiment for flavouring curries, confectioneries and spirits, and for pickling.
- It is not only applied as part of folk medicinal system but also for manufacture of branded medicines in China.
- Star anise has carminative, stomachic, stimulant, expectorant, anti-spasmodic, anti-microbial, aromatic, galactagogue and diuretic properties.

Tamarind

Botanical name: *Tamarindus indica Linn*
Family name: Leguminosae.

Indian names are as follows:

Hindi, Punjabi, Urdu: Imli; Assamese: Ttali; Bengali: Tentul; Gujarati: Ambli; Kannada: Amli, Huli; Malayalam: Puli; Marathi: Chinch, Chincha; Oriya: Tentuli; Sanskrit: Yamadutika, Amli, Abdika; Tamil: Puli; Telugu: Chinthappandu, Chinta, Amlika

The pulp of ripe fruit of tamarind is commonly used as condiment, or more precisely as 'acidulant,' in many Indian dishes particularly South Indian dishes. Tamarind fruit pulp is traditionally popular in India as condiment added to many dishes such as Rasham, Sambar, chutneys, curries, etc.

The ripe fruit, on an average, comprises about 55% tamarind pulp, 33% seeds and about 12% fibre. A typical sample of tamarind pulp shows the following:

Moisture: 18.2%
Free acid (tartaric): 9.8%
Combined acid: 6.7%
Total sugars as invert: 38.2%
Protein: 2.8%
Pectin: 2.8%
Fibre: 19.4%
Total ash: 2.8%
Calcium: 0.17%
Phosphorus: 0.11%
Iron: 0.011%
Vitamin A: 100 I.U./100 g
Niacin: 0.2 mg/100 g
Calorific value: 283 calories/100 g

Of the reducing sugars present, 70% is glucose and 30% is fruit sugar, i.e. fructose. Only a trace of sucrose is present. The pectin present in pulp is of good quality having a jelly grade of 180–200.

The composition of the seed kernel is:

Moisture: 0.1%

Protein: 7%

Fat: %

Fibre: 0.6%

Non-fibre carbohydrates: 5%

Other components: 4%

The constituents of tamarind are citric, tartaric and malic acids, potassium, bitartrate, gum, pectin, some grape sugar, and parenchymatous fibre. Technology is now available for manufacture of pectin out of this pulp. It is also possible to manufacture tartarates and alcohol from this pulp.

- Ayurvedic practitioners and folk doctors frequently used it as a medicine as this ripe fruit is considered as appetizing, mild laxative, tonic to the heart, anthelmintic, heals wounds and fractures, and rectifies disorders of Kapha and Vayu. They used tamarind leaves for treating burns, sprains and swelling.
- It is used to treat bronchial disorders and gargling with tamarind water is recommended for a sore throat.
- Being highly acidic, it is a refrigerant (cooling in the heat) and febrifuge (for fighting fevers).
- The pulp, leaves, and the bark also have medical applications. For example, in the Philippines, the leaves have been traditionally used in herbal tea for reducing malaria fever.
- Its leaves are cooling and antibilious beneficial in the treatment of bilious vomiting, flatulence and indigestion.
- The chief use of the seeds lies in the manufacture of textile sizing powder.
- The kernel is used as creaming agent for rubber latex, soil stabilizer, and as pectin substitute.
- Tamarind is an excellent brass and copper polish.

Following are some of the commonly used spices which come under the root category:

Galangal Root

Botanical name: *Alpinia galanga (Linn) Willd*

Family: Zingiberaceae

Indian names are as follows:

Hindi and Bengali: Kulanjan; Gujarati: Kolanjan; Kannada: Rasmi, Sugandha vachi; Malayalam: Araatta, Perasatta; Marathi: Baripankijar, Koshikulinjan; Punjabi: Kulanjan; Sanskrit: Kulanja, Kulanjana; Sindhi: Kathi, Kunjar; Tamil: Sangandam Tittiram; Telugu: Peddumparashtram, Kachoramu; Urdu: Kulanjan.

Galangal is the dried rhizome or root of the plant. It is slightly pungent, with an aroma similar to that of rhizome. Galangal oil is steam-distilled oil which is a pale yellow to olive-brown liquid with eucalyptus-cardamom-ginger-like odour and warming camphoraceous-like bitter taste. It consists of methyl-cinnamate, cineol, some camphor and probably d-pinene.

- Apart from being used as a spice, it has more elaborate use in various medicinal preparations in rheumatism and catarrhal affections, especially in bronchial catarrh.
- The rhizome and its essential oil are useful in respiratory trouble.
- Galangal is an aromatic stimulant, carminative and stomachic. It is used against nausea, flatulence, dyspepsia, rheumatism, catarrh and enteritis.
- Its antibacterial quality is used in veterinary and homeopathic medicine.
- Galangal tea is a good remedy for treating gas in digestive system, reducing fat, and treating inflammation in the respiratory track.

Garlic

Botanical name: *Allium sativum*

Family: Lilliaceae

Indian names are as follows:

Hindi: Lasum, Lassan, Lahsun; Assamese: Naharu; Bengali: Rasun; Gujarati: Lasan; Kannada: Belluli; Kashmiri: Rahan; Malayalam: Velluli; Marathi: Lusoon; Oriya: Rasuna; Punjabi: Lassan, Lasum; Sanskrit: Lashuna; Tamil: Ullipundu, Vellaip-pundu; Telugu: Velluri; Urdu: Lessun, Lashun.

In 1858 Louis Pasteur noted the antiseptic properties of garlic. In the 1940s, a Nobel Prize winning chemist Dr. Arthur Stoll discovered the compound allicin which he felt was key in garlic's bacterial battling capabilities. As a clove is crushed or sliced the enzyme allinase triggers a series of complex chemical reactions. One of the resulting chemicals, allicin, is generally regarded as one of the key players in garlic medicine. Other substances such as adenosine and ajoene also may be of a great significance.

Fresh peeled garlic cloves have the following composition:

Moisture: 62.8%

Protein: 6.3%

Fat: 0.1%

Total ash: 1.0%

Fibre: 0.8%

Carbohydrates: 29.0%

Calcium: 0.03%

Phosphorus: 0.31%

Iron: 0.001%

Vitamin C: 13 mg/100 g

Nicotinic acid: 0.4 mg/100 g

Calorific value: 142 calories/100 g

Before garlic is crushed, the intact cell contains S-2-propenyl-L-cysteine S-oxide or alliin which can be found in the cell cytoplasm. Within the cell there are vacuoles that contain an enzyme known as alliinase. When the cell is crushed, the enzyme is released. The enzyme transforms the natural product alliin into an intermediate that reacts with itself to form a compound known as allicin. Allicin has been described as an odoriferous, unstable antibacterial substance that polymerizes easily and must be stored at low temperature. When heated, it breaks down to give a variety of compounds, including the diallyl disulfide, which is obtained when oil of garlic is distilled from the raw material.

- Garlic and garlic oil is used practically all over the world for flavoring various dishes.
- According to the Unani and Ayurvedic systems as practiced in India, garlic is carminative, stimulant, and thus aids in digestion and absorption of food. It is an anthelmintic and antiseptic.
- Garlic in high amount may interfere with some antiviral and antidiabetic medications, as well as with other drugs, such as acetaminophen, that are broken down by the same liver enzymes as garlic. It may increase the activity of drugs that lower blood sugar.
- Garlic in human subjects has demonstrated an increased resistance of LDL to oxidation. This suggests that suppressed LDL oxidation may be one of the powerful mechanisms accounting for the antiatherosclerotic properties of garlic.
- The emerging mechanistic basis for the antiproliferative function of allicin, therefore, involves the activation of the mitochondrial apoptotic pathway by glutathione depletion and by changes in the intracellular redox status.
- Raw garlic, not cooked or dried, is most beneficial for health, since heat and water inactivate sulfur enzymes, which can diminish garlic's antibiotic effects. In clinical trials, garlic seems to lower blood pressure and cholesterol and kill parasites in the body.
- Garlic has inhibitory and reverse effect on gastric carcinoma and precancerous lesion.
- Evidence suggests beneficial effects of the regular dietary intake of garlic on mild hypertension and hyperlipidemia.
- Purified extracts of garlic can inhibit the formation of blood clots and provide protection against atherosclerosis by lowering cholesterol and triglyceride levels.

Ginger

Botanical name: *Zingiber officinale*
Family: Zingiberaceae.
Indian names are as follows:
Hindi: Adrak; Bengali: Ada; Gujarati: Adu; Kannada: Shunti, Ardraka; Malayalam: Inji; Marathi: Ale; Oriya: Oda; Punjabi: Adrak; Sanskrit:

Ardraka, Shoont; Tamil: Inji; Telugu: Allam; Urdu: Adrak, Adhrak

Ginger takes its name from the Sanskrit word *stringa-vera,* which means "with a body like a horn".

The composition of dry ginger is given below:

Moisture: 6.9%

Protein: 8.6%

Fat: 6.4%

Fiber: 5.9%

Carbohydrates: 66.5%

Ash: 5.7%

Calcium: 0.1%

Phosphorous: 0.15%

Iron: 0.011%

Sodium: 0.03%

Potassium: 1.4%

Vitamin A: 175 I.U./100 g

Vitamin B$_1$: 0.05 mg/100 g

Vitamin B$_2$: 0.13 mg/100 g

Niacin: 1.9 mg/100 g

Vitamin C: 12.0 mg/100 g

Calorific value: 380 calories/100 g

The aroma of ginger is pleasant and spicy and the flavour penetrating, slightly biting due to antiseptic or pungent compounds present in it. On steam distillation, it yields 1.0 to 3.0% of pale yellow, viscid oil. The oil possesses the aromatic odour but not the pungent flavour of the spice. The primary known constituents of ginger root include gingerols, zingibain, bisabolenel, oleoresins, starch, essential oil (zingiberene, zingiberole, camphene, cineol, borneol), mucilage, and protein.

Ginger oleoresin is manufactured on a commercial scale as it is in great demand by the various food industries. Ginger oleoresin is obtained by extraction of powdered dried ginger. Unlike volatile oil, it contains both the volatile oil and the non-volatile pungent principles for which ginger is so highly esteemed.

- According to the Ayurvedic and Unani system of medicine, ginger is considered to be carminative, stimulant and given in dyspepsia and flatulent colic. With honey and basil leaves, it acts as an excellent expectorant.
- Ginger has been shown to be effective for pregnancy-induced and postoperative nausea and vomiting.
- Ginger helps relieve indigestion, gas pains, diarrhea and stomach cramping.
- Ginger's therapeutic properties effectively stimulate circulation of the blood, removing toxins from the body, cleansing the bowels and

kidneys, and nourishing the skin.

- Other uses for ginger root include the treatment of asthma, bronchitis and other respiratory problems by loosening and expelling phlegm from the lungs.

Onion

Botanical name: *Allium cepa*

Family names: Liliaceae

Indian names are as follows:

Hindi, Punjabi and Urdu: Piyaz; Assamese: Piyaz; Bengali: Penyaz; Gujarati: Dunzari; Kannada: Nirulli; Konkani: Kandu; Malayalam: Bawa; Marathi: Kanda; Oriya: Piyaza; Sanskrit: Palandu; Sindhi: Dungari; Tamil: Vengayam, Irulli; Telugu: Nirulli.

Onions are used for cooking or as salad. Pungent varieties are used as condiment for flavouring a number of food items. The onion is an edible bulb. There are many variations of colour, shape and size. The colour varies from white to red to purple, the shape from spherical to almost conical, and the diameter at the largest point from 10 mm (1/2 in) to 8 cm (3 in) or more. Onions should be firm.

Composition of onion is as follows:

Moisture: 86.8%
Protein: 1.2%
Fat: 0.1%
Carbohydrates: 11.6%
Calcium: 0.18%
Phosphorus: 0.005%
Iron: 0.7 mg/100 g

The bulb and fresh herb yield 0.005% of an essential oil, which has an acrid taste and unpleasant odour. The chief constituent of the crude oil is allyl-propyl disulphide. Onions contain an essential oil and organic sulphides. The scales of onion contain catechol and protocatechuic acid. The pink coloured peel on the onion has preference for natural dye, it gives fast colour on cotton, silk and woolen garments or fabrics.

- Onion is considered as a flavouring spice.
- Onion is said to possess stimulant, diuretic, antiseptic and expectorant properties and is considered useful in flatulence and dysentery.
- Onion's antiseptic properties are used for wound healing, skin complaints (acne), insect bites, hemorrhoids, boils, urinary system, toothache, earache and respiratory complaints.
- The raw juice is diuretic and the whole onion is an appetite stimulant and digestant.
- It is a valuable remedy for cholera.
- Onion is noted for its easily assimilating iron content, hence beneficial in treating anemia.

- Onion has the property to liquefy phlegm and prevents its recurrence.
- It has been used as a vermifuge. It is believed to stimulate the liver and is beneficial to the heart and nervous system.

Turmeric

Botanical name: *Curcuma longa*
Curcuma domestica
Curcuma aromatica
Family name: Zingiberaceae

Indian names are as follows:
Hindi: Haldi; Bengali: Halud, Pitarus; Gujarati: Haldhar, Haldi; Kannada: Arishina; Konkani: Halad; Malayalam: Manjal; Marathi: Halad, Halede; Meitei: Yaingang; Oriya: Haladi; Punjabi: Haldar, Haldhar, Haldi; Sanskrit: Haladi, Haridra, Harita; Tamil: Manjal; Telugu: Pasupu; Urdu: Haladi.

Turmeric is one of the most popular spices of India. It is also popular for its medicinal value.

Turmeric has the following composition:

Moisture: 5.8%
Protein: 8.6%
Fat: 8.9%
Carbohydrates: 63.0%
Fibre: 6.9%
Total ash: 6.8%
Calcium: 0.2%
Phosphorus: 0.26%
Iron: 0.05%
Sodium: 0.01%
Potassium: 2.5%
Vitamin A (carotene): 175 I.U./100 g
Vitamin B_1: 0.09 mg/100 g
Vitamin B_2: 0.19 mg/100 g
Vitamin C (ascorbic acid): 49.8 mg/100 g
Niacin: 4.8 mg/100 g
Calorific value (food energy): 390 calories/100

By steam distillation of crushed turmeric tubers volatile oil of orange yellow colour can be extracted. The dried rhizomes yield 5 to 6%, while fresh ones give 0.24% essential oil. About 58% of the oil composed of turmerones (sesquiterpene ketones) and 9% tertiary alcohols. Oleoresin can be extracted from ground turmeric by solvent extraction followed by vacuum concentration.

- Turmeric is an ancient spice, used from antiquity as dye and a condiment. In India it is commonly used for dyeing wool, silk and cotton.

- It is a stomachic, carminative, tonic, blood purifier, vermicide, and an antiseptic. It is used for cancer patients. Curcumin has been shown to be active against *Staphlococcus aureus.*
- It is said to be anti-oxidant, due to the phenolic character of curcuma. It is considered useful both for internal and external applications.
- It is taken with warm milk to act as expectorant.
- It is applied externally to get relief from sprains and pains. Used as an inhalation to get relief from sore throat and congestion.
- In small pox, it is applied as paste with gingerly oil and neem leaves. The juice of raw rhizome is used as an anti-parasitic for many skin affections. Burnt turmeric is used as tooth powder to relieve dental troubles.
- In beauty care, women have used turmeric paste since very ancient times. Today it finds use as an antiseptic and an antitanning.

Following are some of the commonly used spices which come under the bark category:

Cinnamon

Botanical name: *Cinnamomum zeylanicun Blume*
Family name: Lauraceae

Indian names are as follows:
Hindi: Dalchini, Darchini; Bengali, Gujarati, Marathi, Oriya, Punjabi, Urdu: Dalchini; Kannada, Malayalam: Lavangpattai; Sanskrit: Darushila; Tamil: Sanna-lavangapattai.

Cinnamon consists of layers of dried pieces of the inner bark of branches and young shoots from the evergreen tree Cinnamomum zeylanicum which is obtained when the cork and the cortical parenchyma are removed from the whole bark.

Composition may vary according to the quality and region. The following range of variation may be seen:

Moisture: 5.40 to 11.4%
Volatile oil: 0.3 to 2.8%
Fixed oil: 0.3 to 1.9%
Fibre: 25.6 to 30.5%
Carbohydrates: 16.6 to 22.6%
Protein: 3.0 to 4.5%
Total ash: 3.4 to 6.0%
Ash insoluble in acid: 0.02 to 0.6%.

The primary chemical constituents of this herb include cinnamaldehyde, gum, tannin, mannitol, coumarins, and essential oils (aldehydes, eugenol, pinene). Volatile oil is also prepared from cinnamon leaves, fruits and roots. Cinnamon bark contains 0.5 to 1.0% volatile oil. It is extracted by steam distillation. This oil is light yellow in colour when freshly distilled and changes to red on storage. It contains cinnamaldehyde up to 60 to 75%; eugenol and benzaldehyde, etc.

- Cinnamon is extensively used as a spice or condiment. It is used for flavouring confectionery, liquors, pharmaceutical preparations, soaps and dental preparations. It is also used in candy, gum, incense and perfumes.
- It is aromatic, astringent, stimulant and carminative and also possesses the property to cure nausea, vomiting and diarrhea.
- Cinnamon is predominantly used as a carminative addition to herbal prescriptions. It is used in flatulent dyspepsia, dyspepsia with nausea, intestinal colic and digestive atony associated with cold and debilitated conditions.
- The cinnamaldehyde component is hypotensive and spasmolytic, and increases peripheral blood flow.
- The essential oil of this herb is a potent antibacterial, anti-fungal, and uterine stimulant.
- The various terpenoids found in the volatile oil are believed to account for Cinnamon's medicinal effects.
- Common cold can be effectively cured with the use of cinnamon.
- Studies have determined that Cinnamon may reduce blood sugar, cholesterol, and triglyceride levels by as much as 20%.

Following are the few of the other miscellaneous spices commonly used:

Pepper

Botanical name: *Piper nigrum*

Family name: Piperaceae

Indian names are as follows:

Hindi: Kali Mirch; Bengali: Gol Morich, Kalo marich; Gujarati: Kala Mari; Kannada: Kare Menasu; Kashmiri: Marutis; Malayalam: Karumaluku, Nallamaluku; Marathi: Kali Mirch, Mire; Oriya: Gol Maricha; Punjabi: Kali Mirch; Sanskrit: Ushana, Maricha, Hapusha; Tamil: Milagu; Telugu: Miriyalu; Urdu: Kali Mirch, Siah Mirch.

There are many varieties of black pepper, they differ slightly in their physical and chemical characteristics, colour, size, shape, flavour and bite. White and black peppers are prepared from the berries of the same plant or species. The only difference is that for preparing black pepper, spikes are harvested when berries are fully mature, but unripe, i.e. when green or greenish yellow, but for preparing white pepper, the harvesting of berries is delayed until they become ripe, i.e. yellowish red or red. White pepper is prepared by removing the outer pericarp.

Analysis of 23 types of black pepper from Kerala, South and North Kanara, Coorg and Assam gave the following ranges of value:

Moisture: 8.7 to 14.1%

Total nitrogen: 1.55 to 2.60%

Nitrogen in non-volatile ether extract: 2.70 to 4.22%
Non-volatile ether extract: 3.9 to 11.5%
Volatile ether extract: 0.3 to 4.2%
Alcohol extract: 4.4 to 12.0%
Starch (by acid hydrolysis): 28 to 49%
Crude fibre: 8.7 to 18%
Crude piperine: 2.8 to 9.0%
Piperine (spectrophotometrically): 1.7 to 7.4%
Total ash: 3.9 to 5.7%
Acid insoluble ash (sand): 0.03 to 0.55%.

The alkaloid piperine is considered to be the major constituent responsible for the biting taste of black pepper. Other pungent alkaloids, occurring in pepper in small amount, are chavicine, piperidine and piperetine.

The characteristic aromatic odour of pepper is due to the presence of a volatile oil in the cells of pericarp. On steam distillation, crushed black pepper yields 1.0 to 2.6% (up to 4.8%) of the volatile oil. Oil of pepper consists of chiefly of the terpenes, l-phellandrene, caryophyllene, and perhaps dipentene. The characteristic odour of the oil has been attributed to the presence of small amount of oxygenated compounds (about 0.5% of the oil).

- Black pepper constitutes an important component of culinary seasoning and an essential ingredient of numerous foodstuffs.
- In ancient periods it is considered as a powerful remedy for various disorders of the anatomical system and prescribed it as an effective cure for dyspepsia, malaria, delirium, hemorrhoids, etc.
- They hold the properties such as stomachic, carminative, aromatic stimulant, antibacterial, diaphoretic.
- It stimulates the taste-buds causing reflex stimulation of gastric secretions, improving digestion and treating gastrointestinal upsets and flatulence.
- Pepper calms nausea and raises body temperature, making it valuable for treating fevers and chills.

Clove

Botanical name: *Eugenia caryophyllus*
Syan: Syzygium aromaticum
Family name: Myrtaceae
Indian names are as follows:
Hindi: Laung; Bengali: Labanga; Gujarati: Lavang; Kannada: Lavanga; Malayalam: Grambu; Marathi: Luvang; Oriya: Labanga; Punjabi: Laung; Sanskrit: Lavanga; Tamil: Kirambu, Lavangam; Telugu: Lavangalu.
The clove is the air-dried unopened flower bud obtained from a handsome, medium-sized, evergreen, straight trunked tree that grows in Kerala and Tamil Nadu.

The composition of clove are given below:

Moisture: 5.4%
Protein: 6.3%
Volatile oil: 13.2%
Non-volatile ether extract (fat): 15.5%
Crude fibre: 11.1%
Carbohydrates: 57.7%
Mineral matter: 5.0%
Calcium: 0.7%
Phosphorus: 0.11%
Iron: 01%
Sodium: 0.25%
Potassium: 0.2%
Vitamin B_1: 0.11 mg/100 g
Vitamin B_2: 0.04%
Niacin: 1.5%
Vitamin C: 80.9 mg/100 g
Vitamin A: 175 I.U
Calorific value: 430 calories/100 g

The clove buds, stem and leaves, on steam distillation yield essential oils 15 to 17%, 4.5 to 5.5% and 1 to 2% respectively.

- The primary chemical constituents include eugenol, caryophyllene, and tannins.
- Eugenol, has been found to be a weak tumor promoter, making clove one of many healing herbs with both pro- and anti-cancer effects.
- Clove is very aromatic, has a fine flavour and imparts warming qualities.
- It is used as a culinary spice as the flavour blends well with the sweets and savory dishes.
- It is highly valued in medicine as carminative, aromatic and stimulant. It is also used in flatulence and dyspepsia.
- This is used as an essential oil in medicine for its antiseptic and antibiotic properties in toothache.
- Traditional Chinese physicians have used cloves from a long time to treat indigestion, diarrhea, hernia, and ringworm, as well as athlete's foot and other fungal infections.
- India's traditional Ayurvedic healers have used cloves to treat respiratory and digestive ailments.
- The medieval German herbalists used cloves as part of anti-gout mixture.

- Clove contains antioxidants that help prevent the cell damage that causes cancer.
- Dentists have used clove oil as an oral anesthetic. They also used it to disinfect root canals.

Asafetida

Botanical name: *Ferula asafetida*
Family name:Umbellifereae
Indian names are as follows:
Hindi, Bengali, Gujarati, Marathi, Punjabi and Urdu: Hing; Sanskrit: Badhika, Agudhagandhu; Kannada: Hinger; Kashmiri: Yang; Malayalam and Tamil: Perugayam; Oriya: Hengu; Telugu: Inguva, Ingumo.
Asafoetida is extracted from the Ferula plants which have massive taproots or carrot-shaped roots. It is an oleo gum-resin. The components to which asafoetida owes its character are believed to be due to ferulic ester and volatile oil consisting of different sulfur compounds.
Asafoetida contains

Resin: 40 to 64%
Gum: about 25%
Volatile oil: 10 to 17%
Ash: 1.5 to 10%

An analysis of asafoetida shows that it consists of

Carbohydrates: 67.8% / 100 g
Moisture: 16.0%
Protein: 4.0%
Fat: 1.1%
Minerals: 7.0%
Fibre: 4.1%
Calorific value is 297.

Its mineral and vitamin contents include substantial calcium besides phosphorus, iron, carotene, riboflavin and niacin.
The oil of asafoetida is obtained by steam distillation of the gum resin. The yield varies from 3 to 20%.

- Asafoetida is extensively used in Indian medicine and cookery for ages.
- In cookery for flavouring curries, sauces and pickles in conjunction with garlic and onion.
- Asafoetida oil has been analyzed to have antibiotic and sedative properties.
- In Ayurvedic, Siddha and Unani asafoetida is considered as effective remedies for many diseases and disorders such as spasmodic disorders, respiratory disorders like whooping cough, asthma and bronchitis, flatulence and distension of the stomach.
- Inhalation of this gum prevents hysterical attacks.

Chillies

Botanical name: *Capsicum annuum*
Family name: Solanaceae

Technically, chilli peppers are a fruit. Once dried, they are considered a spice. The medicinal properties that chillies include are stimulant, sialagogue (an agent which stimulates the flow of saliva), rubefacient, carminative, anticoagulant, and digestive. The active ingredient in chillies is a compound called capsaicin, which gives it that unique sting.

- Dried chillies can be used in curries, sauces, pickles, chutneys and pastes.
- Since ancient times, chillies have been used externally to relieve pain and internally to cure disease such as yellow fever, common cold, etc.
- Capsaicin ointments have been found to relieve the pain of arthritis and shingles.
- Capsaicin has a positive effect on blood cholesterol, and also works as an anticoagulant.
- Chillies are high in beta carotene and nearly twice the recommended daily allowance for vitamin C.

UNIT III

NORMAL DIETARY REQUIREMENTS

18 Normal Dietary Requirements

The recommended dietary allowance for many years was the most widely publicized of the definitions of nutrient sufficiency. It was based on available scientific knowledge and deliberation by experts. The first attempt to recommend dietary allowances of energy, protein, iron, calcium, vitamin A, thiamin, ascorbic acid and vitamin D for Indians was made by the nutrition advisory committee of the Indian Research Fund Association (now ICMR) in 1944, following the recommendations of the League of Nations in 1937. Alongside, a typical balanced diet based on habitual Indian diet was also formulated to provide all the nutrients to meet the Recommended Dietary Allowances (RDA) of an Indian reference man.

The recommended allowances for proteins and energy were revised by a Joint Expert Consultation of the FAO, World Health Organization (WHO) and United Nations University (UNU) in 1985.

Recommended Dietary Allowances (RDA) is defined as the nutrient present in the diet which satisfies the daily requirement of almost all individuals in a population. These simply in addition of safety factor amounting to the estimated requirement to cover the variation among individuals, losses during cooking and the lack of precision inherent in the estimated requirement.

Recommended dietary allowances = Requirements + safety factor

Man need a wide range of nutrients to lead a healthy and active life and these are derived through the diet he consumes daily. The components of his diets must be chosen judiciously to provide all the nutrients he needs in adequate amounts and in proper proportions. RDA of an individual depends on many factors such as age, sex, physical work and physiological stress.

- *Age:* An adult requires more total calories than a child due to larger size of the body and increases in activity. A growing child requires more calories and protein per kilogram of body weight than an adult.
- *Sex:* Females require fewer calories than males as BMR is lower and size of the body is smaller.

- *Physical work:* Sedentary workers require less calories and B-vitamins than hardworking person.
- *Physiological stress:* During pregnancy and lactation period the requirement of nutrients are increased.

Adequate intake (AI) is a nutrient recommendation based on observed or experimentally determined approximation of nutrient intake by a group of healthy people when sufficient scientific evidence is not available to calculate an RDA.

GENERAL PRINCIPLES OF DERIVING RDA

A number of approaches have been used in arriving at the nutritional requirements of an individual and the RDA for a population. The general principles are:

1. ***Dietary intakes:*** This approach has been used in arriving at the energy requirements of children. Energy intakes of normally growing healthy children are utilized for this purpose.

2. ***Growth:*** The requirements of any particular nutrient or the breast milk intake, for satisfactory growth have been utilized for defining requirements in an early infancy.

3. ***Nutrient balance:*** The minimum intake nutrient for equilibrium (intake = output) the adults, and nutrient retention consistent with satisfactory growth in children, have been used widely for arriving at the protein requirements.

4. ***Obligatory loss of nutrients:*** The minimal loss of any nutrient or of its metabolic product (viz. nitrogenous end products in the case of proteins) through normal routes of elimination, viz. urine, faeces and sweat, is determined on a diet devoid of or very low in the nutrients (for example, a protein-free diet). This information is used to determine the amount of nutrient to be consumed daily through the diet to replace the obligatory loss. In infants and children, growth requirements are added to the above maintenance requirement.

5. ***Factorial approach:*** In this approach, the requirements for different functions are assessed separately, and added to arrive at the total daily requirement. This is the basis of arriving at energy requirements. Earlier, this was the approach employed for assessing the protein requirement.

6. ***Nutrient turnover:*** Data from turnover of nutrients in healthy persons, using isotopically labelled nutrients have been employed in arriving at requirements of certain nutrients. Earlier, radio isotopic labelled compounds were utilized and currently compounds labelled with a stable isotope are being increasingly used to determine the turnover of nutrients in the body. Stable isotopes are particularly useful in infants, children and in women during pregnancy and lactation where radio isotopes are contraindicated.

7. ***Depletion and repletion studies:*** This approach has been employed in arriving at the requirement of water-soluble vitamins. The levels of vitamin or its coenzyme in serum or tissue (erythrocytes, leucocytes) are used as a biochemical marker of the vitamin status. Requirements of ascorbic acid, thiamine, riboflavin, niacin and pyridoxine have been established employing this approach. The subjects are first fed a diet very low in the nutrient under study till the biochemical parameters reach a low level after which response to feeding graded doses of the nutrient is determined. The level at which response increases rapidly is an indication of requirement.

Reference Indian Adult Man

Reference man is between 20 and 39 years of age and weighs 60 kg. He is free from disease and physically fit for active work. On each working day he is employed for 8 hours in occupation that usually involves moderate activity. While not at work he spends 8 hours in bed, 4–6 hours sitting and moving about, and 2 hours in walking and in active recreation or household duties.

Reference Indian Woman

Reference woman is between 20 and 39 years of age and healthy, and weighs 50 kg. She may be engaged in 8 hours in general household work, in light industry or in any other moderately active work. Apart from 8 hours in bed, she spends 4–6 hours sitting or moving around in light activity, and 2 hours walking or active recreation or household chores (Table 18.1).

Table 18.1: Reference body weights (kg) of Indians of different age groups

	Age (years)	*Male*	*Female*
Infants	0–½	5.4	5.4
	½–1	8.6	
Children	1–3	12.61	11.81
	4–6	19.20	18.69
	7–9	27.00	26.75
	10–12	35.54	37.91
Adolescents	13–15	47.88	46.66
	16–18	57.28	49.92
Adults	·20–50	60	50

Indian Standards for Heights and Weights

Body weight and height of the children reflect their state of health and growth rate, while adult weight and height represent what can be attained by an individual with normal growth. In recommending nutrient intakes, desirable heights and weights of both children and adults, rather than the prevailing ones, are considered necessary since the RDA is intended for a healthy and well-nourished population.

Presently available anthropometric data on well-to-do Indian children indicate that their heights and weights correspond to National Centre for Health Statistics (NCHS) standards, up to the age of 14 years in the case of boys and 12 years in the case of girls. However, the committee recommends that anthropometric data should be collected on healthy, well-nourished children of high income group from different parts of our country so that reliable Indian standards can be drawn up for heights and weights of Indian children. The weights and heights of children aged between 0 and 18 years that are used for computing requirements are given in Table 18.2.

Table 18.2: Mean values of heights and weights of well-to-do Indian children

Age (year)	Boys		Girls	
	Height (cm)	Weight (kg)	Height (cm)	Weight (kg)
1+	80.07	10.54	78.09	9.98
2+	90.01	12.51	87.93	11.67
3+	98.36	14.78	96.21	13.79
4+	104.70	16.12	104.19	15.85
5+	113.51	19.33	112.24	18.67
6+	118.90	22.14	117.73	21.56
7+	123.32	24.46	122.65	24.45
8+	127.86	26.42	127.22	25.97
9+	133.63	30.00	133.08	29.82
10+	138.45	32.29	138.90	33.58
11+	143.35	35.26	145.00	37.17
12+	148.91	38.78	150.98	42.97
13+	154.94	42.88	153.44	44.54
14+	161.70	48.26	155.04	46.70
15+	165.33	52.15	155.98	48.75
16+	168.40	55.54	156.00	49.75
17+	173.00	57.91		
18+	172.05	58.38		
19+	172.14	58.90		
20+	171.75	59.64		
21+	172.40	59.74		
22+	171.63	60.14		

Data from 1+ to 4+ age group were collected in Hyderabad and for the remaining age group, it was taken from different parts of the country.

Source: A report of the expert group of the Indian Council of Medical Research, 2000, nutrient requirements and recommended dietary allowances for Indians, ICMR.

Table 18.3: Summary of RDA for Indians (1989)

Group	Particulars	Body wt (kg)	Net energy (kcal/d)	Protein (g/d)	Fat (g/d)	Calcium (mg/d)	Iron (mg/d)	Vit.A µg/d Retinol	β-carotene	Thiamin (mg/d)	Riboflavin (mg/d)	Nicotinic acid (mg/d)	Pyridoxin (mg/d)	Ascorbic acid (mg/d)	Folic acid (µg/d)	Vit. B12 (µg/d)
Man	Sedentary work		2425							1.2	1.4	16				
	Moderate work	60	2875	60	20	400	28	600	2400	1.4	1.6	18	2.0	40	100	1
	Heavy work		3800							1.6	1.9	21				
Woman	Sedentary work		1875							0.9	1.1	12				
	Moderate work	50	2225	50	20	400	30	600	2400	1.1	1.3	14	2.0	40	100	1
	Heavy work		2925							1.2	1.5	16				
	Pregnant woman	50	+300	+15	30	1000	38	600	2400	+0.2	+0.2	+2	2.5	40	400	1
	Lactation 0–6 months	50	+550	+25	45	1000	30	950	3800	+0.3	+0.3	+4	2.5	80	150	1.5
	6–12 months		+400	+18						+0.2	+0.2	+3				
Infants	0–6 months	5.4	108/kg	2.05/kg				350	1200	55 µg/kg	65 µg/kg	710 µg/kg	0.1			0.2
	6–12 months	8.6	98/kg	1.65/kg		500				50 µg/kg	60 µg/kg	650 µg/kg	0.4			
Children	1–3 years	12.2	1240	22	25	400	12	400	1600	0.6	0.7	8	0.9		30	
	4–6 years	19.0	1690	30			18	400	1600	0.9	1.0	11	1.6	40	40	0.2–1.0
	7–9 years	26.9	1950	41			26	600	2400	1.0	1.2	13			60	
Boys	10–12 years	35.4	2190	54	22	600	34	600	2400	1.1	1.3	15	1.6	40	70	0.2–1.0
Girls	10–12 years	31.5	1970	57			19			1.0	1.2	13				
Boys	13–15 years	47.8	2450	70	22	600	41	600	2400	1.2	1.5	16	2.0	40	100	0.2–1.0
Girls	13–15 years	46.7	2060	65			28			1.0	1.2	14				
Boys	16–18 years	57.1	2640	78	22	500	50	600	2400	1.3	1.6	17	2.0	40	100	0.2–1.0
Girls	16–18 years	49.9	2060	63			30			1.0	1.2	14				

Many national and international bodies have set dietary reference standards (RDA) (Table 18.3). Originally, the primary aim of these standards was to help prevent nutritional deficiency and ensure nutritional adequacy within a population. However, the sole use of the RDA as a dietary reference standard has a few limitations.

i. Because an RDA covers the needs of virtually everyone, it overestimates the needs of many. In more, affluent societies, it is becoming increasingly apparent that while nutrient deficiency remains a problem in some sectors of the population; surplus intakes lead to health problems for many others.

ii. It tends to be assumed that the term 'recommended' means the same as 'required'. This is not the case. The nutrient 'requirement' is the amount sufficient to meet individual needs and prevent deficiency. The amount 'recommended' is a generous allowance that includes a safety factor to take account of individual variability.

iii. There are close interrelationships between metabolisms of nutrients. Establishment of the requirements for a particular nutrient is complicated by numerous interrelationships with other nutrients in the diet. The body does not work in water tight compartments. There is always multi-nutrient relationship. Certain relationships are well established like calcium and vitamin D and certain others not so well understood. Interrelationships can be of several types:
   - Precursor interrelationship—tryptophan to niacin.
   - Chemical combination or reaction—vitamin C and iron.
   - Noncompetitive metabolic interrelationship—folic acid and iron.
   - Competitive interrelationship—zinc and copper.
   - Exchange interrelationship—vitamin E and selenium. The level of intake of one nutrient can influence the requirement of the other. A few examples are given in Table 18.4.

Table 18.4: Dietary components that influence nutrient requirement

Nutrient	Influence by dietary components
Protein	Requirement related to calories when the latter are deficient.
Essential amino acids	Utilization curtailed if any essential amino acid is deficient.
Phenylalanine	Requirement inversely related to tyrosine intake.
Methionine	Requirement inversely related to cystine intake.
Valine, leucine, isoleucine	Requirement of each is increased by excess of other branched chain amino acids.
Vitamin E	Requirement proportional to intake of polyunsaturated fat.
Thiamine	Requirement proportional to calorie intake.
Niacin	Requirement inversely related to tryptophan intake.
Vitamin B$_6$	Requirement increases by protein intake.

Contd.

Table 18.4: Dietary components that influence nutrient requirement (*Contd.*)

Nutrient	Influence by dietary components
Folacin	Requirement increases by alcohol intake.
Calcium	Urinary excretion increases by high protein intake. Absorption of calcium decreases by fats.
Non-haeme iron	Absorption improved by vitamin C or sulphur containing amino acids.
Copper	Absorption decreased by calcium, requirement increased by excess dietary zinc.

DIETARY REQUIREMENTS FOR SPECIFIC NUTRIENTS

Energy

The energy allowances recommended are designed to provide enough energy to promote satisfactory growth in infants and children and to maintain constant body weight and good health in adults. Among the factors which influence the energy needs are age, body size, activity and in a limited way climate and altered physiological status such as pregnancy and lactation.

Units of Energy

The unit of energy which has been in use in nutrition for a long time is the kilocalorie (kcal). However, recently the International Union of Sciences and the International Union of Nutritional Sciences (IUNS) have adopted 'Joule' as the unit of energy in place of kcal. These units are defined as follows:

A joule is defined as the energy required to move 1 kg mass by 1 meter by a force of 1newton acting on it. One Newton is the force needed to accelerate 1 kg mass by 1 m per sec^2.

The unit kcal is defined as the heat required to raise the temperature of 1 kg of water by 1°C from 14.5°C to 15.5°C.

$$1 \text{ kcal} = 4.184 \text{ kJ (kilo joules)}$$
$$1000 \text{ kcal} = 4184 \text{ kJ} = 4.18 \text{ mJ (mega joules)}$$
$$1 \text{ kJ} = 0.239 \text{ kcal}$$

Deriving Estimates of Energy Requirments of Adults

Energy requirements are best determined by measurements of energy expenditure. Energy expenditure from a physiological point of view is made up of three major components:

  i. Basal metabolic rate (BMR)
 ii. Regulatory thermogenesis, which is categorized into obligatory and facultative components and includes the metabolic response to food ingested, i.e. the use of energy in digesting, absorbing, storing and disposing of ingested nutrients as well as the response of the body to stimuli such as cold, stimulants and drugs.

iii. Physical activity, which includes both the cost and quantum of the activity as well as the types of activity, viz.

   a. Essential economic or occupational activities and

   b. Discretionary activities, while include household tasks, socially desirable activities and activities aimed at maintenance of physical fitness.

For all practical purposes, the components of energy expenditure related to regulatory energy output or thermogenesis are known to merge into measurements related to the cost of physical activity. Consequently the new simplified approach has only two principal components of energy expenditure: BMR and physical activity. Assessment of energy requirements is then based on specifying the needs for the basal metabolic rate and then considering all physical activity costs as effectively occurring in the fed state (i.e. inclusive of the energy costs of thermogenesis) (Table 18.5).

Table 18.5: Comparison of energy cost of some common activities in terms of BMR units

Activity	Energy cost of activities in BMR units	
	Indian data	International data
Sitting quietly	1.20	1.25
Standing quietly	1.40	1.33
Sitting at desk	1.30	1.36
Standing and doing lab work	2.0	1.95
Harvesting	3.6	3.5
Hand saw	7.4	7.5
Typing (sitting)	1.58	1.69
Walking 3 MPH	3.71	3.77

The modified equations applicable to Indians as recommended by the ICMR Committee are given in Table. 18.6. Basal metabolic rates calculated using these equations for Reference Indian man (60 kg) and woman (50 kg) will be 1517 and 1169 kcal per 24 hours respectively.

Guidelines for the use of recommended dietary allowances of energy:

1. Energy allowances represent only the average requirement and no allowance is to be made for any safety margin, in contrast to other nutrients (such as protein), since excess intake of energy has undesirable consequences.

2. Energy requirement for adults are given in terms of a Reference Man and Woman. Energy requirement of other individuals of different body weights and age have to be calculated as suggested. In computing average energy requirement of a population also, weighted averages will have to be used.

3. Energy requirement of adults should be related to energy expenditure rather than to intake. In case of children below 10 years of age, however, energy requirements are related to intakes for satisfactory growth.

Table 18.6: Equations for predicting BMR (kcal/24 hrs.)

Sex	Age (years)	Prediction equation Proposed by FAO/WHO/UNU	Proposed by ICMR expert group for Indians*	Correlation coefficient	S.D
Male	18–30	15.3 × B.W. (kg) + 679	14.5 × B.W. (kg) + 645	0.65	151
	30–60	11.6 × B.W. (kg) + 879	10.9 × B.W. (kg) + 833	0.60	164
	>60	13.5 × B.W. (kg) + 587	12.8 × B.W. (kg) + 463	0.79	148
Female	18–30	14.7 × B.W.(kg) + 496	14.0 × B.W. (kg) + 471	0.72	121
	30–60	8.7 × B.W. (kg) + 829	8.3 × B.W. (kg) + 788	0.70	108
	>60	10.5 × B.W. (kg) + 596	10.0 × B.W. (kg) + 565	0.74	108

*5% lower than that proposed by FAO/WHO/UNU (1985)

4. For malnourished children, the recommended intakes for the actual age should be used and no adjustments for the actual body weights should be made.

Protein

Dietary proteins provide amino acids for the synthesise of body proteins and other biologically important nitrogenous compounds in the body. Adequate protein is essential during growth when new tissue proteins are being synthesized. In the adult, dietary protein is essential to synthesize new proteins that will replace those which are constantly being broken down. During pregnancy and lactation, additional proteins are required for the synthesis of foetal tissue proteins and milk proteins respectively. Dietary proteins should supply the eight essential amino acids (EAA) in the proper proportions needed by the body. The other twelve amino acids present are not considered essential since the body can synthesise them from other carbon and nitrogen sources. Since most of the body nitrogen is derived from proteins, protein and nitrogen requirements are used interchangeably.

Protein requirements have been determined by the following methods like such as:

a. N balance
b. Obligatory N loss and
c. The factorial method.

Although the factorial method was used earlier, greater reliance is currently placed on the N-balance method which reflects physiological reality and provides a true estimate of requirements of body proteins.

Protein Quality

An important factor in relation to defining protein needs is the quality of protein, since the efficiency of utilization of a dietary protein depends upon its ability to supply the required amount of essential amino acids (EAA). Animal proteins in general are of higher quality since they contain EAA, an important determinant of protein quality, in the right proportions. Egg protein in particular is used as a reference against which the qualities of other proteins are compared. Vegetable proteins are generally of poorer quality than animal proteins, not only because of lower digestibility but also because of their deficiency in one or the other of the essential amino acids, like lysine, methionine, and, etc. The relative biological quality of the mixture of vegetable proteins which are present in Indian diets that are based on cereals and pulses is only about 65 compared to the 100 of egg proteins.

Taking into consideration the available data on protein requirements in relation to the 1978 ICMR recommendations and the 1985 FAO/WHO/UNU recommendations, the present ICMR expert group has adopted the following principles in fixing the protein requirements of Indians:

1. Nitrogen balance data (both short term and long term) obtained under appropriate conditions should form the basis of arriving at minimum maintenance nitrogen requirements.
2. Daily protein requirements in different age groups should be expressed on a g/kg body weight basis. The safe level of requirement is given by the Mean ± 2SD of the mean requirements.
3. Requirements for protein should be derived by a two-step process. First, the level of requirement according to age has to be chosen and next the actual amount has to be calculated by multiplying with the standard body weight for that age. Only during adolescent and adult periods have requirements to be indicated according to sex.
4. The coefficient of variation of 12.5% which was used by the 1985 FAO/WHO/UNU committee should be used for all groups. This figure covers both intra-individual and inter-individual variations.
5. Nitrogen values of 8 mg/kg body weight for adults and 10 mg/kg for children as suggested by the 1985 FAO/WHO/UNU expert consultation are accepted for miscellaneous endogenous losses.
6. As in earlier ICMR recommendations, the requirement for protein should be given in terms of the average quality of the Indian diet, proteins from which are considered to have NPU of 65%.
7. In computing the protein requirements of children, the body weight standards are to be used as the reference values of weight for age.
8. The deliberations of the WHO/FAO/UNU expert group bring out the fact that the theoretical growth requirements based on factorial gains in nitrogen for children below 10 years of age have to be increased by a factor of 50% to obtain the physiological growth requirements. Similarly during pregnancy (second half), actual nitrogen retentions are 50% higher than the computed accretions of tissue nitrogen, though the FAO/WHO/UNU group disregarding this fact and recommended only the additional requirement of 925 g protein during pregnancy obtained by the factorial method. If 50% additions are used in calculating the growth requirement of children, a similar correction seems logical in arriving at the protein requirements for foetal growth in pregnancy.
9. For adults 0.5 g per kg body weight of (milk) protein is adequate. For other groups the minimum protein requirements as suggested by the FAO/WHO/UNU consultation are accepted.

In arriving at the RDA for protein in terms of the proteins actually present in Indian dietaries, a value of 65 NPU that has been found in several experimental studies has been used.

Protein Calorie Ratio of Diets

It is useful to consider together the protein and energy requirement on habitual Indian diets. The protein requirement can be expressed as the ratio of protein calories to total dietary calories (PE%). A comparison of this PE % value with the protein energy % of the diet will indicate whether diets can fulfill protein needs if an adequate quantity of the diet is eaten to meet the energy requirement. This concept is useful because in many population groups enough diet is not consumed to meet energy needs, resulting in energy deficits. The ratio of protein requirement, expressed as the ratio of protein calories to the energy requirements is given in Table 18.7 for various population categories. It will be seen that a PE % between 8 and 12 would meet the protein requirement of any group provided its energy needs are met.

Table 18.7: Protein energy ratios

Group	Recommended protein intake g/day	Recommended energy intake kcal/day	Protein energy ratio (%)
Reference adult			
(Moderate activity)			
Man	60	2900	8.3
Woman	50	2200	9.1
Pregnant woman	65	2500	10.4
Lactating woman (0–6 m)	75	2750	10.9
Preschool children:			
1–3 years	21	1240	6.8
4–6 years	29	1690	6.9
7–9 years	40	1950	8.2
Adolescents:			
13–15 years Boys	67	2450	10.9
Girls	62	2060	12.0
16–18 years Boys	75	2640	11.4
Girls	60	2060	11.7

Fat

Fat is a major nutrient and has several functions. Fat in the diet also helps in the absorption of β-carotene and other fat soluble vitamins. Dietary fat must also provide essential fatty acids (EFA) which are the functional components of membrane lipids and have other important metabolic function.

Quality of Fat

Besides being a concentrated source of energy, fats are also a source of essential fatty acids (EFA). Fats are made up of fatty acids which include saturated fatty acids like palmitic and stearic, monounsaturated fatty acids like oleic and polyunsaturated fatty acids like linoleic and linolenic. The latter two cannot be synthesized in the body and have to be supplied through dietary fat. Dietary fat with an equal proportion of saturated, monounsaturated and polyunsaturated fatty acids components have been considered as desirable.

Fats like ghee, hydrogenated fats and coconut oil are comparatively saturated and are poor source of EFA. Other edible oils are better source of EFA, their levels ranging from 10% in Palmolein to 25% in groundnut oil, 50% to 70% in cottonseed, corn, sunflower, soyabean and safflower oils. Linolenic acid content is found to be high in mustard/rapeseed (13%) and soyabean (5%). Essential fatty acid composition of commonly consumed edible oils and fats are given in Table. 18.8.

Table 18.8: Linoleic, linolenic acid content of edible oils (g/100 g)

Oil	Linoleic	Linolenic	Total EFA
Ghee	1.6	0.5	2.1
Coconut	2.2	–	2.2
Vanaspathi	3.4	–	3.4
Palmolein	12.0	0.3	12.3
Rape/mustard	13.0	9.0	22.0
Groundnut	28.0	0.3	28.3
Rice bran	33.0	1.6	34.6
Sesame	40.0	0.5	40.5
Cotton seed	50.3	0.4	50.7
Corn oil	50.0	2.0	52.0
Sunflower	52.0	Trace	52.0
Soyabean	52.0	5.0	57.0
Safflower	74.0	0.5	74.5

EFA Requirements

The desirable amount of linoleic acid to be consumed by a normal adult person has been placed at 3 en%. The requirements of linoleic acid during pregnancy and lactation are higher, i.e. 4.5 and 5.7 en% respectively. The EFA requirement of children is placed at 3 en% (Table 18.9).

a. Contains 20% EFA, about 6% would be from cereals and pulses and rest from milk, nuts, spices, etc.

b. EFA at least 20%.

c. Average for males and females.

Table 18.9: Fat requirement of Indians

Group	EFA requirement en%	Invisible fat en%	Minimum visible fat en %	g/day	Suggested desirable visible fat intake g/day	en%
Adults	3	10	5	12	20	9
Older children	3	10	5	12	22	9
Young children	3	10	5	8	25	15
Pregnant women	4.5	10	12.5	30	30	12.5
Lactating women	5.7	10	17.5	45	45	17.5

The invisible fats present in many Indian food materials have high linoleic acid content (rice 50%, wheat 55%, Bengal gram 65%, red gram 58% and linolenic acid contents of about 3%). The invisible fats in spices have a particularly high content of linolenic acid (5.4%). As a result, average Indian diet predominately based on cereals and some pulses including the diets of poor income groups carry sufficient linoleic acid levels and a proportion of linolenic acid as well.

Upper Limit of Fat

Although a minimum amount of fat is essential to provide EFA, fat intake above a certain level is also undesirable, being associated with health hazards like cardiovascular disease and obesity. Studies relating fat intake to cardiovascular diseases, suggest that an intake of fat energy at 30% or more of total calories is undesirable particularly in sedentary individuals. Since in India some 10–15% of this can come from invisible fat, visible fat intake should be kept below 20 en%. This means that daily visible fat intake should be kept below 50 g/day.

Minerals

Minerals that are important in human nutrition are calcium, phosphorus and magnesium and the electrolytes, sodium and potassium. Besides these macro elements, the body needs several other trace elements. These are known to be essential in many enzyme reactions and for many body functions. After reviewing the available information, the expert committee recommended dietary intakes of the main minerals and several trace elements.

Calcium and Phosphorus

Calcium is required by adult man for replacing Ca lost from the body through urine, stools, bile and sweat. About 20–30% of the Ca in the diet is absorbed and such absorption is greatly facilitated by vitamin D. Additional Ca is required during growth for skeletal development and during lactation for milk secretion. Long-term calcium balance studies among population groups consuming moderate levels of calcium indicate that calcium balance can be achieved with intakes of 300–500 mg/day. It was suggested that an

Table 18.10: Indian foods rich in calcium

Foods	Calcium mg/100 g	Foods	Calcium mg/100 g
Cereals/Millets		*Green leafy veg.*	
Ragi	344	Agathi	1130
Amaranth seeds	510	Amaranth	397
Rajkeera seeds	223	Fenugreek	395
Pulses/Megumes		Rape leaves	370
Bengal gram whole	202	*Milk and milk products*	
Horsegram whole	287	Cow milk	120
Rajmah	260	Buffalo milk	210
Nuts and oilseeds		Cheese	790
Gingelly seeds	1450	Khoa	956
Mustard seeds	490	*Fish and sea foods*	
Cumin seeds	1080	Hilsa	180
Poppy seeds	1584	Rohu	650

elemental Ca : P ratio of 1 : 1 may be maintained in most age groups, except in infancy where the ratio suggested is 1 : 1.5 (Table 18.10).

Iron

Iron requirements are derived by using the factorial approach which takes into account the basal loss in case of men, basal loss + menstrual loss in case of women and basal loss + growth requirement in case of children. Dietary iron requirements are prescribed at a level of absorption of 3% in adult men from habitual diets based on mixed cereals.

Iodine

The minimal requirement of iodine of adults of both sexes is considered to be in the range of 50–75 µg/day. However, the safe allowance of iodine for both sexes is set at 150 µg/day.

Trace Elements

Desirable daily intakes of some trace elements suggested for an adult are: chromium 65 µg, copper 2.2 mg, manganese 5.5 mg, zinc 15.5 mg and molybdenum 500 µg.

VITAMINS

Vitamin A: The recommended level of vitamin A (retinol) for an adult is 600 µg. In terms of β-carotene, it will be 2400 µg, the conversion and bioavailability factors used being 1 µg β-carotene = 0.25 µg retinol. In diets containing both retinol and β-carotene, the vitamin A content can be expressed as follows.

a. Retinol content in µg = µg retinol + 0.25 µg β-carotene, if retinol and β-carotene are expressed in µg.
b. Retinol content in µg = vitamin A International Units (IU) × 0.3 + β-carotene in IU × 0.15, if vitamin A and β-carotene are expressed in International Units.

Thiamine, riboflavin and nicotinic acid: The daily allowances for these vitamins are related to energy intake. The basic allowances per 1000 kcal are: thiamine 0.5, riboflavin 0.6 mg and nicotinic acid 6.6 mg niacin equivalents.

Niacin allowance also takes into account the contribution of tryptophan, assuming that 60 mg dietary tryptophan yield 1 mg of niacin in the body.

$$\text{Niacin equivalents} = \text{Niacin content} + \frac{\text{Tryptophan content in mg}}{60}$$

Folic acid: Allowance for folic acid is given in terms of the free folate (L. casei activity) present in foods. RDA of folate in pregnancy will be 300 µg in addition to the normal requirement of 100 µg. Since such high levels of folate cannot be obtained through diet alone, therapeutic supplementation becomes necessary in pregnancy.

Vitamin B_{12}: Recommended intake of vitamin B_{12} is 1 µg/day. Since this vitamin is entirely derived from animal foods, there is justification for including some animal foods in the daily diet.

Vitamin C: The recommendations for adults are 40 mg/day. For infants, the RDA is 25 mg/day.

Vitamin D: No recommendation for dietary vitamin D is made since adequate vitamin D can be obtained through exposure to sunlight in India. In conditions of inadequacy, vitamin D medicinal supplements may be given.

Vitamin B_6: Recommended intakes in mg/day are: Adults 2.0, pregnant and lactating women 2.5, infants 0.3 in the first 6 months and 0.4 in the 6–12 months period and children 0.9–2.0 at various age levels.

FOOD GROUPS

Foods have been classified into different groups depending upon the nutritive value, for the convenience of planning meals. Food groups such as "Basic four", "Basic five", or "Basic seven" can be used for planning meals as per the convenience. The "Basic Five Food Groups" are suggested by Indian Council of Medical Research (ICMR), a more practical system of food grouping. It helps in choosing a variety of foods and to make our diet more interesting and also to meet our nutritional requirements.

FIVE FOOD GROUPS SYSTEM

The five food group plan permits an individual to plan a menu to achieve nutrient intake as specified by RDA. The five food groups suggested by ICMR are given in Table 18.11.

Table 18.11: Five food groups and their major nutrients

Food groups	Main nutrients
1. *Cereal grains and products:*	
Rice, wheat, ragi, bajra, maize, jowar, barley, rice, flakes, wheat flour	Energy, protein, invisible fat, vitamin B_1, vitamin B_2, folic acid, iron, fibre
2. *Pulses and Legumes:*	
Bengal gram, black gram, green gram, red gram, lentil (whole as well as dhals), cowpea, peas, rajmah, soyabean, beans.	Energy, protein, invisible fat, vitamin B_1, vitamin B_2, folic acid, calcium, iron, fibre
3. *Milk and meat products:*	
Milk, curd, skimmed milk, cheese, chicken, lever, fish, egg, meat.	Protein, fat, vitamin B_2, calcium
4. *Fruits and Vegetables:*	
Fruits: Mango, guava, tomato, papaya, orange, sweet lime, watermelon.	Carotenoids, vitamin C, fibre, invisible fat, vitamin B_2, folic acid, iron
Vegetables (green leafy): Amaranth, spinach, gogu, drumstick leaves, coriander leaves, fenugreek leaves.	Carotenoids, vitamin B_2, folic acid, calcium, iron, fibre
Other vegetables: Carrots, brinjal, ladies finger, beans, capsicum, onion, drumstick, cauliflower.	Carotenoids, folic acid, calcium, iron, fibre
5. *Fats and sugar:*	
Fats: Butter, ghee, hydrogenated fat, cooking oils like groundnut, mustard, coconut.	Energy, fat, essential fatty acids
Sugar: Jaggery and sugar.	Energy

The five food group system can be used by health professionals for the following purposes:

- *Tool for nutritional assessment and screenings:* A brief dietary history system can disclose inadequacies of nutrient from any of the five groups. The information can be the first clue for the possibility of the subject may be the risk of developing 7 nutritional deficiencies.
- *Tool for nutritional counseling:* The dietary history based on the five food group system allows a health team to counselor teaches a patient about nutrition.
- *Explaining therapeutic diets to the patient:* Therapeutic diets are scientifically based on nutrient composition and groups which can be used in menu planning.
- *Food labelling and surveillance system:* Food groups can be used for food labelling and for nutrition surveillance system.

THE FOOD GUIDE PYRAMID

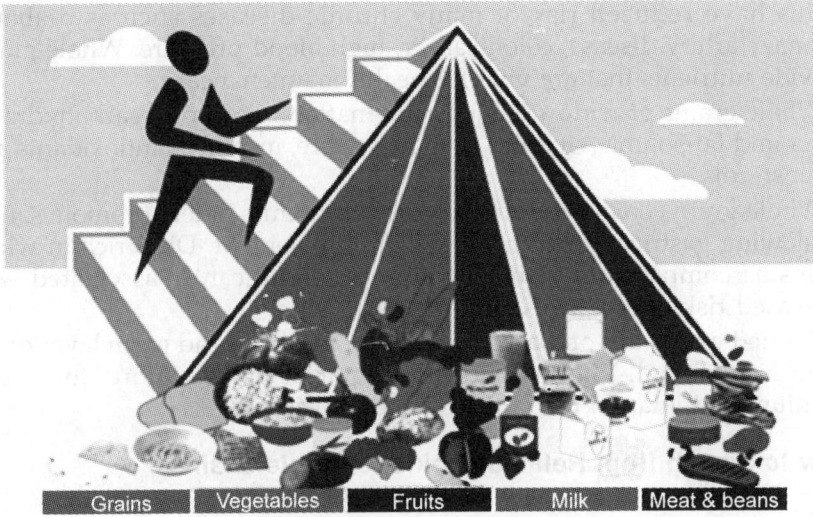

Fig. 18.1: Food guide pyramid

Grains

- Grains are an integral part of Indian diet providing basic energy, proteins, iron, fibre and many micronutrients.
- Different grains provide different proteins, carbohydrates, fibre and many nutrients. In vegetarians it is important to combine a grain with a pulse or two different grains to provide total proteins.
- Whole grains are preferred to refined grains.

Whole grains are more nutritious and disease preventing than refined grains. Freshly made refined grain products such as boiled rice, idli, upma, dosa, etc. are better than packed refined grain products (pasta, noodles). Rotis are better than buns.

Whole Grains and Products

Wheat: Roti, parantha, bahkri, puri, dhalia, whole bread, buns and biscuits.

Maize: Roti, bhutta, cornflakes, corn soup.

Other whole grains: Ragi balls, roti, porridge, dosa, bajra-roti, jowar-roti, buck wheat (kutu)-roti, poori, oatflakes, oatmeal.

Refined Grains and Products

Wheat: Bread, buns and biscuits, naan, rumali roti, white bread, buns, biscuits, noodles, spaghetti, pastas, bakery items, suji upma, etc.

Rice: Boiled rice, dosa, idli, poha, iddiappam, puttu, pointabhat, komal chaul, pithaguri.

Grains Can be Whole or Refined

Eating whole grains provide many health benefits. People who eat whole grains have reduced risk of many chronic diseases such as diabetes, coronary artery disease, colon cancer, high blood pressure. Whole grains provide nutrients that are vital for health maintenance.

Whole grains provide a unique combination of complex carbohydrates, water and fat-soluble vitamins, minerals, fibre, insoluble antioxidants and phytosterols.

Whole grain cereal products have low glycemic index; promote satiety by slowing gastric emptying due to its fibre content. Diets rich in whole grains as compared to refined grains are significantly associated with decreased risk of cardiovascular diseases.

Refined grains are prepared by milling. The bran and germ layer of the grain is removed. This reduces linoliec acid content, fibre, folic acid, selenium and vitamin E and many other nutrients.

How to Switch from Refined Grains to Whole Grains

Tips

- Get the wheat ground from a nearby chakki rather than buying readymade flours.
- Switch from polished rice to partially polished rice.
- Read label of products for words like "whole grain" or "whole wheat". In India, foods labelled with "stone ground", "100% wheat", "bran" are usually not whole grain products.
- Draining the excess of water while cooking of rice depletes them of valuable vitamins and it should be avoided.
- Idlis and dosas made with brown rice are preferable to those made from white rice. ·

Remember all freshly made grain preparations are better than packeted preparations. There is no substitute for fresh food.

Vegetables

- The colours of life
- Include a variety and plenty of seasonal, locally available fresh vegetables everyday in your daily diet (ensure a minimum intake of 500 g of fruits and vegetables).

White: Cauliflower, cabbage, radish, turnip, onions, garlic, mushroom, tapioca, vegetable marrow (safed kaddu), sweet potato, potato, yam, jack fruit, colocassia, ginger, lotus stem.

Green leafy vegetables: Amaranthus, bathua, spinach, fenugreek (methi), mustard, coriander, mint, curry leaves, drumstick leaves, lettuce agathi, ponnagani, gogu, shepu (soy saag), raddish leaves, cabbage leaves, cauliflower leaves, knoll-khol leaves, colocassia leaves.

Yellow: Pumpkin, squash, yellow capsicum.

Red: Carrot, beetroot, turnip, tomatoes, red peppers, raddish.

Other green vegetables: Ash gourd, ridgegourd, bottle gourd, snakegourd, bitter gourd, capsicum, broccoli, knoll knoll, drumsticks, tinda, chow chow marrow, bell pepper, sundakai, french beans, broad beans, double beans, cluster beans, cucumber, ladiesfinger, shallots, raw papaya, parwar, plaintain, kovai.

Purple: Brinjal, karonda.

Habitual consumption of a variety of fresh vegetables everyday reduces the risk of hypertension, stroke, coronary heart disease, cancer, diabetes and other chronic diseases.

Vegetables have a unique combination of nutrients like folate, vitamins, minerals, fibre, anti-oxidants and are relatively low in calories. All these work together to protect the body from disease. They have a high water content and low energy density which also assists in weight control. It is recommended that all age groups should consume a minimum of 300–400 g of vegetables everyday (along with a minimum of 200–250 g fruits everyday). Opt for a variety of seasonal, locally available and cheap vegetables. Locally available berries and greens are desirable.

Fruits

* Savour the rainbow on your plate.
* Eat a variety of fresh fruits everyday
* Colourful fruits and vegetables provide a wide range of vitamins, minerals, and phyto-chemicals.
* Fruits have a unique combination of micro and macro nutrients which protect against many diseases.

Red and orange: Apple, orange, strawberries, cherries, tangerine (kinow), papaya, pomegranate, watermelon, raspberries, plums, zizyphus (ber), tomatoes, loquat, bael fruit, litchi, passion fruit.

Yellow: Mango, sweet lime, lemon, musk melon, peaches, pineapple, wood apple, apricots, figs, jackfruit ripe.

Green: Grapes, pears, guava, gooseberry, kiwi fruit, star fruit.

Purple: Purple grapes, phalsa, jamoon, black currants, plums.

Brown: Sapota (chikoo), dates.

White: Banana, custard apple, water-chestnut

Fruits are irreplaceable by any other food items. They contain the magic and unique combinations of micro and macronutrients and anti-oxidants and many other ingredients that we are yet to discover!

Daily regular consumption of fruits leads to lower risk of high blood pressure, stroke (paralysis), coronary artery disease, cancer, diabetes and other chronic diseases. It also enhances the body's immune system, prevents acute diseases and delays ageing. It lowers blood pressure in persons already having high blood pressure.

It is recommended that all age groups should consume a minimum of 200–300 g of fruits daily (along with a minimum of 250 g or more of vegetables). Preferably include a variety of fruits which are seasonal, cheap and easily available. Locally available seasonal cheap berries are also very beneficial. Try and include more of citrus fruits.

The beneficial effects of fruits and vegetables are due to a unique combination and the presence of:

- Antioxidants and micronutrients such as vitamins A, C, E, and selenium (yellow, orange, purple, green fruits and vegetables) and fibre.
- The high potassium which has protective effect on blood pressure, reduces the risk of developing kidney stones and may help to decrease bone loss.

Oils and Nuts

- Meet most of your fat requirements from nuts, fish and vegetable oils.
- Limit solid fats. Use a mixture of oils rather than one oil or eat foods cooked in different oils. But beware, oils are calorie dense and their intake should be limited in quantity.
- Remember, vegetable oil is zero cholesterol, but they are not free of fatty acids.
- The caloric content, all cooking oils, butter and fats are the same, i.e. 9 kcal/gm

Fats and Oils

Body needs fat to function properly. This is provided from three sources: Invisible fat in food that we eat, like pulses, grains etc; visible fat which is used to cook the food or put in the food; and fat which is made endogenously in the body.

Dietary fats and oils are combination of glycerol with fatty acids. The major kinds of fatty acids in the foods are saturated, monounsaturated, polyunsaturated and trans fatty acids. It contains the same amount of calories—about 120 calories per tablespoon. Visible dietary fats carry fat-soluble vitamins—vitamins A, D, E and K—from your food into your body.

SATURATED FATTY ACIDS

Saturated fats (SFA) are usually solid at room temperature. Since our body manufactures its own saturated fat, we don't need to include any in our diet. It is found mainly in animal foods and dairy products (exceptions: palm oil, coconut oil). Saturated fats increases total cholesterol, LDL-C (bad), and triglycerides.

MONOUNSATURATED FATTY ACIDS

Monounsaturated fat (MUFA) is found in animal products and vegetables. Monounsaturated fat is believed to lower total cholesterol with no change or slight increase in HDL-C (good). It is cardio-protective, lowers blood glucose and triglycerides in type II diabetes. It may also offers protection against certain cancers, like breast cancer and colon cancer. The major fatty acid composition of MUFA is oleic acid.

Oils high in monounsaturated are best for cooking (frying). For example, groundnut, mustard, canola, rapeseed, olive oil. They have high oxidation thresholds: Meaning, they remain stable at higher temperatures and are not easily transformed into hydrogenated or saturated fats.

Monounsaturated fatty acids (MUFA) are liquid at room temperature but start to solidify on refrigeration.

POLYUNSATURATED FATTY ACIDS

Polyunsaturated fatty acids (PUFA) are liquid at room temperature and in the refrigerator. PUFA are not manufactured by our body and must be obtained in our diet and are hence called essential fatty acids.

These healthy fats include the family of omega 3 and omega 6 fatty acids.

Omega 6 is the commonest PUFA in the diet. The richest natural source of omega-6 (Linoleic) is safflower oil. Other good sources include sunflower, corn, soybean and wheat germ oil.

Omega 3 is much less widely available. It is further divided into alpha-linoleic acid, eicosapentaenoic acid (EPA) and docosahexaenoic acid (DHA). The best natural source of linoleic acid is flax seed oil. EPA and DHA are found in fatty fish such as mackerel, herring, salmon, and tuna.

Polyunsaturated fat helps to reduce total cholesterol, LDL-C (bad) and triglycerides more significantly than MUFA, with a slight drop in HDL-C. When omega 6 fatty acids are consumed in excess, it is shown to increase the risk of cardiovascular disease, cancer, and inflammatory and autoimmune diseases. Hence when consumed in the correct ratio (3 : 1 omega-6 to omega-3), polyunsaturated essential fatty acids offer a wide range of specific benefits.

Health benefits of omega-3 and omega-6 fatty acids are:
- Anti-thrombotic and anti-arrhythmic properties and hence have shown protection against cardiovascular disease.
- Anti-carcinogenic properties.
- Anti-inflammatory properties which protect against diseases such as rheumatoid arthritis, gingivitis and asthma.
- Help to regulate blood glucose levels by increasing insulin sensitivity.
- Seems to lower the risk of Alzheimer's disease and may also benefit conditions such as attention deficit disorder, dyslexia and dysphasia.
- Skin complaints such as eczema and psoriasis.

Milk and Milk Products

- Milk and milk products provide essential calcium and other nutrients.
- Go for low fat or fat-free milk. Drink a minimum of 250–500 ml of low fat pasteurized milk or consume milk products instead. If your diet doesn't contain other sources of calcium, then drink/eat 750 ml of low fat milk and milk products everyday.
- If you can't have milk, then include other sources of calcium into your daily diet.

People who have a daily diet rich in milk and milk products throughout their lifecycle, have a higher bone mass than those who don't. Thus regular daily consumption of skimmed milk or skimmed milk products can reduce the risk of osteoporosis in later life. Nutrients in milk are calcium, potassium, vitamin-D and protein. The calcium in the milk is very easily absorbed in the intestines. In the absence of other sources of dietary calcium, 750 ml of skimmed milk should be consumed.

During childhood and adolescence and throughout life adequate intake of milk and milk products along with weight bearing exercises (walking, playing outdoor games, etc.) is important to enhance and maintain bone strength and density.

Since milk is a rich source of total protein and calcium, it is an important component of a balanced healthy diet. In case standardized and pasteurized milk is not available,.milk should be boiled, cooled and consumed after eliminating the top creamy layer. In persons who have abnormal lipid profile only skimmed milk and its products are recommended. Consumption of condensed and sweetened milk products, which are calorie dense, should be restricted.

Whole milk contains both saturated and unsaturated fatty acids. Hence whole milk and its products are important contributors to dietary fat and cholesterol and its excessive consumption leads to rise in blood cholesterol levels and coronary heart disease.

Composition of Cows and Buffalos Milk (Table 18.12)

Table 18.12: Cows and buffalos milk

Milk	Total caloric value/100 ml	Cholesterol (mg)	Saturated fatty acids (g)	Proteins (g)	Calcium (mg)
Cow	67	14	2	3.2	120
Buffalo	117	16	4	4.3	210

* The bioavailability of calcium in the milk is very good which means calcium will be absorbed.

Pulses (Dals), Fish, Meat

- Pulses (dals) in the Indian diet are the primary source of protein. It's important to eat dal everyday more so in vegetarians.

- Each dal has a unique combination of amino acids. Dal needs to be combined with grains or another dal to provide total protein to the body.
- In non-vegetarians pulses can be substituted with fish, chicken and meat.

Husked (With Chilka)

Bengal gram (white), bengal gram (black), black gram, cow pea, rajma, broad beans, soy bean, peas, moth, masoor dal, green gram dal.

De Husked (Dhuli)

Tuar dal, chana dal, black gram dal, masoor dal, moong dal.

Pulses provide vegetable protein, complex carbohydrate, dietary fibre, vitamins, minerals and isoflavones.

Indian diet consists of a variety of pulses and legumes, which differ, in their amino acid composition, fibre content, and in micronutrients. All pulses have low glycemic index and are rich in soluble fibre. Include a variety of dals in your daily diets. All freshly made dals are healthy and nutritious.

Dehusking or milling of dals decreases their nutritive value and fibre content. Hence husked dals are preferred to dehusked dals. Shift from refined dals to whole dals.

Fish

Fish (fresh water and sea fish) are excellent source of proteins, omega-3 fatty acids, vitamins (A and D), minerals (iodine, phosphorus and calcium). Based on site of storage of fat, fish can be classified into fatty or oily fish and lean or white fish.

Fatty fish such as herring, salmon, mackerel, hilsa, purava, and seer that store fat in the *muscle* are rich sources of omega-3 fatty acids-eicosapentaenoic acid (EPA) and docosahexaenoic acid (DHA). The protective effects of fish on coronary artery disease are probably mediated by these fatty acids.

Lean fish like pomfret, murrel, katla, rohu, bhetki that store fat in the *liver* are high in protein, vitamins, minerals, and low in fat. These fishes can be used as meat substitutes. They have their own anti-thrombotic properties in spite of low fatty acid content.

Fish should be eaten either in boiled/ baked/grilled/steamed form for better health benefits as frying the fish brings change in its fatty acid composition and its beneficial effects are destroyed. Hence it is recommended that at least 200–300 g of fish should be taken in a week. Prefer fish to fish oil supplements and capsules.

Balanced Diet

"Balanced diet is one which contains different types of foods in such quantities and proportions so that the need for calories, proteins, minerals, vitamins and other nutrients is adequately met and a small provision is made for extra nutrients to withstand short duration of leanness".

A balanced diet should provide around 60–70% of total calories from carbohydrate, 10–12% from protein and 20–25% of total calories from fat, and also should provide bioactive photochemical such as dietary fibre, antioxidants and nutraceuticals.

NUTRITIONAL CLASSIFICATION OF FOODS

Nutritionally food can be classified into three categories:
I. Energy-yielding foods,
II. Body-building foods,
III. Protective foods.

ENERGY-YIELDING FOODS

This group includes foods rich in carbohydrates, fats and protein.
- One gram of carbohydrate gives 4 calories.
- One gram of protein gives 4 calories.
- One gram of fat gives 9 calories. They may be broadly divided into two groups. They are,
  1. Cereals, pulses, roots and tubers.
  2. Pure carbohydrates like sugars and fats.
     - Cereals provide, in addition to energy, the greater part of the proteins, certain minerals and vitamins.
     - Pulses provide protein and B vitamins besides energy.
     - Roots and tubers mainly provide energy and to some extent minerals and vitamins.
     - Pure carbohydrates like sugars provide only energy (empty calories).
     - Fat provide concentrated source of energy.

Body Building Foods

Foods rich in proteins are called body building foods. These may be broadly divided into two groups:
a. Milk, egg, meat and fish, rich in proteins of high biological value.
b. Pulses, oilseeds and nuts and low-fat oilseed flours rich in proteins of medium nutritive value.

Protective Foods

Foods rich in proteins, vitamins and minerals are termed protective foods.
Protective foods are broadly classified into two groups:
a. Foods rich in vitamins, minerals and proteins of high biological value, e.g. milk, eggs, fish and liver and
b. Foods rich in certain vitamins and minerals only, e.g. green leafy vegetables and some fruits.

Low-cost Balanced Diet

The nutrition expert group of the Indian Council of Medical Research (ICMR) has recommended certain dietary allowances for balanced diets. However, diet surveys in different parts of the country have shown that the content of different nutrients in Indian diets is considerably lower than the recommended levels. An attempt has, therefore, been made here to suggest nutritious low-cost menus within the economic means of the people.

The menus suggested are meant mainly for the lower income groups of people. Modifications in these menus needed to bring them into closer conformity with the recommendations for the ideal diet have also been indicated at the end of this section. These modifications will naturally put up the cost of the dietaries. However, for the higher income groups who can afford the increased cost, these modified menus are recommended.

In drawing up these menus, the following principles have been followed:

As a result of extensive diet surveys, considerable information on the dietary pattern and practices of the population has been collected. In suggesting menus, care has been taken to include mainly foods which are in common use in the locality and which are, therefore, not 'foreign' to the people. The recipes suggested are again generally based on the prevalent cooking practices in the community. It is, therefore, expected that the popularization of these menus will not involve drastic changes in the dietary habits of the people and will, therefore, not encounter significant psychological 'resistance'. This would mean that the propaganda and nutrition education required will be minimal.

While rice is the major staple cereal of a considerable part of the south, an attempt has been made here to replace a part of the rice, preferably half of it, with wheat, millets and tubers. Recent researches have shown that such combinations apart from lessening the demand on rice may also be beneficial from the nutritional standpoint. Different preparations based on wheat, millet and tapioca have also been suggested with a view to popularizing the consumption of these foods among the predominantly rice-eating South Indian communities. Emphasis has also been laid on the need for the inclusion of foods other than cereals like pulses, fish, vegetables and fruits. It is further recommended that generous amounts of fish or pulses should be taken whenever tapioca forms the staple food.

Since these menus are mainly meant for the low income group, they have been so framed that the number of courses per meal is minimal and the cooking procedures are simple. In addition, a number of alternatives in the exchange lists are provided so that there will be no monotony in the diets and there will be reasonable variety.

The menus are suggested for an adult and are based on 425 g cereals, 70 g pulses or fish, 100 g of leafy vegetables, 75 g of other vegetables, 30 g of oil, 30 g sugar or jaggery, 115 g of milk and about 30 g of fruits per day. The calorific value will work out to about 2400 with a protein intake of about 60–70 g per day. All other nutrients will be supplied in reasonable amounts to satisfy at least the minimal requirements. However, diets suggested here are not necessarily the ideal for the community. They could be considered to be the nutritious low-cost diets possible under the prevalent socio-economic conditions.

For persons who can afford the extra cost daily one egg can be included. In addition, intake of milk can be increased from 115 ml to 200 ml for vegetarians and about 30 g meat or fish can be included for non-vegetarians. These will provide variety and avoid monotony in the diet (Table 18.13).

Table 18.13: Balanced diets for pre-school children (low cost) (ICMR Nutrition expert group)

Foodstuffs	1 to 3 years		4 to 6 years	
	V (g)	NV (g)	V (g)	NV (g)
Cereals	150	150	200	200
Pulses	50	40	60	50
Green leafy vegetables	50	50	75	75
Other vegetables, roots and tubers	30	30	50	50
Fruits	50	50	50	50
Milk	300	200	250	200
Fats and oils	20	20	25	25
Meat, fish an eggs	–	30	–	30
Sugar and jaggery	30	30	40	40

UNIT IV

PREPARATION, PRESERVATION AND STORAGE OF FOOD

19

Cooking

Cooking not only improves the taste, smell and appearance of foods but it may also improve its digestibility. Cooking may also improve the keeping qualities of food by killing moulds, yeasts and bacteria that promote decay though cooking needs to be distinguished from the use of heat treatment to preserve food.

Cooking may be simply defined as the heat treatment of foods carried out to improve the palatability, digestibility and safety of foods

Table 19.1 summarizes the principal methods of cooking food and it also indicates the different ways in which heat can be used for cooking. The source of heat may be the result of combustion of wood, coal, gas or oil by electric heating elements contained in hot plates or electric ovens, or by a microwave cooker.

Table 19.1: Methods of cooking

Method	Examples	Description	Method of heat transfer
Dry heat	1. Baking and roasting	Cooking in an oven or other closed vessel.	Hot air and reflected radiant heat
	2. Grilling and broiling	Direct heating.	Radiation and some convection
Moist heat	1. Boiling	Cooking in boiling water.	Conduction
	2. Steaming	Cooking directly by stem (or in a steam-heated vessel).	Conduction (and convection)
	3. Pressure cooking	Cooking by steam under pressure.	Conduction
	4. Stewing and simmering	Cooking in water below its boiling point.	Conduction
Hot fat	1. Frying	Food partly or completely immersed in heated fat.	Conduction
	2. Braising	Brief frying in shallow fat followed by stewing.	Conduction
Microwave		Food subject to microwave radiation in an oven.	Heat generated in food.

Water or steam and air or fat or combinations of these are used as cooking media. Moist heat involves water and steam. Air or fat are used in dry heat. Foods can also be cooked by microwaves.

MOIST HEAT METHODS

Boiling: Boiling is a common method of moist heat cooking, it utilized the fact that because water has a high specific heat, it is an efficient heat, reservoir and therefore is a convenient medium in which to transfer heat to food. Boiling is cooking foods by just immersing them in water at 100°C and maintaining the water at that temperature till the food is tender water is said to be boiling when large bubbles are seen raising constantly on the surface of the liquid and then breaking rapidly. Water receives heat by conduction through the sides of the utensil in which the food is cooked and passes on the heat by connection currents which equalize the temperature and become vigorous when boiling commence. When foods are cooked by boiling, the food should be brought to a vigorous boil first, and the heat is then turned down, as violent boiling throughout tends to break out the food. Further temperature of water cannot be increased because continued vigorous boiling results in excessive evaporation of water and waste of fuel. Foods are also likely to get burnt at the bottom and form a dry crust at the top.

Advantages

1. Boiling is a simple method which does not need skills and equipment.
2. Uniform cooking can be done.
3. Easy method of cooking and safe and simple
4. It is appropriate for large-scale cookery.

Disadvantages

1. Vegetables when cooked by boiling results in an inevitable loss of mineral elements and vitamins.
2. Although a little or no carotene is lost when vegetables are boiled considerable amounts of thiamine, and ascorbic acid are destroyed as both these vitamins are water soluble and easily destroyed by heat.
3. By boiling minerals such as sodium, potassium, calcium get leaches into water.
4. The loss of minerals and vitamins increases as the amount of water used increases. For example, in a series of experiments it was found that cabbage which lost 60% ascorbic acid when cooked in a small volume of water, lost 70% when cooked in larger amount. This water can be reused to prepare dishes like sambhar, rasum, dhall. Time-consuming procedure and fuel gets wasted.

Simmering

When foods are cooked in a pan with a well fitting lid at temperature just below the boiling point 80–99°C of the liquid in which they are immersed, the process is known as simmering. It is an useful method when foods are cooked for a long time. One can use this method to prepare soups, custards, halwa, kheer, etc.

Advantages

1. Foods get cooked well.
2. Scorching or burning is prevented.
3. Losses due to leaching are minimum.

Disadvantages

1. There is a loss of heat sensitive nutrients, due to long period of cooking.
2. Time and fuel get wasted. ,

Stewing

Stewing involves cooking food in hot water, the temperature of which is kept below its boiling point; the changes which occur in stewing are, therefore similar in characters to those which occur during boiling though they occur at a slower rate. Stewing being a slow method of cooking involves considerable loss of soluble matter. This method is generally used for cooking cheaper cuts of meals along with some root vegetables and legumes, all put in the same cooking pot and cooked in stock or water. The larger cooking time and lower temperature enable tougher meat fibres to become soft. A few fruits and vegetables can also be stewed. It is suitable for cooking tough meat.

Advantages

1. This process makes the dish attractive and nutritious since liquid is discarded.
2. Because of low temperature used, protein is also lightly coagulated and is therefore, in its most digestible form.
3. It exerts a tenderizing effect on protein food because insoluble tough collagen is converted into soluble gelatin by prolonged contact with hot water, therefore it is suitable for cooking tough meat.

Disadvantages

Time and fuel get wasted since it is a long-time cooking method.

Steaming

This method of cooking includes using the steam produced from boiling water. As the contact between the food and water is less than in boiling, there is smaller loss of soluble matter.

Three types of steaming get done:

1. *Wet steaming:* In this procedure food will have direct contact with steam, e.g. idly, dhokla, idiappam, etc.

2. *Dry steaming:* In this kind of cooking double boilers are used. Double boiling is cooking in a container over hot water. Food is usually kept in one utensil and water in the other utensil, e.g. custards.

3. *Waterless cooking:* In this method the steam originates from the food itself. Cooking food wrapped in aluminium foil or in a plastic bag is a form of waterless cooking. In this case, there is the advantage of preventing the transmission of flavour from or to the sealed food.

Advantages

1. Cooking time is less
2. Steamed foods are easily digestible and texture will be soft.
3. Nutritionally good since there is no contact between food and water. Leaching will not happen.

Disadvantages

Limited recipes can be done by this method.

Pressure Cooking

The rate of cooking in steaming may be increased by the use of steam under pressure, this being the principle of the pressure cooker. Pressure cooking is a device to reduce the cooking time by increasing the pressure so that the boiling point of water is automatically raised. While water boils at 100°C at normal atmospheric pressure, it boils at 121°C at a pressure of 1.07 kg/cm^2 which is the pressure at which food is cooked in a kitchen pressure cooker.

In cooking by the steam, the food is heated as a result of steam condensing on the food, and the release of the large quantity of heat (latent heat) contained in the steam. This continues until the heated food reaches the same temperature as steam.

Advantages

1. Nutrient loss is less by this cooking.
2. It takes less time and fuel gets saved.
3. Food get cook thoroughly.
4. Flavour loss will be less, taste will be good.

Disadvantages

Usage of equipment and procedure to use should be well known, otherwise accident can happen.

Dry Heat Methods

Dry heat methods of cooking use higher temperatures than moist heat method. In this either air or fat is used as the medium of cooking.

Air as medium of cooking: Grilling, roasting and baking take place in air.

Grilling or Broiling

Grilling consists of placing the food below or above a red hot surface. When under the heater, the food is heated by radiation only. This results in the browning of many foods, then the heat is more slowly conducted through the surfaces of the food downward. As heating is most superficial, grilled foods are usually reversed or toasted. If the food is above the heater, heat is transmitted to the food through convection current as well as radiations with consequent increased efficiency.

Advantages

1. Quick method of cooking
2. Less fat required
3. Fuel and time saved
4. Flavour gets enhanced
5. Grills may be situated in view of customers.

Disadvantages

1. Should pay more attention to prevent charring.
2. More suitable for expensive cuts of meats
3. Requires skill.

Pan Broiling or Roasting

Pan broiling is the cooking of food by exposing it to direct heat. In this case, cooking takes place by conduction through direct contact of food with the hot broiler some radiation cooking also takes place in broiling.

Advantages

1. Reduces the moisture content of food and improves storage life of food.
2. Roasted foods are easy to powder.
3. Improves the texture and flavour of food.
4. It is an easy method of cooking.

Disadvantages

Constant attention is needed.

Baking

Food gets cooked by hot air. Basically the food is cooked partially by dry heat and partially moist heat, if the food is high in moisture content. In baking, the oven atmosphere should be moist initially so that the moisture condenses on the cold dough.

This helps in heat transfer and plays a part in the formation of crust. The oven is insulated to prevent the outside temperatures from causing fluctuations in internal temperatures of the equipment. Baking involves heat transfer from the heat source in the oven by radiation, conduction and convection. Heat is transferred directly into the container of the food through which it is conducted to the food. Temperatures that are normally maintained in the oven are 120–260°C. Foods prepared by baking are custards, pies, pizzas, buns, biscuits, bread, cakes, fish, meat and chicken varieties.

Advantages

1. It uses less oil than frying method.
2. Less possibility of the production of less toxic byproducts (free radicals).
3. Baked foods tend to be more "savoury" due to partial caramelisation process that the food undergoes.

Disadvantages

1. The equipment and procedures to be done need to be handled by skilled person.
2. It requires more energy to cook.

Cooking in fat: Fat is used at medium for cooking in sauteing, shallow fat frying (pan frying) and deep fat frying.

Sauteing

Sauteing is the cooking of food in a slightly greased pan. Only thin pieces of food are cooked this way, e.g. dosa. This prevents food from sticking to the pan. The heat is transferred to the food mainly by conduction. The food is to be turned from one side to the other to complete the cooking. The product obtained in cooking by this method is slightly moist, tender but without any liquid or gravy. Foods cooked by sauteing are generally vegetables used as side dishes in a menu.

Shallow Fat Frying

In this method, food is cooked in a larger amount of fat, but not enough to cover it. Heat is transferred to the food partially by the convection currents of the food. This prevents local burning of food by keeping away the intense heat of the frying pan. As in sauteing, even in this case, the food must normally be turned over to ensure some degree of uniform cooking. Both sauteing and pan frying are really a type of baking.

Deep Fat Frying

Deep fat frying is similar to boiling. Food is cooked by vigorous convection currents and cooking is uniform on all sides of the foods. As fat can be heated to a much higher temperature than the boiling point of water, cooking can be rapidly completed in deep fat frying. In most foods, this high temperature results in rapid drying out of the surface, and the production of a hard, crisp surface, usually brown, and the absorption of a fair amounts of fat, which raises the calorific value of the food substantially.

Fats should not be heated to the smoking point as they decompose at the point to fatty acids and glycerol, followed by the decomposition of glycerol to acrolein which causes irritation to the eyes and nose.

Advantages

1. Quick method of cooking
2. Texture and taste get improved.
3. Increases the calorific value.

Disadvantages

1. More attention is needed while cooking food to avoid charring of food.
2. While cooking, one has to be careful to avoid accidents.
3. Oily food takes time to get digest.
4. Repeated use of heated oils may produce harmful substances and reduce the smoking point.

Effects on Nutrients by Dry Heating Cooking Methods

Dry heat methods of cooking use higher temperature than moist heat methods and loss of nutrients which are sensitive to heat is correspondingly greater. Apart from mineral salts, which are stable to heat, all nutrients are affected to some extent by dry heating.

Fat: Fats are stable to moderate heating and although they darken, little breakdown occurs unless they are heated to high temperatures when they start to decompose with the formation of acrolein, which has an unpleasant acid odour.

Carbohydrates: Carbohydrates are affected by dry heat. Starch is converted into pyrodextrins which are brown in colour and which contribute colour to toast and bread crust, sucrose is converted into dark-coloured caramel in a complex multistage reaction that involves its initial breakdown into monosaccharides and its final polymerization into coloured substances.

Vitamins

Dry heat cooking destroys those vitamins which are unstable to heat, notably ascorbic acid, which as we have already noted, is destroyed at quite low temperature, the B vitamins, thiamine, is the most readily destroyed while riboflavin is relatively stable, a little being lost provided that the pH of the food is below 7. Nicotinic acid is stable to heat and any losses that occur due to leaching into the liquid lost from the food during heating.

Proteins

Proteins are externally sensitive to heat but their nutritive value is not significantly affected unless they are heated to a fairly high temperature, such as occurs in roasting. Loss of nutritive value depends not only on the cooking temperature but also on the time of cooking and the pressure of other nutrients, particularly carbohydrates. Amino acids are only destroyed at high temperatures such as employed in roasting and even then the loss of protein is small and confined to the surface of the food. A much greater loss of nutritive value results from a change in protein structure which affects the linkages between amino acids in such a way that they become resistant to enzymic hydrolysis. Amino acids affected in this way—notably aspartic acid, glutamic acid and lysine cannot be released by enzymes during digestion and are therefore unavailable to the body.

When protein and carbohydrate exist together in the same food, an additional loss of nutritive value may occur due to non-enzymic browning also called the Maillard reaction. Reaction occurs between amino groups projecting from a protein chain or peptide or amino acid and the carbonyl group of a reducing substance such as glucose. The first of which is an addition reaction between the amino acid and carbonyl groups and the last is a polymerization to form a brown substance. Several amino acids undergo this reaction, notably lysine and methionine. The reaction results in the formation of substances which cannot be hydrolyzed by enzymes, and the proteins affected are thus unavailable to the body.

Non-enzymic browning occurs particularly at high temperature and at pH values of seven and above: A certain amount of moisture are also necessary. The reduction in nutritive value of protein due to non-enzymic browning has been studied intensively in terms of the loss of lysine during cooking, e.g. it has been found that bread loses 10–15% lysine during baking, a further 5% during staling and a further 5–10% during toasting. Apart from producing some loss in the nutritive value of proteins during dry heat cooking, non-enzymic browning is also responsible for producing some desirable changes in the flavour, colour and aroma of food during roasting, baking, and toasting. For example, it improves the quality of bread during baking and toasting and of nuts and coffee beans during roasting.

COMBINATION OF COOKING METHODS

Braising: Food may also be prepared by combination of media. Braising is a combined method of roasting and stewing in a pan with a tight fitting lid. Preparation of uppuma, for example, involves the use of combination of fat and water media, some components (onions) of the preparation are first browned in a small quantity of fat followed by the cooking of semolina in water, e.g. chicken biryani, vermicelli payasam, vegetable cutlet, meat balls, samosa.

Microwave Cooking

Microwave cooking, which was first recognized as valuable for cooking food in 1947, is becoming more and more popular because it is a convenient and very quick method of cooking food. Microwaves do not require any medium for transfer of heat in cooking. They are generated by an electric instrument called magnetron microwaves which have a high frequency of

2,450 mj (or 2,450 million times) per second. The microwaves can be absorbed, transmitted or reflected when they impinge on substances. They pass through paper, glass and some plastics without absorption; and are reflected by metals and absorbed by food. When food is kept in the cavity of a microwave oven for cooking, microwaves generated by the magnetron strike the food and the metal walls are reflected and bounce back so that they disperse through the oven. This is accomplishing a uniform heating of food. Microwaves penetrate food to a depth of 2.5 to 7.5 cm, up to this limit of penetration of the microwaves, the food gets heated and cooked. Thus, food will heat up inside and outside at the same time. When the thickness of food is large, microwave will heat it up throughout at the same time to the depth of their penetration and the portion of food beyond it will be heated more slowly by conduction. Food, for cooking in a microwave oven, should not absorb or reflect them. This is achieved by using paper containers, such as paper plates or cups, or utensils made of plastic, glass or chinaware, which do not contain metalic substances.

Precautions to be taken while Microwave Cooking

1. Do not dry meats, herbs, fruits and vegetables in the oven.
2. Do not leave open unattended while in use.
3. Do not heat narrow mouthed containers as the liquid may boil over even after cooking has stopped.
4. Do not attempt to deep fry in microwave oven. Cooking oils may burst into flames. Microwave utensils may not be able to withstand the temperature of the hot oil and could shatter.
5. For even cooking place in the oven equal distances apart.
6. Do not heat eggs with their shell in microwave oven. Pressure will build up and the eggs will explode.
7. Potatoes, apples, eggyolks, and whole vegetables must be pierced before microwave cooking to prevent bursting.

Advantages

1. The most important advantage of microwave cooking is the speed with which cooking may be accomplished resulting in a considerable saving of time in cooking.
2. Microwave heating also saves time in heating refrigerated or frozen foods. The latter can be defrosted in minutes instead of hours.
3. During cooking, only food gets heated, the oven does not get heated and utensils do not become hot, except when the cooking period is relatively long and some heat is conducted from the food to the container.
4. The flavour and texture of prepared food do not change when reheated in microwaves.
5. Electrical energy required for microwave cooking is less than that required by the traditional method.
6. Preserves the natural colour of fruits and vegetables.

Disadvantages

1. Due to the short period of time of cooking, the food does not become brown on the surface as many foods do when they are roasted or baked in a conventional oven, unless microwave has a browning unit.
2. The short cooking time may not give a chance for the blending of various flavours to develop as in the conventional methods of cooking.
3. Microwave cooking cannot be employed for simmering or stewing for tenderizing foods, as also for deep-fat frying.
4. The operator should be careful in operating the microwave oven since any exposure to microwave oven causes physiological abnormalities.

20 Food Preservation

IMPORTANCE OF FOOD PRESERVATION

Food preservation can be defined as the science which deals with the process of prevention of decay or spoilage of food and helps it to be stored in a fit condition for future use.

Preservation of food material has played a vital role avoiding widespread starvation and it continues to do so till date, even in industrially developed world. Food supply has to keep pace with the needs of the population. There is always shortage of food in developing countries like India because of demand of increasing population. Therefore, it is important to improve and expand facilities for storage and preservation of food.

- Delay in the use of fresh foods alters their freshness, palatability, and nutritive value but by preserving these foods, spoilage can be avoided. Thus perishable foods can be made available throughout the year by preservation.
- By preservation and proper storage of food, it can be saved for future use at the time of scarcity, natural drought, etc.
- Preservation of food also helps in stabilizing the prices of the food by making the availability of seasonal foods throughout the year.

CLASSIFICATION FOR FOOD PRESERVATION

Foods have been preserved for centuries by various techniques. Various methods for the preservation of foods based on techniques which eliminate moisture and other factors causing food spoilage have been devised and practiced. For purpose of food preservation, foods are classified into perishable, semi-perishable and non-perishable.

1. *Perishable foods:* The perishable foods are those which deteriorate quickly after harvesting such as tomatoes, mangoes, papayas, peaches, plums and other juicy fruits, also some juicy vegetables and meat, fish and poultry. These foodstuffs have a high degree of moisture content and are highly susceptible to spoilage.

2. *Semi-perishable foods:* They have much less moisture content. Semi-perishable commodities are those that do not require refrigeration, but

still have a limited shelf life. They include things such as potatoes, onions, pumpkins and salamis. These items are usually kept on shelves in the storeroom complex, where they get plenty of air circulation around them. Potatoes need to be kept away from light as they will start sprouting.

3. *Non-perishable foods:* Non-perishable foods are "shelf-stable" items that do not spoil or decay. They can withstand months of shelf life.

Most canned foods such as vegetables and fruits are considered to be non-perishable, provided that they are properly processed and the containers show no signs of leakage. Other foods include dried peas and beans and grain products such as wheat, barley and oats are also considered non-perishable. Some foods are vacuum-packed like tuna and tofu and can remain on the shelf for a long period of time. Big blocks of processed American cheese, often used in macaroni and cheese and melted dips, can remain on the shelf almost indefinitely. Pastas, including macaroni and spaghetti, will store for indefinite periods of time.

PRINCIPLES OF FOOD PRESERVATION

Food spoilage may be caused due to chemical and biological factors. Inherent enzymes present in food may cause spoilage under certain conditions. Growth of bacteria, molds or yeasts already present or inoculated in food while processing causes more serious spoilage than enzymes. To prevent spoilage of food, various methods of preservation are available which are based on certain principles.

The basic principles of food preservation primarily involves the process of inhibiting:

1. The growth and activity of microorganism.
2. Activity of endogenous enzymes.
3. Invasion and spoilage by insects and rodents.

1. *Inhibiting the growth and activity of microorganism:* This can be achieved by
    - Keeping out microorganism (asepsis)
    - Removing the microorganism, e.g. by filtration
    - Hindering the growth and activity of microorganisms, e.g. by the low temperature, drying, anaerobic conditions, chemical or antibiotics.
    - Killing the microorganism, e.g. by heat, or radiation.

2. *Inhibit the activity of endogenous enzymes:* This can be achieved by:
    - Destruction or inactivation of food enzymes, e.g. by blanching.
    - Prevention or delay of purely chemical reactions, e.g. prevention of oxidation by use of antioxidants.

3. Invasion and spoilage by insects and rodents

Food if not packed and stored properly, may be attacked by insects, worms, etc. which damage the products and make them unfit for human consumption. This can be prevented by the use of chemicals. So keeping quality of products can also be retained by using proper packaging material.

Based on these principles, various methods of preservation are developed. These methods can be broadly divided into two categories on the basis whether the activity of microorganisms is being stopped or killed by that method.

Bacteriostatic Methods

Growth of microorganisms can be prevented by changing the environmental conditions. Such conditions are called bacteriostatic conditions in which number of microorganism remain static.

These conditions can be created by removal of water, use of acid, use of oil, smoking, freezing, etc.

1. *Asepsis:* Asepsis means keeping out microorganisms (absence of infection). If there is protective covering around the food, the microbial decomposition of food is delayed or prevented. If nature covering like shell of nuts, skin of fruits and vegetables husk of corn, shells of eggs, and the skin, membrane of fat on meat or fish or damaged decomposition spreads from outer surface to inner surface.

   Packaging of food is widely used application of asepsis. Use of clean vessels and hygienic surroundings prevents spoilage of milk during collection and processing.

2. *Removal of Microorganisms:* Removal of microorganisms may be accompanied by
   – Filtration
   – Centrifugation (sedimentation of classification)
   – Washing and Trimming

   a. *Filtration:* In filtration, the liquid is filtered through a sterilized "Bacteria Proof" filter made up of asbestos pads, sintered glass, unglazed porcelain membrane pads, etc. and the liquid is forced through it by positive or negative pressure. This method is successful with water, fruit juice, beer, soft drinks, wine, etc.

   b. *Centrifugation (or) sedimentation:* In this method only some of the microorganisms are removed but not all. It is used mainly in water and milk. Centrifugation at high speed removes most of the spores.

   c. *Washing and trimming:* Washing raw fruits removes soil organisms that might be resistant to heat. Trimming away helps in removing the spoiled portion of food that may be helpful in food preservation.

3. *Maintenance of anaerobic condition:* A condition in which no or only a minimal amount of air or oxygen is present is termed anaerobic. Lack of oxygen prevents growth of any surviving bacteria. During canning, spores of some aerobic organisms may survive the high temperature but in sealed cans they are unable to grow due to the absence of oxygen.

Completely filled container, evacuation of the unfilled space or replacement of air by some inert gas (N_2 or CO_2) produces anaerobic condition. Fermentation also helps in maintenance of anaerobic condition.

4. *Drying:* Presence of excess moisture in food leads to food spoilage. Food preservation by drying is the oldest and simplest method practiced from ancient times. Drying of food involves removal of water under controlled conditions in such a way the microorganisms cannot grow and enzyme activity is controlled. Dried foods contain moisture to the extent of 1–5%, and they have storage stability at room temperature of a year or longer. There are many methods of drying. Some are particularly suited for liquids, others for solid foods or mixture containing food pieces.

The common drier types used for liquid and solid foods may be categoried as the air-convection driers, drum or roller driers and vacuum driers. In the air-convection method, hot air supplies the heat for evaporation. If liquid, the food may be sprayed or poured into pans or on belts.

Drum or roller driers are limited to be used with liquid foods, puree and mashes that can be applied as thin films.

Vacuum driers are employed to lower the temperature of drying. Freeze driers are vacuum driers where, at an extremely low temperature water vapour directly forms ice without going through the liquid state. The above division of drier is not rigid, since many driers are combination, e.g. a drum drier can be operated in vacuum or by blowing high-velocity heated air.

5. *Salting:* Salt used in high concentration (15–20%) helps to increase the keeping quality. Presence of salt at high concentration prevents the water from being available for bacterial growth. Salt reduces the solubility of oxygen in moisture, it ionizes to heal chlorine ion which is harmful to organisms and it also sensitizes the cell against CO_2. Effectiveness of salt varies with its concentration and temperature.

The effects of salts are:

   a. Causes high osmotic pressure and hence plasmolysis (shrinking) of cell.

   b. Dehydrates food by drawing out and tying up moisture as it dehydrates microbial cells.

   c. Ionizes to yield the chloride ion, which is harmful to organisms.

Examples of salting preparation of tamarind, raw mango, amla, fish, and meat.

6. *Sugaring:* Addition of sugar binds the moisture and prevents growth of microorganisms and helps to preserve the food. Sugar acts by osmosis; sugar used at high concentration (65%) or above can preserve the food for a long time. Example of food preserved by sugaring are sweetened condensed milk, jams, jellies, marmalades and candies.

7. *Pickling:* Pickling was widely used to preserve meats, fruits and vegetables in the past, but today it is used to almost exclusively to produce "Pickles" or pickled cucumbers, onions and sauces. Pickling uses the salt combined with the acid, such as acetic acid (vinegar). Vinegar or acetic acid checks aerobic and anaerobic fermentation. It possesses germicidal and antiseptic properties. It is more effective against yeast and bacteria than moulds. Its effectiveness increases with a decrease in pH, examples of some of the fruits and vegetables which lend themselves to pickling are raw mangoes, limes, amla, ginger, turmeric and green chillis.

8. *Fermentation:* This is one of the oldest method of preservation. Any other methods of preservation, such as drying, salting, sugaring, pickling, etc. have the common objective of decreasing the number of microorganisms in food or holding them against further multiplication. In fermentation, multiplication of microorganisms and their metabolic activities are encouraged. However, the organisms that are encouraged to grow and multiply are the select groups whose metabolic products help food preservation.

The term fermentation means the breakdown of carbohydrate material by microorganisms (or enzymes) under anaerobic conditions. In the fermentation of foods, a complex mixture of carbohydrates, proteins, fats, etc. undergo modifications simultaneously under the action of a variety of microorganisms and enzymes present. Thus, the carbohydrates and carbohydrate-like materials undergo fermentation, proteinaceous material undergo proteolysis or "putrefactive" breakdown and lipids "lipolytic" breakdown. The nature and extent of these changes depend upon the food, types of microorganisms present and conditions affecting their growth and metabolic pattern. The preservative effect of fermentation is caused by the chemicals excreted by the microorganisms. The principal chemicals involved are acids (especially lactic acid) and alcohol. These inhibit the growth of common pathogenic organisms in foods.

The list of foods produced by fermentation is extremely long and includes the following: Cheese, curd, butter, all alcoholic beverages, pickles, sauerkraut, vinegar, bread, idli, soya sauce, coffee, tea and cocoa.

The benefits of fermentation are:
- It produces flavour and textural changes.
- More nutritious than unfermented, synthesize several vitamins and other growth factors.
- Indigestible carbohydrates like cellulose and hemicelluloses are converted into digestible carbohydrates such as sugars and their derivatives.

9. *Cheese Making:* This is used in preserving the milk for a long period. In this process, the milk in cheese becomes something completely unlike

milk, but cheese has its own interesting and delicious properties. Cheese making is a long and involved process that makes use of bacteria enzymes and naturally formed acids to solidify milk proteins and fats and preserve them.

10. *Smoking:* In smoking foods are exposed to smokes by burning some special kinds of wood. It has two main purposes—adding desired flavouring and preserving. Most meat is smoked after curing to aid its preservation. Preservation action is provided by such bactericidal chemicals in the smoke as formaldehyde and creosote, and by the dehydration that occurs.

11. *Cold preservation:* Preservation of food by cold storage with the development of mechanical refrigeration system made cold preservation of food, food processing, storage and distribution widespread. It has become possible to transport perishable foods for a long distance, and make seasonal food available at all time of the year. Low temperatures are used to retard the chemical reaction and action of food enzymes. The rate of chemical reaction, enzyme action and microbial growth is directly related to the temperature; lower the temperature, the lower is the reaction. Freezing generally prevents the growth of most food-borne microorganisms and refrigeration temperature makes growth rate slow. Low temperature employed can be:

  a. Cellular storage temperature (about 15°C): It is used to store foods such as root crops, potatoes, onions, apples, etc. for a limited period.

  b. Refrigerated or chilling temperature (0°C to 5°C): Foods kept at this temperature slows down the microbial activities and chemical changes resulting in spoilage. Mechanical refrigerator or cold storage is used for this purpose, e.g. meat, poultry, eggs, fish, fresh milk and milk products, fruits, vegetables, etc. can be preserved for two to seven days.

  c. Freezing (–18°C to – 40°C): In freezing water in food turns into ice and makes unavailable for reaction to occur and for micro-organisms to grow. Most perishable foods like poultry, meats, fish, ice creams, peas, vegetables, juice concentration, etc. can be preserved for several months at this temperature. Freezing is cheaper than canning and frozen products of better quality than canned products, but for storage of frozen products uninterrupted supply of electricity is essential. In vegetable enzymes action may still produce undesirable effects on flavour and texture during freezing. Hence, heating like blanching should be done to destroy the enzymes before the vegetables are frozen.

12. *Heat preservation:* This is very commonly used method of food preservation. The microorganisms are killed by heat due to denaturation of proteins and inactivation of enzymes. Most bacteria, yeasts and moulds show a growth optimum between 16°C and 38°C

(Mesophiles). Such organisms, in general, do not grow below 5°C and above 45°C. Some organisms grow in the range of 66 – 82°C (Thermophiles). Most bacteria are killed in the range of 82 – 93°C. However, bacterial spores and certain other heat-resistant forms can withstand prolonged exposure to 100°C. Some organisms endure this temperature for 5½ hours. However, they last only minutes at 120°C and are destroyed in moist heat at 100°C in about 15 min. The thermal death of microorganisms in dry air is due to oxidation. Therefore, a high temperature is required for their destruction. In wet heat, cell death is due to coagulation consisting of reactions between proteins and water; this is also accelerated by raised temperatures.

The heat treatment required to kill microorganisms or their spores varies with the kind of organisms, its state and the environment during heating. The heat treatment selected depends on:

– Kinds of organisms to be killed.
– Other preservative method to be employed.
– Nature of food to be preserved.
– Effect of heat on the food.

The temperature and exposure period depend on the food to be treated. Food such as milk or certain soft vegetables cannot be heated for a long period of time without undergoing a change in appearance and shape. More intensive the heat treatment, more effective it will be for destruction of microorganisms. Various heat treatments used to prevent spoilage of foods might be classified as:

– Pasteurization temperature (below 100°C)
– Heating at about 100°C
– Sterilization temperature (100°C or above)

Pasteurization

Pasteurization is a heat treatment that kills a part but not all the microorganisms present and usually involves the application of temperatures below 100°C. This process serves two objectives:

• It destroys pathogenic organisms associated with the food.
• Extends the products shelf-life by decreasing the microbial population and inactivating some enzymes.

There are three methods of pasteurization:

• Bottle or "Holding" pasteurization
• Overflow method.
• Flash pasteurization

    a. *Bottle or "Holding" pasteurization:* This method is commonly used for the preservation of fruit juices at home. The extracted juice is strained and filled in bottles. The bottles are then sealed air-tight and pasteurized.

    b. *Overflow method:* Juice is heated to a temperature of about 2.5°C higher than the pasteurization temperature, and filled in hot sterilized bottles.

The sealed bottles are sterilized at a temperature of 2.5°C and then cooled.

c. *Flash pasteurization:* The juice is heated rapidly to a temperature of about 5.5°C higher than the pasteurization temperature and kept at this temperature for about a minute. This method has been developed specially for canning of natural orange juice, grape and apple juice. The advantages are loss of flavour is minimum, and vitamins are not destroyed.

The choice of temperature and time of pasteurization will be influenced by the consideration of the purpose of the process and the chemical and physical composition of food. Thus, milk is pasteurized at 62.8°C for 30 minutes, to inactivate pathogens and whole egg at 64.4°C for 2–5 minutes, to control the dissemination of *Salmonella spp.* The other foods which are usually pasteurized are beer, wines, fruit juices, etc.

Pasteurized products are not sterile. They contain vegetative organisms and spores still capable of growth. Pasteurized foods must be stored under refrigeration.

The spore-forming bacteria found in tomato juice, however, require heating at a higher temperature for a much longer duration. Acid fruit juices require a lower temperature and less time for pasteurization than the less acid ones. Juices and milk can be pasteurized in two ways.

i. *HTST (high temperature – short time) method:* HTST, using a temperature of 130°C and above for short times, for example, milk is heated to 72°C and kept at this temperature for 15 seconds.

ii. *LTLT (low temperature – long time) method:* In this method the product is heated at lower temperature for a longer time. For example, milk is heated at 62.8°C for 30 minutes.

Boiling or Heating at About 100°C

Cooking of rice, vegetables, meat, fish, etc. at home is usually done by boiling the food with water and involves a temperature around 100°C. Blanching of fresh vegetables before freezing or drying also involves heating at about 100°C. This method does not destroy the spores of *C. botulinum* in non-acid foods.

Sterilization

The complete destruction of microorganisms is known as sterilization. This is achieved when organisms are exposed at 121°C to wet heat for 15 min. Canned foods which are commercially sterile have a shelf-life of two years or more. Since the heat required for complete sterilization of food also adversely affects the properties of foods, the heat treatment given should be just enough to destroy the pathogenic organisms and toxins, and ensure desired storage life.

Canning

Canning is the process in which the foods are heated in hermetically sealed (air tight) jars or cans to a temperature that destroys microorganism and inactivates enzymes that could be a health hazard or cause the food to spoil.

Aseptic Canning

Aseptic canning is an application of high temperature processing. In normal canning, heat transfers from the outside of the container to the inside will require several minutes or even hours depending upon the container size to reach the sterilization temperature. The time of sterilization can be shortened to seconds or even fraction of a second in aseptic canning. The basic principle of this method is that food is pumped continuously through a plate-type or tubular heat exchanger which heats it very quickly to a high temperature holding it at that temperature for time required and then cooling. Food temperature employed may be as high as 150°C and sterilization takes place in 1 or 2 seconds. Such a rapid sterilization at high temperature is referred to as ultra-high-temperature (UHT) sterilization. The sterile food is quickly cooled, placed in aseptic containers and the lids are sealed while in a sterile environment. The food canned aseptically retains the nutrients and the sensory attributes will be good. Such types of foods if stores for one year may lose only 25% ascorbic acid from fruits and vegetables, 20–30% of thiamine from meat but riboflavin content is not affected. Carotene content losses in fruits and vegetables are small even after months of storage.

13. *Food concentration:* Foods are concentrated for the same reason that they are dried—preservation and reduction in weight and bulk. Relatively a few liquid foods are preserved by concentration, mainly because of the reduction in water activity (a_w) and development of osmotic pressure which retard the microbial growth and enzymatic reactions. Concentration of food is usually done for reasons like: Reduction in volume and weight, reduction in packaging, storage and transport costs, better microbial stability and convenience. Examples of food preserved by concentration are tomato paste, fruit juice concentrate, soup and condensed milk. The main requirement to improve processing of these products is to control the rate of heating to prevent localized burning of the product, particularly when it has become thickened towards the end of boiling.

14. *Food additives:* Food additives are defined as *non-nutritive substances added intentionally to food, generally in small quantities to improve its appearance, flavour, texture or storage properties.* There are five main uses for food additives.

  i. To maintain product consistency.

  ii. To improve or maintain nutritional value.

  iii. To maintain palatability and wholesomeness.

  iv. To provide leavening or control acidity/alkalinity.

  v. To enhance flavour or impart desired colour.

There are over 3000 different chemical compound used as food additives. There are two categories of food additives: Enrichment substances and the Technological additives.

Enrichment Substances: These improve the nutritional value of food and used as a tool in reducing deficiency disease. For example, iodine is added to salt to avoid goiter and vitamins—A, D, E and K are added to hydrogenated fats to avoid health effects due to deficiency of these nutrients.

Technological Food additives: These are mainly used to increase the shelf life (preservative and antioxidants), or to give it a better taste (sweeteners and flavouring agents), or to change its consistency (emulsifiers and thickeners). Technological additives can be divided into sub-groups. Most of the additives are present in nature as natural constituents, for example, fruits and vegetables. However, some of them are now produced synthetically. Other additives that are produced synthetically are not present in nature. Semi-synthetic additives are natural compounds that have been chemically modified. Nevertheless, all these food additives, except for the flavouring agents, are pure compounds that have been evaluated for safety and their use and intake are regulated (Table 20.1).

Table 20.1: Food additives

Preservatives	Sodium benzoate in fruit drinks, potassium meta bisulfate in fruit products, sorbic acid in cheese, sodium and calcium propionates in breads and cakes, nitrates and nitrites in meats.
Antioxidants	Butylated hydroxy anisole (BHA), butylated hydroxyl toluene (BHT), propylgallate (PG), tocopherols in oily or fried foods, ascorbic acid, SO_2 in fruit products.
Sequestrants (chelating agents)	Polyphosphates, citric acid—to remove elements from the food.
Surface-active agents (emulsifiers)	Lecithin, mono- and di-glycerides and bile acids—to stabilize oil in water.
Stabilizers and thickeners	Gums, gelatin, carboxy methyl cellulose, pectin, egg yolk, etc. in jellies, chocolate milk drinks, pie fillings and cake toppings.
Bleaching and maturing agents	Oxides of nitrogen, chlorine dioxide in bleaching and maturing flour.
Food colours	Natural sources: Annatto, caramel, carotene, saffron; synthetic sources: Coal tar dyes.
Non-nutritive sweetners	Saccharin, cyclamates, etc.
Flavouring agents and flavour enhancers	Monosodium glutamate (MSG), 5' - nucleotides

Food Irradiation

Food irradiation is another sterilizing technique in which the foods are bombarded by high-energy rays called gamma rays, (wavelengths < 2Å) or by fast moving electrons emitted from excited radioactive elements and accelerated negatively charged particles, electrons (β-particles), which are emitted from a hot cathode. Gamma rays are very similar to X-rays, except that they have much greater penetrating power. An electron beam can be accelerated to very high speed and increased energies so that it can penetrate foods, by passing it through electronic devices.

Ultraviolet radiations are also employed in preservations, but they have a very low degree of penetration and are employed to inactivate microorganisms on the surface of food and to treat air, water and the surface of food processing equipment to reduce the number of microorganisms cobalt-60 or cesium-137 or electron-producing machines are the principal sources of ionizing radiations used for food irradiation. The unit of radiation is in terms of rads (kilorad or megarad). UV irradiation is being applied commercially in the following processes of food:

- Tenderizing or aging of meat
- Curing and wrapping of cheese.
- Prevention of surface mould growth on bakery products.
- Air purification in bottling and food processing.
- Treatment of knives for slicing bread.
- Treatment of bread and cakes.
- Sanitizing of utensils used for eating.
- Prevention of growth of film of yeasts on pickles, vinegar.
- Killing of spores on sugar crystals and in syrup.
- Treatment of air in storage and processing rooms.

  Effects of radiations on nutrients:
- Irradiation produce molecular changes in starch, converting it into sugar.
- It produces denaturation and coagulation of milk protein, e.g. casein.
- Losses of amino acids also occur ranging from 5 to 7%, e.g. tryptophan, methionine, phenylalanine, whereas there is an increase up to 60% in valine content of irradiated foods.
- Lipids are very sensitive to radiations. Auto-oxidation of lipids increases peroxide value and develops rancidity.
- During irradiation $2/3^{rd}$ of vitamin B_1 is found to be lost and only 37% of B_1 is retained.
- Frozen foods if irradiated, then vitamin C losses are very less.
- Vitamin K is sensitive to radiation and is destroyed in appreciable quantity during irradiations.

Uses of Radiations

- Used for sterilization of foods in hermetically sealed packs.
- Poultry products, seafoods and various fruits such as apples, mangoes, banana, etc. can be irradiated and preserved at low temperature for a long period.
- Prevents sprouting of potatoes, onions, etc. helps in long storage are of great economic value.
- It helps in delayed ripening in fruits, therefore, exports of fruits to foreign countries without deterioration in quality is done.
- Prevention of insect infestation in dry foods and food products—ionizing radiations are lethal to different stages of insects and also to eggs. Nuts, dried fruits and processed cereal foods can be preserved for a long period after disinfestations by radiation treatment.

21   Food Adulteration

Adulteration of food consists of substituting it wholly or in part by any cheaper or inferior substance or of removing any of its constituents, wholly or in part, which affects adversely the nature, substance or quality of food.

Under the PFA act, the definition of "food adulteration takes into account not only the intentional addition or substitution or abstraction of substances which adversely affects the nature, substance, and quality of foods, but also their incidental contamination during the period of growth, harvesting, storage, processing, transportation and distribution". To put it in simple terms, let us take an example of milk under the PFA act, a trader is guilty if he sells milk to which water has been added (intentional addition) or the cream of the milk has been replaced by cheap vegetable or animal fat (substitution) or simply the cream has been removed and the milk is sold as such, with low fat content (abstraction) unintentional contamination of the milk, due to carelessness on part of the trader is also considered as adulteration under the law. For instance, if the cans in which the trader is transporting or storing the milk, had been earlier treated with the chemicals like washing soda or boric acid or some detergent and not been washed thoroughly with water, residues of the chemicals may get mixed with the milk. Such milk would be considered adulterated. In addition, food is also considered to be adulterated, if it does not conform to the basic quality standards. For instance, the maximum amount of moisture allowed in a milk powder sample is 4%. If a sample is found to have greater moisture levels, it is considered to be adulterated.

Adulteration of foodstuffs is commonly practiced in India by the trade. In order to protect the health of consumer, the Government of India promulgated the prevention of Food Adulteration Act (PFA Act) in 1954, the Act prohibits the manufacture, sale and distribution of not only adulterated foods but also foods contaminated with toxicants and misbranded foods. A Central Food Laboratory established under the Act is located at Kolkata for the purpose of reporting on suspected food products.

The Central Food Technology Research Institute, Mysore has been recognized as another laboratory for the testing of adulterated foods for the southern region. A central committee for food standards has been constituted under the Act and has been charged with the function of advising the central government on matters relating to the food standards.

Provisions have been made in the Act for the appointment of food inspectors by the state governments and their powers have been defined. The state government will set up food testing laboratory and will appoint public analysis with adequate staff to report on suspected foods.

It is evident that according to PFA Act of 1954, food adulteration includes:

1. Intentional addition, substitution or abstraction of substances which adversely affect the quality of foods.
2. Incidental contamination of foods with deleterious constituents such as toxins, insecticides, pathogenic, bacteria and fungi, etc. due to ignorance, negligence or lack of proper storage facilities and
3. Contamination of the food with harmful microorganisms during production, storage and handling.

INTENTIONAL ADULTERANTS

Intentional adulterants and methods of identification of adulterants in different foods are given in Table 21.1.

Table 21.1: Simple methods for detecting adulterants

Sl.No.	Food	Adulterant	Method of detection
1.	Milk, milk product, powdered spices	Starch	Mix sample in a test tube with water, add a few drops of iodine solution. A blue colour indicates the presence of starch.
2.	Milk	Water	Measure the specific gravity with a lactometer by immersing it in milk kept in a deep vessel. The normal values lie between 1.028–1.032. But this is not a foolproof method, as, in addition to water, sugar or urea may have been added to the milk to increase its specific gravity.
3.	Milk	Developed acidity	Place a test tube containing 5 ml of the milk sample in a boiling water bath and hold for about 5 minutes. Remove the tube and rotate in an almost horizontal position. The film of milk on the side of the test tube is examined for any precipitated particles. Formation of clots is indicative of developed acidity in the milk due to microbial spoilage. Such milk is unsuitable for consumption.
4.	Milk, milk powder	Neutralizers like carbonates	To about 5 ml milk in a test tube add 5 ml of alcohol and a few drops of rosalic acid solution and mix the contents of the test tube. A rose red colour is obtained in the presence

Contd.

Table 21.1: Simple methods for detecting adulterants *(Contd.)*

Sl.No.	Food	Adulterant	Method of detection
			of a carbonate, whereas pure milk shows only a brownish colouration.
5.	Ghee, butter	Margarine or vanaspati	In one tea spoonful of completely melted sample, add 5 ml concentrated hydrochloric acid. Shake for 5 minutes, add a pinch of sugar or furfural. Appearance of pink colour in the acid layer indicates added vanaspati.
6.	Oils and fats, black pepper	Mineral oil	To 2 ml of oil sample taken in a flask, add 20 ml of 0.5 ml normal alcoholic potash. Heat for 30 minutes and add 20 ml hot water. If turbidity appears, mineral oil is present.
7.	Sweetmeats, ice cream and beverages, sella rice, pulses, spices	Metanil yellow	Extract colour with lukewarm water from food sample and add a few drops of concentrated hydrochloric acid. A magenta colour indicates the presence of metanil yellow.
8.	Pulses, whole and split, besan	Kesari dal	Kesari dal is wedge shaped, with a slant on one side and a square face on the other side. Physical examination can detect the adulterant.
		Metanil yellow	Put the sample in dilute hydrochloric acid. Pink colour develops indicating the presence of the adulterant.
9.	Mustard seeds	Argemone seeds	Argemone seeds have a rough surface and mustard seeds are smooth. Upon pressing, mustard seeds are yellow inside while argemone seeds are white.
10.	Black pepper	Papaya seed	Papaya seeds are comparatively shrunken, oval and greenish brown to brownish black in colour.
11.	Tea leaves, sugar	Iron filings	Easily separated using a magnet.
12.	Silver foil	Aluminium foil	To metal foil add 2 drops of concentrated nitric acid in a test tube. The silver foil will completely dissolve, whereas the aluminium foil remains undissolved.
13.	Honey	Sugar solution	A cotton wick dipped in pure honey, when lighted, burns smoothly. If water is present, it will not allow the honey to burn. Even if it does, a crackling sound is produced. (The test is for water which is there in the sugar solution added as an adulterant to honey).
14.	Coffee	Chicory	Sprinkle coffee powder on the surface of water in a glass. Coffee floats while chicory

Contd.

Table 21.1: Simple methods for detecting adulterants (*Contd.*)

Sl.No.	Food	Adulterant	Method of detection
			starts sinking leaving a trail of colour, due to a large amount of caramel.
15.	Tea	Artificial colour (coal tar dyes)	Put the tea leaves on a moistened blotting paper. Artificially dyed tea will impart colour to the moistened blotting paper immediately.
16.	Cardamom	Talc Powder	The sticking of talc on finger touch will indicate its presence. The talc powder sticking to the finger when tested will give an aromatic flavour which confirms extraction of essential oil.
17.	Coffee powder	Tamarind powder	Sprinkle a little coffee powder on a bloating paper and spray a little potassium hydroxide solution. It adulterated with tamarind powder, a brown colour spreads around the particles.
18.	Chilly or Turmeric powder	Colouring matter, (e.g. metanil yellow)	To a little powder in a test tube, add little quantity of ether and shake well. Let it stands. Transfer the extract into another test tube and add a few drops of concentrated HCl. A dark pink colour confirms adulteration.
19.	Jalebi	Metanil yellow	Put the sample in dilute hydrochloric acid. Pink colour develops indicating the presence of the adulterant.
20.	Khoa	Starch	Add tincture of iodine. Indication of blue colour shows the presence of starch.
21.	Saffron	Dyed tendrils of maize cob	Genuine saffron will not break easily like artificial one, the colour dissolve in water if artificially coloured.
22.	Wheat, bajra and other foodgrains	Ergot (a fungus containing a poisonous substance)	a. Purple black longer size grains in bajra show the presence of ergots b. Put some grains in a glass containing 20% salt solution. Ergot floats over the surface while sound grains settle down.
		Dhatura	Dhatura seeds resemble chilly seeds with blackish brown colour which can be separated out by close examination.
23.	Wheat flour	Maida	When dough is prepared from resultant wheat flour, more water has to be used and chapatis prepared out of this will blow out. The taste of chapatis prepared out of wheat is somewhat sweetish, whereas those prepared out of adulterated wheat flour will

Contd.

Table 21.1: Simple methods for detecting adulterants (*Contd.*)

Sl.No.	Food	Adulterant	Method of detection
			taste insipid.
24.	Common salt	White powdered stone, chalk	Stir a spoonful of simple salt in a glass of water. The presence of chalk will make the solution white and other insoluble impurities settle down.

INCIDENTAL CONTAMINATION IN FOOD CAN ALSO OCCUR BY THE MICROORGANISMS

Raw foods such as meat, fish, milk and vegetables grown on sewage purchased from the market are likely to be contaminated with harmful microorganisms. These are generally destroyed during cooking or processing of the food. Some of the microorganisms may survive due to inadequate heat processing. Further, some of the foods, if consumed in the raw state may cause food poisoning. Recent studies have shown that food grains, legumes and oilseeds when stored in humid atmosphere are infected by pathogenic fungus which can cause serious illness. The pathogenic microorganisms commonly contaminating foods and responsible for causing serious illness are listed in Table 21.2.

Table 21.2: Food-borne disease caused by some pathogenic organisms (*Contd.*)

	Microorganism	Foods commonly involved	Ill-effects and diseases
Bacterial	Bacillus cereus	Cereal products	Nausea, vomiting, abdominal pain
	Cl. Botulinum toxins	Defectively processed meat and fish and honey	Botulism (muscular paralysis, death due to respiratory failure)
	Cl. perfringens (welchii)	Defectively processed precooked meat	Nausea, abdominal pain and diarrhoea
	Salmonella	Defectively processed meat, fish and egg products, raw vegetable growns on sewage	Salmonellosis (vomiting, diarrhoea and fever)
	Shigella sonnei	Foods kept exposed for sale in unhygienic surroundings	Bacillary dysentery
	Staphylococcus aureus	Foods kept exposed for sale in unhygienic surroundings	Increased salivation, vomiting, abdominal pain and diarrhoea
	Streptococcus pyogenes	Foods kept exposed for sale in unhygienic surroundings	Scarlet fever, septic, sore throat
Fungal	Aspergillus	Corn and groundnut	Liver damage and cancer

Contd.

Table 21.2: Food-borne disease caused by some pathogenic organisms (*Contd.*)

Microorganism	Foods commonly involved	Ill-effects and diseases
flavus (Aflatoxin)	infected with *Aspergillus flavus*	
Claviceps purpurea (Ergot)	Rye and pearl millet infested with ergot	Ergotism (burning sensation in extremities peripheral gangrene)
Fusarium sporotrichiodis	Cereals and millets infected with fusarium	Alimentary toxic aleukia Liver damage
Penicillium islandicum	rice	
Parasitic *Trichinella spiralis*	Pork and pork products	Nausea, vomiting, diarrhoea, colic and muscular pains (Trichinosis)
Ascaris lumbricoides	Raw vegetables grown on sewage farms	Ascariasis
Entamoeba histolytica	Raw vegetables grown on sewage farms	Amoebic dysentery
Ancylostoma duodenale (Hookworms)	Raw vegetables grown on sewage farms	Epigastric pain, loss of blood in anaemia

Foods can become contaminated with toxic metals or chemicals such as compounds of lead, mercury, arsenic, antimony, DDT, BHC, etc. due to the following causes
1. Accidental mixing of the food with toxic chemicals used as rat poisons such as arsenic oxides, barium carbonate, lead arsenate and others.
2. Accidental contamination with pesticides and insecticides.
3. The presence of some toxic chemicals or minerals in certain marine foods, (e.g. mercury).
4. Presence of excessive amount of certain food additives.

Toxic Metals

Lead is a toxic element and contamination of food with lead can cause toxic symptoms. For example, turmeric is coated by illiterate manufacturers in India with lead chromate, lead brings about pathological changes in the kidneys, liver and arteries. The common signs of lead poisoning are nausea, abdominal pain, anaemia, insomnia, muscular paralysis and brain damage. Fish caught from waters contaminated with mercuric salts contain a large amount of mercury. The organic mercury compound—methyl or dimethyl mercury is the most toxic. The toxic effects of methyl mercury are neurological. When the brain is affected, the subject becomes blind, deaf and paralysis of the various muscles makes him a cripple. The other elements which are toxic in small closes are cadmium, arsenic, antimony, cobalt, etc. Toxic effects in human subjects due to consuming foods contaminated with these elements (Table 21.3).

Pesticides

Organic pesticides such as DDT, BHC, and Malathion, etc. are toxic compounds. The PFA Act has prescribed maximum limits for the presence of these pesticides in foods. If the pesticides are present in a greater amount, they are likely to cause toxic effects.

Food Additives

The PFA Act has prescribed safe maximum limits for the presence of food additives such as metabisulphite benzoic acid and sorbic acid in processed foods.

Solvent Residues

Hexane is the solvent permitted for the solvent extraction of oil from oilseed cakes. A safe limit of 170 ppm has been prescribed for hexane in solvent extracted edible oilseed flour.

Animal Feed Additives

Special additives such as diethyl stilbisterol and antibiotics are added to animal and poultry feeds in the USA and other western countries. These are present in the meat of animals fed on feeds containing these chemicals. Stilbisterol even in small dose can cause leukemia and cancer. Antibiotics can cause drug resistance and hardening of arteries.

Table 21.3: Toxic effects of some metals and chemicals

Name	Foods commonly involved	Toxic effect
Arsenic	Fruits sprayed by lead arsenate	Dizziness, chills, cramps, paralysis leading to death
Barium	Foods contaminated by rat poison (barium carbonate)	Violent peristalsis, muscular twitching and convulsions
Cadmium	Fruit juices, soft drinks, etc. in contact with cadmium plated vessels	Excessive salivation, liver and kidney damage, prostrate camcer, multiple fractures (painful 'Ital-Itai' disease reported from Japan due to cadmium poisoning)
Cobalt	Water, beer	Cardiac failure
Copper	Acid foods in contact with tarnished copperware	Vomiting, diarrhoea, abdominal pain
Lead	Some processed foods	Paralysis, brain damage
Mercury	Mercury tungicide treated	Paralysis, brain damage

Contd.

Table 21.3: Toxic effects of some metals and chemicals (*Contd.*)

Name	Foods commonly involved	Toxic effect
	seed grains or mercury contaminated fish	
Tin	Canned foods	Colic vomiting, photophobia
Zinc	Foods stored in galvanised ironware	Dizziness, vomiting
Pesticides	All types of food	Acute or chronic poisoning causing damage to liver, kidney, brain and nerves leading to death
Diethyl stilbisterol	Present in meat of stilbisterol fed animals and birds	Teratogenesis, carcinogenesis
Antibiotics	Meat from animals fed antibiotics	Drug resistance, hardening of arteries, heart disease

New Adulterants

In the fast changing food scenario in India along with increased food production and availability and stringent international food trade laws and norms, the traders try new ways and means of cheating the consumers and food control authorities by adulterants which are not likely to be detected by analysts. The newer adulterants identified are included in Table 21.4.

Table. 21.4: Newer adulterants

S.no.	Food	Newer food adulterants
1.	Legumes/pulses	Toxic lentils (imported), leucaena leucocephala seeds
2.	Milk	Veterinary drug residues
3.	Flour	Mouldy wheat flour
4.	Bakery products	Animal fat
5.	Vanaspathi	Industrial contaminants like ortho nitroaniline

22 Selection and Storage of Food

Selection of food is a very important task. Selection alone will not help but the person should know the storage space, type of storage available and the way the foods should be stored. Now we shall see about the selection and storage of a few foods.

CEREALS AND PULSES

Selection

i. Free from infestation, stones (or) other adulterants.
ii. Standardized bread qualities such as ISI, AGMARK, etc.
iii. The grains shape, colour size should be well.
iv. No undesirable odour present.

Storage

i. The store room must be dry and well ventilated.
ii. Mostly cereals and cereal flours are stored in jute/poly bags/tins.
iii. Any opened bags should be immediately emptied into metal bags, plastic bins, polythene bags, or cans with tight fittings lids.
iv. Bags should not be placed closed to the wall.

Wheat Flour

Poor flour will be grey (or) dull in colour. The first flour comes from the first streams. This is called "Patent Flour". The sack used should be off flavours because the flour can absorb odours.

VEGETABLES

Selection of Vegetables

Tomatoes

- It should be pink firm, ripe depend upon the length of time, there to be held.
- The selection is based on flavour, firmness, colour and size.
- Free from other delay, injury, dirt, puffiness, disease worms and other decay.

- The best fruits are those that have ripened on the plant. A sign of naturally ripened tomato is a faint flesh of green at the stem end.
- Ripened artificially have much less flavour.

Beans

- Beans should be tender, fresh, crisp, clean, firm, velvety to touch, seeds should be less than ½ round should break easily with sharp sound.

Cauliflower

- Compact, no insect find, leaves tender, green, leaves should not be rough, and flowers should not be spread out.
- Flower should not be yellow colour, it indicates overmaturity.

Brinjal

- It should be firm, bright, uniform, dark, rich purple (or) green in colour, free of scars, should not be witted, flabby (or) soft, no insect holes present.

Ladies Finger

- Should be young, tender, tips should be broken easily.
- Should not have any holes which indicates infestation, should not be hard while cutting.

Root Vegetables

Carrot

- Carrots should not be less than 3" in length.
- Carrots should not be yellow orange in colour.
- All carrots should be nearly of the same diameter. The carrots should break with a crisp shape when bent.

Onion

- It should be bright and clean, well shaped with dry skin. When shaken, they should give a dry rattle.

Potatoes

- Select good firm, smooth skinned potatoes.
- Deeply set eyes will have higher waste.
- It should be free from scale, mechanical worm (other injury, witted) leathery, discoloured potatoes should be rejected.
- A green colouring is sun burn which given bitter taste.

Greens

Cabbage

- A domestic cabbage is identified by flatness at the top, moderately green coloured and smooth round head.

- It should be fresh, compact without yellow or withered leaves, the leaves should be little and crisp.
- No insect holes (or) burst head.

Green Leafy Vegetables

- The leaves should be bright green without yellowing.
- Greens should be fresh and tender.
- No insects (or) worm damage.
- The stack should be fresh and crisp to sharp when bent.

Storage

- Root vegetables should be emptied from racks and stored in bins (or) racks in a cool place without refrigerator.
- Most green vegetables may be kept fresh and crisp in covered containers (or) plastic bags in the refrigerator.
- If the green vegetables are washed before storing, they should be drained thoroughly as too much moisture can increase the possibility of spoilage decay.
- Seeds such as peas can remain fresh longer if left in pods.
- Salad vegetables can be left in containers and stored in a cool place.
- Canning, dehydration, drying, pickling, salting, and freezing can be done to preserve.

FRUITS

Selection

Apple

- Apples which are raw, eating should be juicy, moderate to low acidity and high sweeteners.
- Skin should be bright, reddish form in colour.
- Free from dirt, blemishes sign of infestation and injury.

Grapes

- Juicy, full covered with a thin skin, tender green (or) purple in colour. No insect holes should be present.

Lime

- Select firm, well formed fruit with well textured.
- Should be with thin skin, free from blemish. Hard dry or broken rinds burses, scales (or) other defects should be avoided.
- Immature fruit will have high acid, low sugar, lack in flavour and juice.
- Citrus fruits must be picked ripe.

Banana

- Ripen fruits will have a bright attractive yellow colour, speckled with brown dots. The fruit should be fresh appearing plump and have good strength of pulp. Examine for size, fullness of fruits, and degree of maturity. Avoid bruised fruit.

Storage

- Hard fruits such as apples, can be left in boxes and kept in cold storage.
- Soft fruits such as rasberries and strawberries should be left in their baskets in a cold room.
- Store fruits are best if placed in trays so that any damaged fruit can be seen and discarded, e.g. cherries, mangoes, plum, and peaches.
- Banana should not be stored into cold place because the skin turns black.
- Preservation can be done by, drying, canning, bottling, jams, jellies, quick freezing and cold storage.

NUTS

Seléction

- Nuts should be of a good size.
- Nuts should be heavy, for their size.
- They should be absent of infestation.

Storage

- Desert nuts those with the shell on are kept in a dry ventilated store.
- Nuts without shells whether ground ribbed, flacked, or whole,are kept in air-tight containers.

EGGS

Selection

- The egg shell should be clean, well-shaped strong, and slightly rough.
- When broken they all to be a high proportion of thick white to thin white.
- The yolk should be firm, round, and of a good even colour.

Storage

- Eggs must be stored in their packing trays, blunt end upwards in a cool but not too dry place a refrigerator of 0.5°C is ideal.
- No strongly smelling foods such as cheese, fish, should be stored near the eggs because the egg shell is porous and the egg will absorb the strong odours.
- Eggs should not be washed before being stored as washing could remove the natural protective covering.

- Eggs are stored point end down.
- Preservation methods like cold storage, frozen eggs, dried eggs, and grease method can be followed.

MILK AND MILK PRODUCTS
Selection

- Milk should be pasteurized
- Milk in well sealed bottles (or) packs.
- No sour odours (or) taste presents.
- It should be uncurdled.
- Condensed milk—easy flouring, slight-brown colour, no lumps.
- Khoa-solid cream coloured balls smooth without cracks, moist free in the mouth.
- Milk and cream should be purchased daily.

Storage

- Poly bags of milk powder and milk should be preferred by refrigerated.
- Fresh milk should be kept in the container in which it is delivered.
- Milk should be kept covered as it absorbs strong smells such as onions or fish.
- Skimmed milk is stored in a cool, dry, ventilated room.
- Dried milk is stored in air tight bins and kept in dry store.

Evaporation condensed (or) dried milk are the process followed for preservation.

Meat
Selection

- Lean meat should be bright red with small flasks of white fat (marble).
- Fat should be firm, brittle in texture, creamy white in colour and odourless.
- Meat is selected for its tenderness, juiciness and flavour.
- Good quality is indicated by a bright-clear typical colour.
- The meat must be moist and not sticky, the flesh must be firm but pliable.
- The quantity of connective tissue binding the fibres together as much to do with the tenderness and eating quality.
- Exercised meat will be more flavourable and tender.

Lamb and Mutton
Selection

- Lamb is tender on year old, after one year it is turned mutton.
- The carcass should be compact and much fleshed.
- The lean flesh of lamb, mutton ought to be joined and of a pleasing dull red colour and of a fine texture.

- The fat should be evenly distributed, hard, brittle fleshy and clear white in colour.
- The bones should be porous in young animal.

Storage

- Fresh meat must be hung to allow it to become tender.
- The time for hanging depends on the temperature of the cold storage. The lower the temperature the long it can be hung.
- The time for hanging at 1°C could be up to 14 days.
- Meat should be suspended on hooks.

POULTRY
Selection

- The breast of the bird should be plump.
- The end of the breast bone must be pliable.
- The flesh should be firm.
- The skin should be white, unbroken and with a faint bluish tinge.
- The legs should be smooth, with small scales and small spurs.
- Old birds have large scales and large spurs on the leg.

Storage

- Fresh poultry must be hung by the legs in a well ventilated room for at least 24 hours otherwise, it will not be tender.
- The inwards are not removed until the bird is required.
- Frozen birds must be kept in a deep freeze cabinet until required; they are then allowed to take out before cooking.
- Canning, chilling, freezing and curing are the few preservation methods for poultry.

FISH
Selection

- The skin looks bright and shiny. The skin on state fish may show sign of wrinkling and shrinking away from flesh.
- The eyes of the fleshy part fish will be convex, the pupil black and the cornea transculant, the eyes should be bright, clear, and bulging.
- The gills of freshly caught fish are bright red as the blood in them oxidizes, they rapidly turn brownish and any mules on turns opaque.
- A fish is spit along the backbone and try lift out the bone. It must be finely to the fish, if the bone lifts out easily, the fish is stale.
- The surface should be firm to touch with no traces of browning or drying around the edges.
- A fish having odour indicates deterioration due to oxidation of poly unsaturated fat and bacterial growth.
- Rancidity can be recognized by sour taste, uncharacteristic of fresh fish.

Storage

- Fresh fish are stored in a box containing ice, in a separate refrigerator or part of refrigerator used only for fish.
- The temperature must be maintained just above the freezing point.
- Frozen fish must be stored in a deep freeze cabinet (or) compartment.
- Smoked fish should be kept in refrigerator.
- Preservation can be done by freezing, canning, salting, smoking and pickling.

FATS AND OILS

Oil Storage

- Should be kept in a cool place.
- If refrigerated some oils coagulate, they return to fluid state in a warm temperature.
- Oils will go rancid if keeps for a long time, hence need to keep in a cool place.

Butter

Selection

- The taste should be creamy and pleasant.
- The texture should be soft and smooth.
- It must smell fresh.
- Colour of pure butter-white (or) very pale yellow.
- Fresh butter should be used fairly and quickly, otherwise it will go rancid.

Cheese

Selection

- The skin of the cheese should not show spots of mild dew, as this is a sign of damped storage.
- Cheese when cut should not give off odour or an over stewing smell, which is an indication of ammonia.
- Hard (or) semi-hard cheese when cut should not appear bright.
- Soft-cheese when cut, should not appear slimy but should have delicate creamy consistency.

Storage

- Should be kept in a cool, dry well ventilated store and whole cheese should be turned occasionally if being kept for any length of time, kept from other foods, which may be spoilt by the smell.

SUGAR

- It should be stored in dry and cool place, when purchased by the sacks; the sugar is stored in covered bins.

SALT

- Stored in a cool and dry store, as it readily absorbs moisture. It should be kept in air tight packets, drums or bins.

COFFEE AND TEA

- Should be kept in air-tight containers in a well-ventilated store—coffee beans should be roasted and ground as they are required.

UNIT V

COMMUNITY NUTRITION

23   Community Nutrition

CONCEPT OF COMMUNITY NUTRITION

The term "community health" has replaced the term "public health" in many countries. It is because of the changing nature of public health which focuses on individual responsibility and community participation, "community health is defined more broadly encomparing the entire gamut of community organized effort of maintaining, protecting and improving the health of the people. It involves individuals and groups to change patterns of behaviour to achieve optimum health".

Nutrition a basic requirement for health and vigour is inadequate in respect to quality and quantity for millions of people. In spite of progress and achievements made in the field of health and welfare, India still has to go a long way in improving the standard of health and reducing health-related problems.

NUTRITIONAL NEEDS FOR SPECIAL GROUPS

Infants

Excluding foetal growth, growth in the first year of life is more rapid than at any other time in the life cycle. At age 6 months as infant has probably doubled the birth weight and at 1 year may have tripled it. To support the rapid growth rate, the need of calories and nutrients is high. Full-term infants have the ability to digest and absorb protein, a moderate amount of fat and simple carbohydrate. They have some difficulty with starch, since amylase, that starch-splitting enzyme, is not being produced at first. However, as starch is introduced, this enzyme begins to function.

Nutritional Requirements

Nutrient needs of infants reflect rates of growth, energy, expended in activity, basal metabolic needs, and the interaction of the nutrients consumed.

Breastfeeding

Infants have to be exclusively breast fed for the first 6 months of life and continue to receive breast milk until the age of 1 year. Breastfeeding is superior to formula feeding because it offers unique nutritional and non-nutritional advantages to both infant and mother.

The infant should be put to breast with half an hour after normal delivery and within four hours after caesarian sections. Prelacteal foods like honey, distilled water or glucose should not be given as these foods will satisfy the thirst and will reduce the vigour to suck and may lead to diarrhoea and helminthic infection.

During the first two or three days watery and yellowish fluid that comes from the mammary gland is called colostrum. It is rich is protein. It is nutritionally rich than when compared to matured human milk. Human milk and colostrum contain antibodies and anti-infective factors that are not present in infant formulas. Breast milk enhances the growth of the bacterium *Lactobacillus bifidus*, which produces an acidic gastrointestinal environment that interferes with the growth of certain pathogenic organisms. Because of these anti-infective factors, the incidence of infections is lower in the breast-fed infants than in formula-fed infants.

Nutritional Factor of Human Milk (Table 23.1 and Fig. 23.1)

Table 23.1: Nutritional factors

Nutrient	Human milk	Cow's milk (values per 100 g)	Buffalo's milk
Water g	88	87.5	81
Energy kcals	65	67	117
Protein g	1.1	3.2	4.3
Carbohydrates g	7.4	4.4	5
Fat g	3.4	4.1	6.5
Calcium mg	28	120	210
Phosphorous mg	11	90	130
Iron mg	–	0.2	0.2
Carotene mcg	137	174	160
Thiamine mg	0.02	0.05	0.04
Riboflavin mg	0.02	0.19	0.1
Vitamin C mg	3	2	1
Caseinogen and lactalbumin ratio	1:2	3:1	–

Energy

Human milk and cow's milk provide equal energy; however, the nutrient sources of the energy are different (Table 23.2).

For an infant 6 per cent of energy should come from protein and this is very well reached in human milk. Carnitine is needed to transport fatty acid within the cell. Newborns do not have a fully developed ability to synthesise carnitine and they must obtain it from breast milk.

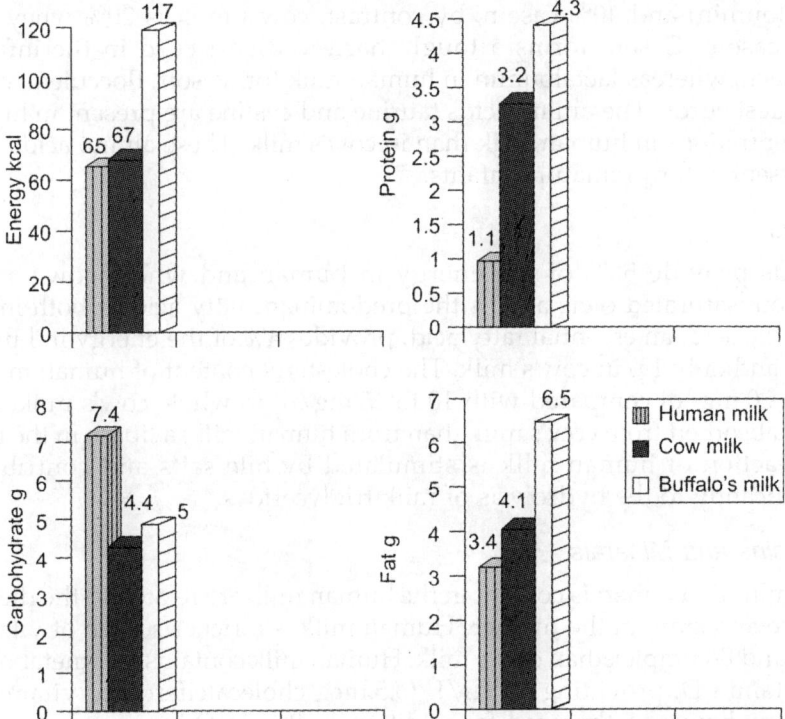

Fig. 23.1: Comparison of macro nutrients of human, cow's and buffalo's milk

Table: 23.2: Calories percentage from protein, fat and carbohydrate in human and cow's milk

Nutrient	Human milk	Cow's milk
Total energy (per 100 ml)	65	67
Protein	7	19
Fat	47	55
Carbohydrates	31	26

Carbohydrate

Lactose which is present in higher levels (42%) in human milk facilitates the absorption of magnesium and calcium and favours amino acid absorption and nitrogen retention. Galactose is present only in milk is essential for the formation of myelin, which in turn is essential for the normal nerve function. High content of galactolipid promote rapid brain growth of infant.

Protein

Protein provides 6% to 7% of the energy in human milk and 20% of the energy in cow's milk. Human milk is 60% whey proteins (mainly lactalbumin) and 40% casein; by contrast, cow's milk is 20% whey and 80% casein. Casein forms a tough, hard-to-digest curd in the infant's stomach, whereas lactalbumin in human milk forms soft, flocculent, easy-to-digest curds. The amino acids taurine and cystine are present in higher concentrations in human milk than in cow's milk. These amino acids may be essential for premature infants.

Lipids

Lipids provide 50% of the energy in human and whole cow's milk. Monounsaturated oleic acid is the predominant fatty acid in both milks. Linoleic acid, an essential fatty acid, provides 4% of the energy in human milk and only 1% in cow's milk. The cholesterol content of human milk is 10 to 20 mg/dl compared with 10 to 15 mg/dl in whole cow's milk. Less fat is absorbed from cow's milk than from human milk; a lipase in the non-fat fraction of human milk is stimulated by bile salts and contributes significantly to the hydrolysis of milk triglycerides.

Vitamins and Minerals

Vitamins and minerals content in the human milk are related to the dietary intake and store in the mother. Human milk is a richer source of vitamin A, E and B-complex than cow's milk. Human milk contains five metabolites of vitamin D, providing 20 IU/L (0.5 mcg cholecalciferol) of vitamin D activity; however, the need for additional vitamin D becomes important by 2 months of age. Approximately 50% of the iron is absorbed from human milk, whereas less than 1% of the iron is absorbed from cow's milk. Iron is more available, in the presence of lactoferrin in human milk. The bioavailability of zinc in human milk is higher than in cow's milk.

Cow's milk contains three times as much as calcium and six times as much as phosphorus as in human milk. Though the calcium content of human milk is less than in cow's milk, calcium phosphorus ratio of 2 : 1 in human milk is favourable.

Low sodium content of human milk is an advantageous to the infant as kidneys have difficulty in handling excess sodium.

Additional fluids in the form of water or juice are not necessary for exclusively breast feed babies even in hot weather, it may interfere with the establishment of lactation. A thirsty baby will demand more breast milk.

Human milk contains a wide range of constituents which play important roles in the development of the gastrointestinal system and protection against infection or anti-inflammatory. They include:

Hormones (thyroid stimulating hormone, thyroxine, growth hormone releasing factor, insulin and prolactin), trophic factors, anti-inflammatory agents, anti-infective agents, cytokines, digestive enzymes, lactoferrin, lysosymes, bifidus factor, macrophages, lymphocytes, oligosaccharides, vitamin B_{12} and folate-binding proteins. It also contains growth regulating factors, growth promoting factors and growth modulators (Table 23.3).

Table 23.3: Immune factors in breast milk

Immune factor	Functions
• β-lymphocytes	– Give rise to antibodies targeted at specific microbes.
• Macrophages	– Kill microbes in the infant's gut; produce lysozyme; activate other components of the immune system.
• Neutrophils	– Ingest bacteria in the infant's gut.
• T-lymphocytes	– Kill infected cells, send chemical messages to mobilize other defences.
• Immunoglobulin antibodies	– Bind to microbes in the infant's gut, preventing them from passing through the mucosa.
• B_{12} binding protein	– Binds B_{12}, preventing use by bacteria for growth.
• Bifidus factor	– Promotes growth of *Lactobacillus bifidus.*
• Fatty acids	– Disrupt membranes surrounding certain viruses, destroying them.
• Fibronectin	– Increases antimicrobial activity of macrophages; facilitates repair of damaged tissues.
• Gamma-interferon	– Enhances antimicrobial activity of immune cells.
• Hormones and epithelial growth factor	– Stimulate epithelial maturation, reducing vulnerability to microorganisms.
• Lactoferrin	– Binds iron, reducing availability for bacteria.
• Lysozyme	– Kills bacteria by disrupting cell walls.
• Mucins	– Adhere to bacteria and viruses, preventing attachment to mucosa.
• Oligosaccharides	– Adhere to microorganisms, preventing attachment to mucosa.

BENEFITS OF BREASTFEEDING

- A sense of security and belonging in the mother and child relationship.
- Superior nutritional composition with high bioavailability of nutrients.
- It is economical and hygienic. Less danger of contamination and gastrointestinal problems.
- Low danger of incorrect formula and overfeeding.
- Less renal solute load to infants and sodium to excrete and no risk of overconcentrating.
- Enzymatic components which improve digestion.
- Provision of immunological, antimicrobial and anti-inflammatory agents.
- Improve neurological and cognitive development.

BENEFITS TO THE MOTHER

- *Help in birth control:* Prolactin which stimulates milk production decreases the synthesis of ovarian hormones.
- Breastfeeding helps in regaining the normal size of the uterus and decrease postpartum bleeding due to the secretion of oxytocin.
- Breastfeeding helps the mother to loss the extra weight accumulated during pregnancy.
- Risk of breast cancer and ovarian cancer is higher in women who have not breast-fed their children.

Artificial Feeding/Bottle Feeding

No milk or formula feed can be a real substitute for mother's milk. But, at times, formula feeding by bottle may be preferred by some mothers. In conditions like, mothers are unwilling, unavailable or unable to breast feed, if the infant is too week or have cleft palate or harelip are usually fed a formula based on cow's milk.

Even when bottle feed is given, the baby should be cradled in the arm. The close human touch and warmth are important. When the infant is obviously satisfied, extra milk should not be forced, regardless of the amount remaining in the bottle. Any remaining should be thrown away and not refrigerated for reuse.

Disadvantages

- Bottle-fed infants are susceptible to folate deficiency because heating can destroy milk folacins. Total serum homocysteine level appears to be a sensitive indicator of folate deficiency in children on a poor diet, with HIV infection, and with antifolate drug treatment.
- Regular unmodified cow's milk can cause gastrointestinal bleeding.
- Its renal soluble load is too heavy for the infant's renal system to handle, leaving too small a margin of safety for maintaining water balance during illness, diarrhoea, or hot weather (Table 23.4).

Table 23.4: Undesirable effect of cow's milk on human infant

Composition	Undesirable effect
• Low level of lactose	• Reduced calcium absorption.
• High protein	• In small infants as the gut is not matured enough, there is a chance for unsplit protein to escape into the circulation and cause sensitization.
• Cow's milk protein intolerance	• Lactoglobulin or alpha casein may cause diarrhoea, respiratory allergy and eczema.

Contd.

Table 23.4: Undesirable effect of cow's milk on human infant (*Contd.*)

Composition	Undesirable effect
• Low osmolarity	• There is an increase additional load on immature kidney. Due to increased demand for water to excrete of this solute load, there is a chance for dehydration and constipation.
• High levels of tyrosine and aromatic amino acids that are not utilized	• Lead to azotemia and acidosis.
• SDA high	• Increased energy waste.
• High fat	• Infantile obesity.
• Low amount of iron and poor availability. Enteric loss of blood. Low vitamin C.	• Iron deficiency anaemia.
• High phosphate	• Decreased iron and calcium absorption.

Weaning

Solid food additions to infant's diet are called beikost. This is done after 6th month of age. Earlier use may contribute to allergies. As solid food is gradually added, the amount of milk consumed is reduced accordingly.

The introduction of solids into an infant's diet begins the weaning process in which the infant transitions from a diet of only breast milk or formula to a more varied one. Weaning should proceed gradually and should be carefully chosen to complement the nutrient needs of the infant, promote appropriate nutrient intake, and maintain growth. Weaning is a mandatory process, since,

- Increasing needs of calories and protein of growing children cannot be met by the diminishing output of mother's milk.
- Milk is a poor source of vitamin C and D and supplementation is essential.
- Iron stores in liver of the infant would last only up to 4–6 months. Hence iron-rich foods should be given at least from six month onwards.

Weaning to the infants can be started with liquid supplements and then gradually increases it to solid mashed supplements. Examples of liquid supplements are milk, fresh fruit juices, strained soups from green leafy vegetables, etc.

Examples of solid mashed supplements which can be started around 7th or 8th month of life are well cooked and mashed rice, ragi, corn and other cereals and pulses, mashed potato, green leafy vegetables, carrots, stewed apples, boiled egg, minced and cooked meat or boiled fish (Tables 23.5 and 23.6).

Table 23.5: Summary of recommendations for weaning (peadiatric group of the British dietetic adapted from the position statement on breastfeeding and weaning on Solid Foods Association, 2004 b)

Food	6 months (26 weeks)	6–9 months	9–12 months	Over 12 months
Starchy foods	1–2 servings/ day	2–3 servings/ day	3–4 servings/ day	1 serving at each meal
	Smooth cereals, e.g. rice based potatoes or millet	Start to introduce more cereals, inclu-ding wholemeal bread, 'lumpier texture' 'finger food', e.g. toast, rice cakes	Starchy foods of normal adult texture	• Starchy foods of normal adult texture • Discourage high-fat foods, savoury snacks and pastry
Vege-tables and fruit	1–2 servings/ day	2 servings/day	3–4 servings/ day	Offer at each meal and some snacks—about 5 small servings/day
	Soft-cooked vegetables and fruit as a smooth puree	• Raw soft fruit and vegetables, (as finger foods) • Cooked furit and vegetables can be a coarser/ mashed texture	• Lightly cooked or raw foods • Small chunks of finger foods • Vitamin C-containing foods (e.g. un-sweetened or-ange juice), if diet is meat free	Adult texture for fruit and vegetables
Meat and alter-natives (e.g. fish, pulses, eggs)	At least 1 serving per day	Minimum 1 serving/day	Minimum 1 serving/day from animal source or 2 from vegetable source	Minimum 1 serving/ day from animal source or 2 from vegetable source
	• Use soft cooked meat and pulses as a puree • Well-cooked eggs	• Soft-cooked, pureed mashed or finely minced meat/fish/ pulses • Well-cooked or hard-boiled	• Minced/ chopped cooked meats/fish/ pulses	• Encourage lean meat • Offer oily fish once a week

Contd.

Table 23.5: Summary of recommendations for weaning (peadiatric group of the British dietetic adapted from the position statement on breastfeeding and weaning on Solid Foods Association, 2004 b) (*Contd.*)

Food	6 months (26 weeks)	6–9 months	9–12 months	Over 12 months
Other advice	• No liver	egg can be used as a finger food • Limit liver to no more then once per week	• Limit liver to no more than once per week	• Limit liver to no more than once per week
	• Encourage savoury rather than sweet foods	• Can have gluten-containing food	• No added salt and limit salty foods	• Allow toddlers to decide themselves how much to eat
	• Introduce cup or beaker	• Introduce cup or beaker	• Discontinue bottles by 12 months, use cups or beakers	• Encourage 3 meals per day
	• No honey	• No honey	• No honey	• Limit crisp and savoury snacks
	• No added salt or salty foods	• No added salt or salty foods		• Do not add sugar to drinks
				• Discourage snacking on foods high in fat, salt and sugar

Table 23.6: Examples of weaning appropriate foods

	Weaning foods	Finger foods
Asian (vegetarian)	• Rice-boiled (mashed) or khichdi (mixture of rice and dal) mixed with yogurt • Rice flakes with milk • Root/green vegetables cooked and mashed • Chappati or roti made into crumbs and soaked in milk • Soft fruits, e.g. banana, papaya, mango – mashed • Puddings made from rice, rice flour, wheat flour, semolina flour	• Chapatti, roti, naan, puri, paratha, pitta bread • soft cooked pieces of root vegetable and potato • Soft fruits
Asian (non-vegetarian)	As above. In addition: • Boiled egg – chopped or mashed • Meat, fish, chicken, pureed and mixed with rice	As above

PREPARATION OF MALTED CEREAL

Soak the cereal overnight. Remove the water and tie in a moist cloth and keep in warm place. After 48 hours when sprout comes out, dry in sun or roast it. Remove the sprout as they may be toxic substances in the sprouts. Make it into flour. During the process of malting, starch is covered to maltose due to increase production of enzyme amylase. This is also called amylase rich food. Due to the conversion of starch into amylose, thinner gruels are made. With this either the infant can consume more gruel or more flour can be added to make thick gruel. This way calorie consumption can be increased. Other cereals such as rice, rice flour, rice flakes, and corn flakes can also be given in the form of porridge.

When a tooth erupts babies can be introduced with solid supplements. Solid foods such as idli, idiappam, bread, chapathi, rice, dhal, chopped vegetables, cooked potato, well-cooked leafy vegetables, skin and seed removed fruits can be given.

TO AVOID POOR WEANING

- Overfeeding and underfeeding should be avoided in order to avoid the consequences of obesity and underweight.
- When introducing new food, one at a time and initially should be very small amount and should be gradually increased, to ensure that there are no adverse reactions to these new food.
- In the beginning, the consistency of new food should be thin and then it can be gradually increased to solid.
- If the baby develops allergy or acute dislike for a particular food, omit that item for a week or two and then try again with very small amount. If the allergy or dislike persists, it is better to forget about the food for a while and substitute another.
- A variety of nutrient dense foods should be provided.
- Start with liquid supplement, then to semi-solid and latter to solid supplement food.
- Select fresh, quality fruits, vegetables and any other ingredients on preparing infant foods.
- Follow hygienic and simple method in preparation.
- Avoid overcooking, which may destroy heat-sensitive nutrients.
- Do not add salt or sugar. Allow the infant to become familiar with the real taste of the food.

24

Nutritional Need for Children

Table 24.1: Recommended dietary allowances of children between 1 and 6 years

Nutrient	Years	
	1–3	4–6
Weight kg	12.2	19.0
Energy kcals	1240	1690
Protein g	22	30
Fat g	25	25
Calcium mg	400	400
Iron mg	12	18
Vitamin A mcg	400	400
β carotene mcg	1600	1600
Thiamine mg	0.6	0.9
Riboflavin mg	0.7	1.0
Nicotinic acid mg	8	11
Pyridoxine mg	0.9	0.9
Ascorbic acid mg	40	40
Folic acid mcg	30	40
Vitamin B_{12} mcg	0.2–1	0.2–1

The period 1 to 3 years (toddler) is a time of transition between infancy and preschoolers. After the rapid growth of the first year the growth rate of children slows. The dramatic decrease in the growth rate is reflected in a disinterest in food, a "physiologic anorexia" due to lower calorie needs.

Body proportions of young children change significantly after the first year. The legs become longer, trunk growth slows substantially, little head growth happens. The child begins losing baby fat. There is less body water and more water inside the cells.

Energy demands are fewer because of the slackened growth rate. However, important muscle development will take place. Muscle mass development at this age accounts for about one half the total weight gain. With increased physical activity and walking, the legs straighten while the abdominal and back muscles tighten to support the erect child. Therefore, more muscle is needed to strengthen the body.

CATCH-UP GROWTH

The child recovering from an illness or undernutrition, who has slowed or ceased growth, will experience a greater than expected rate of recovery. This is referred to as "catch-up" growth, the body strives to catch up to the child's normal growth curve. The degree of growth suppression is influenced by the timing, severity and duration of the insult; that is, a severe illness or deprivation for an extended time during a period of rapid growth has the most dramatic effect. Malnourished infants who did not experience immediate catch-up growth would have permanent growth retardation.

Nutrient requirements, especially for energy and protein, vary depending on the rate and stage of catch-up. Generally, the protein needs increase proportionately more than the energy need when the gain is greater. Milk or a milk-based formula often provides the basis of the diet for young children during catch-up, along with developmentally appropriate foods. Frequent, small feedings are usually better tolerated because total volume and the child's stomach capacity can be limiting factors, energy and nutrients can be concentrated or adjusted by the use of commercial liquid supplements, formula concentration, increased use of fats and oils, etc.

Growth and nutritional status should be monitored frequently and dietary management can be modified as needed. In all cases, medical, social and environmental concerns related to the growth retardation need to be resolved.

The period of 3 to 6 years (preschooler) tends to settle into a regular genetic growth channel as physical growth continues in spurts. Physical activity increases as well as the mental capacities like thinking and exploring of the environment. Energy and protein requirement will be more than the first 3 years of the life.

The school-age period (6 to 12 years) has been called the latent time of growth. The rate of growth slows, and body changes occur gradually.

Energy

The need for kilo calories is not high due to the relatively decreased growth rate after the first year of life. Dietary energy must be sufficient to ensure growth and spare protein from being used for energy but not allow excess weight gain. Minor illness, which occurs frequently in this age group, is a common cause of short-term impaired food intake. Energy requirement increases in the pre-school age since the physical activity and mental observation increases.

Protein

Protein needs are higher than the energy requirement among these groups since there is rapid growth of muscle and tissues. The recommended protein intake is 1.5 to 2 g/kg of body weight. Children most likely to be at risk for inadequate protein intake are those have multiple food allergies, strict vegan diets, or those who have limited food selection because of fad diets, behaviour problems, or limited access to food.

Fat

The percentage of energy from dietary fat is about 50% in a breast feed infant. Later, after the first year of age, fat intake should be gradually reduced from 50% to 30%.

Minerals And Vitamins

- The overall rate of skeletal growth slows but there is more deposit of mineral rather than lengthening of the bones. The increased mineralization strengthens the bone to support the increasing weight. Calcium is needed for adequate mineralization and maintenance of growing bone in children.
- The accretion of calcium in the body is not uniform throughout the growth period, but relatively greater during childhood. Milk is the best source of calcium. Hence including 1 to 2 glasses of milk per day is recommended.
- Iron is needed to maintain adequate haemoglobin levels in an increasing blood volume as the body size increases. The toddlers between 1 and 3 years of age are at high risk for iron deficiency anaemia. To meet this increased demand for iron, iron-rich foods such as rice flakes, egg yolk, greens, dates, etc. should be included.
- Zinc is essential for growth; a deficiency results in growth failure, poor appetite, decreased taste acuity, and poor wound healing. The best sources of zinc are meats and sea food; some children may regularly have a low intake which may lead to deficiency. Therefore, food choice should be done carefully in order to meet all the essential nutrients.
- Vitamin A, the main food sources of vitamin A are milk and vegetable. Since only a limited number of foods are rich sources of vitamin A and young children tend not to consume large quantities of vegetables, a supplementary source of vitamin A is required in this age group.
- Vitamin D is necessary for the calcium absorption. If children did not reach the dietary intake and thus relay on exposure to sunlight.
- The daily allowances of B-vitamin requirements are based on energy intake. The allowances per 1,000 kcals are (same as an adult) 0.5 mg thiamine, 0.6 mg riboflavin and 6.6 mg niacin equivalents.

DIETARY GUIDELINES

- About 2 to 3 cups of milk/day are sufficient for the young children (1–3 years). Excess milk intake may exclude many solid foods from the diet which will lead to anaemia.
- Offering the child on increasing variety of foods will help to develop good food habits.
- Toddler should be allowed to eat according to their appetite rather than to specific serving sizes.

- The menu should include a combination of foods from all five foods groups to meet all nutrient requirements.
- Finger foods, such as chopped fruits and vegetables, rice cakes, biscuits, etc. can be given.
- Parents can encourage their children to taste and eat foods by setting an example and eating and enjoying these foods themselves when offering to kids.
- Strong flavour foods can be avoided since children are very sensitive to flavours.
- At times allow the children to feed themselves, this may help them to learn about food and they learn how to eat.

Nutritional Problem in Pre-school Children

Dental Caries

Dental caries are more prevalent among children due to improper care of teeth, high consumption of sugar confectionery and carbonated drinks. The preventative measure is brushing teeth twice per day with a fluoridated toothpaste.

Vitamin A Deficiency

Vitamin A deficiency is a major public health problem. It is the main cause of preventable blindness and severe visual impairment in young child, and increases the risk of severe illness and death from childhood infections such as diarrhoea and measles. The WHO estimates that 100–140 million children are vitamin A deficient and between one-quarter and half a million children become blind every year as a result of vitamin A deficiency.

Vitamin A deficiency is often linked to the nature of the foods available and feeding practices used. Interventions to combat vitamin A deficiency include promoting breastfeeding, fortifying foods, improving dietary diversity and administering supplement of vitamin A.

Pre-school children are at a greater risk of vitamin A deficiency. Children from rural and tribal families belonging to low-income group are more vulnerable to vitamin A deficiency. A great majority of the cases of corneal xerophthalmia occurs between 1 and 3 years, coinciding with the peak-prevalence of severe protein energy malnutrition.

The WHO recommends the following classification of xerophthalmia:
- Night blindness (XN)
- Conjunctival xerosis (XIA)
- Bitot's spot (XIB)
- Corneal xerosis (X2)
- Corneal ulceration/keratomalacia (<1/3 corneal surface (X3A))
- Corneal ulceration/keratomalacia (>1/3 corneal surface (X3B))
- Corneal scar (XS)
- Xerophthalmia fundus (XF)

Iron Deficiency

Iron deficiency is most common nutrient disorders of childhood. Iron deficiency is associated with frequent infections, poor weight gain, and developmental delay and behaviour disorders. Iron deficiency in young children is usually of dietary origin due to the early introduction of cow's milk as a main drink before 12 months of age or over-dependence on milk where it replaces iron-rich or iron-enhancing foods.

Obesity

BMI should normally decrease between the ages of 1 and 5 years but in obese children this decrease may not be seen. Adequate physical activity, proper food choice and lifestyle will help in preventing obesity in this age group.

PEM

World Health Organization (WHO) defined PEM as "Protein Energy Malnutrition is defined as a range of pathological conditions arising from coincident lack of varying proportions of protein and calorie, occurring most frequently in infants and young children and often associated with infection".

Protein energy malnutrition is the deficiency of macronutrients (energy and protein) in the diet.

ECOLOGY OF PEM

A. Poverty contributes the major part in percentage of malnutrition.
B. Low birth weight
C. Inadequate breast milk
D. Improper weaning
E. Faulty practice of feeding food
F. Frequent chronic infections
G. Quantity and quality less diet
H. Ignorance and poor socioeconomic states (Fig 24.1)

CLASSIFICATION OF PEM

The term PEM is used to describe a wide range of clinical conditions ranging from the very clinically detectable forms to the mildest forms in which growth retardation is the major manifestation (Table 24.2).

Kwashiorkor

Kwashiorkor is an African word, meaning a "disease of the displaced child" who is deprived of adequate nutrition. This mostly occurs in children between the ages of 1 and 3 years.

The important clinical signs and symptoms of kwashiorkor are as follows:

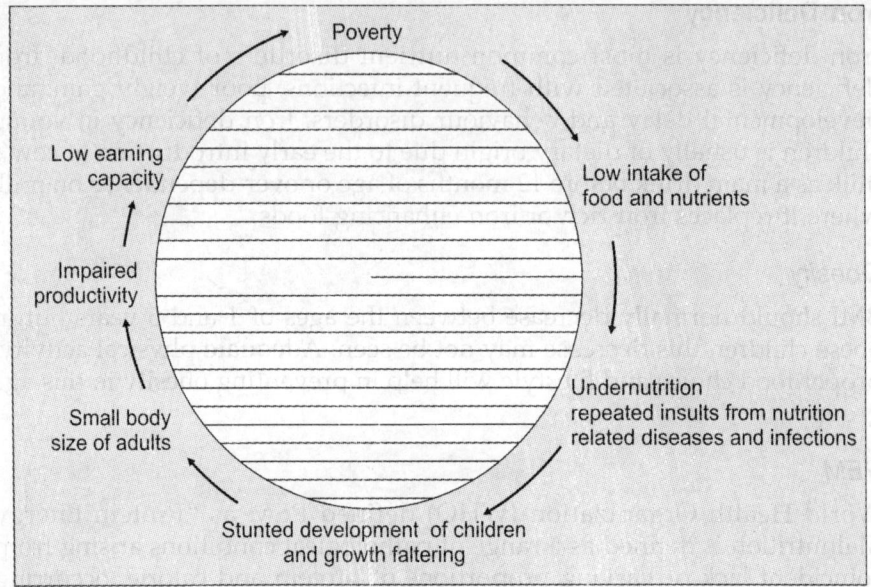

Fig. 24.1: The vicious cycle of poverty

Table 24.2: Classification of PEM (FAO/WHO)

Type of PEM	Body weight as percentage of standard	Oedema	Deficit in weight for height
Kwashiorkor	80–60	+	+
Marasmic kwashiorkor	<60	+	++
Marasmus	<60	0	++
Nutritional dwarfing	<60	0	Minimal
Underweight child	80–60	0	+

Growth Failure

Growth retardation is the earliest manifestation of kwashiorkor. This is manifested by decreased body length and low body weight in spite of retention of water in the body (oedema) and presence of subcutaneous fat in some children. The thinness of the child is masked in the presence of oedema. The child's arms and legs will appear thin as a result of wasting.

Oedema

Oedema refers to accumulation of fluid in the tissues and usually begins with a slight swelling in feet gradually spreading up the legs. Later, hands and face also have oedema. Puffiness in face due to oedema is known as moon face. The oedema is mainly due to hypoalbuminmia and also due to high sodium and low potassium levels in serum. Copper could play an important role in the aetiology of oedema in kwashiorkor. Plasma copper and its carrier protein ceruloplasmin and RBC superoxide dismutase are significantly decreased. This suggests that oedema formation could be due to lower levels of copper and its metalloenzyme superoxide dismutase.

Mental Change

Mental development is affected. The child will be unusually apathetic with absolutely no interest in the surroundings. The child will irritable easily and prefers to stay at one place and in one position.

Hair Change

The hair loses its health and become thin. The colour of the hair become coppery red colour may be generated or localized with alternate bands of pigmentation and depigmentation referred to as "flag sign". You can easily pluck small tufts of hair without causing any pain just by passing your hands through the hair which is referred as easy pluckability.

Skin Change

Dermatosis is very common. Dark pigmented patches, akin to sun-baked and blistered paint known as 'flaky-paint' dermatosis is present.

GASTROINTESTINAL TRACT

Loss of appetite (anorexia) and vomiting are common. Diarrhoea occurs in most cases.

MICRONUTRIENT DEFICIENCIES

Anaemia occurs due to the deficiency of iron and folic acid. It may be aggravated by parasitic infection which prevents the absorption of nutrients.

Signs and symptoms of vitamin A deficiency such as xerophthalmia and keratomalacia are widely prevalent. Angular stomatitis and glossitis due to deficiency of riboflavin may be present.

WATER AND ELECTROLYTE IMBALANCE

The total body water and especially the extracellular fluid volume are increased in all forms of PEM. At the same time, there may be clinical signs of dehydration, particularly sunken eyes, loss of skin turgor, dry mucosa. As for the electrolytes, its total sodium is increased although in some cases the serum sodium and osmolarity are seen to be reduced. This is obvious in patients who have oedema and sings of dehydration. As for potassium it is usually deficient and magnesium deficiency is reported (Fig. 24.2).

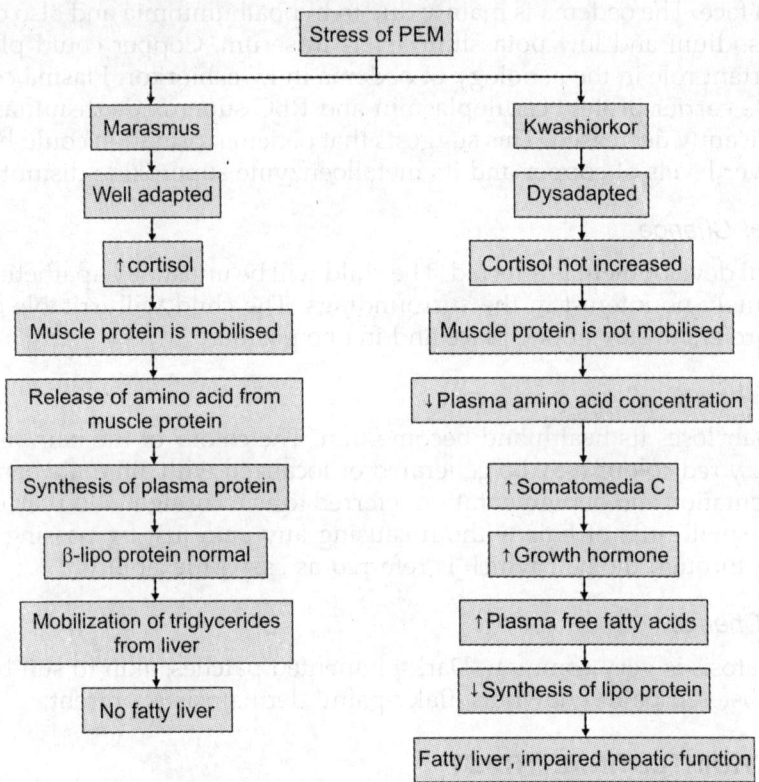

Fig. 24.2: Metabolic change in marasmus and kwashiorkor

Marasmus

Marasmus is principally due to the consumption of diets markedly deficient in both proteins and calories. It is seen most commonly in weaned infants of about 1 year of age in contrast to kwashiorkor which occur more often among children of the age group 2–4 years.

Child reacts to the stress of PEM and secrets cortisol, which mobilises protein from muscle and subcutaneous tissue to amino acid pool resulting in wasting with no oedema and no hepatomegaly. Raised cortisol level lowers growth hormone and so the child is stunted. Marasmus is said to be well adapted to the stress of deficit in protein and calories.

The important clinical signs and symptoms of marasmus are as follows:
- Severe growth retardation
- Extreme emaciation
- Old man's or monkey's face
- Loose and hanging skin folds over arms and buttocks due to extreme muscle wasting.
- The child will be absolutely week that they may not have even energy to cry.

- Oedema and fatty infiltration is absent.
- The hair is thin and dry.
- Irritability, fretfulness and apathy
- Failure to thrive
- Frequent diarrhoeal episode leads to
  - Dehydration
  - Micronutrient deficiencies of vitamin A, iron and B-complex are common

Marasmic Kwashiorkor

Sometimes, in areas where PEM is common, malnourished children exhibit the features of both kwashiorkor and marasmus. Such changes could occur during the transition from one form of severe PEM to another. For example, a marasmic child can develop oedema after a severe bout of infection or a kwashiorkor child, when loses oedema may develop this condition. Such a child is considered as suffering from 'marasmic kwashiorkor'. These children will have extreme wasting of different degrees (representing marasmus) and also oedema (a sign of kwashiorkor).

Nutritional Dwarfing

Nutritional dwarfism is a term used to describe a child who appears normal until it is realized that he or she is short for age. Reduced linear growth occurs in response to undernourished; dental development is less retarded so the facial appearance is inappropriate for the age. As to an adult, the undernourished child is very susceptible to respiratory and gastrointestinal infections leading to an increased mortality in this group.

Underweight Child

Many children in developing countries are underweight, and subclinical PEM is often present if looked carefully using anthropometric criteria. Mild-to-moderate malnutrition can be detected in children by the mid upper-arm circumference (MUAC) (Table 24.3).

Table 24.3: Features of PEM in children

Features	Marasmus	Kwashiorkor
Essential features		
1. Oedema	None*	Lower legs, sometimes face, or generalized*.
2. Wasting	Gross loss of sub-cutaneous fat, "all skin and bone"*	Less obvious; sometimes face blubbery.
3. Muscle wasting	Severe*	Sometimes.
4. Growth retardation in terms of body weight	Severe*	Less than of marasmus.

Contd.

Table 24.3: Features of PEM in children (*Contd.*)

Features	Marasmus	Kwashiorkor
5. Mental changes	Usually none	Usually present.
Variable features		
1. Appetite	Usually good	Usually poor.
2. Diarrhoea	Often (past or present)	Often (past or present).
3. Skin changes	Usually none	Often, diffuse pigmentation; occasional "flaky paint"* or "enamel" dermatosis.
4. Hair changes	Texture may be modified but no dyspigmentation.	Often sparse-straight and silky; dyspigmentation grayish or reddish.
5. Moon face	None	Often.
6. Hepatic enlargement	None	Frequent, although it is not observed in some areas.

*The most characteristic or useful distinguishing features

Treatment

Treatment must involve the provision of protein and energy supplements and the control of infection.

Treatment strategy can be divided into three stages:
1. Resolving life-threatening conditions.
2. Restoring nutritional status without disrupting homeostasis.
3. Ensuring nutritional rehabilitation.
   Criteria for improvement:
1. Disappearance of mental apathy in 4 to 5 days.
2. Disappearance of oedema in 7 to 10 days.
3. Weight gain in 3 to 4 weeks.
4. Rise in serum albumin level in about 2 week's time.

Resuscitation

The severely ill child will require correction of fluid and electrolyte abnormalities, but intravenous therapy should be avoided if possible because of the danger of fluid overload.

WHO/UNICEF	NaCl	3.5 g	
Rehydration fluid-	Na Citrate	2.9 g	
	KCl	1.5 g	dissolved in 1 l of water
	Glucose	20 g	

The oral rehydration solution, formulated by WHO can be safely used for correcting dehydration even in malnourished children.

Depending on the dehydration 70–100 ml ORS/kg body weight can be given. This amount should be given in small quantities at frequent intervals over a period of 4–6 hours.

Diarrhoea is often due to bacterial or protozoal overgrowth. Parasites are also common, appropriate antibiotic therapy can be given. For the most frequent infections such as pneumonia, otitis and skin infections, penicillin is recommended. If the infection does not respond to penicillin, broad spectrum antibiotics must be used. Giardiasis and ascariasis must be treated with appropriate deworming agents.

Refeeding

Careful planning is needed when refeeding a PEM child. During the initial treatment of the acute situation, a balanced diet with sufficient protein and energy is given to maintain a steady state. Large increases in energy lead to heart failure, circulatory collapse and death. A child requires approximately 150 to 200 kcal/kg body weight/day for the existing weight. 5 grams of protein/kg body weight/day should be given for the existing weight. This is often given as milk with additional water, flour, maize or whatever is available locally in a palatable mixture. Attempts should be made to give the feeds as slowly and as often as possible, although anorexia is often a problem and can be exacerbated by excessive feeding. If necessary, fluids and foods should be given by nasogastric tube. The child is then gradually weaned to liquids and then solids by mouth.

Hypothermia and hypoglycaemia occur in severely ill children, often with an accompanying infection, and need to be treated urgently. Because of the cold temperatures, blankets and sometimes additional heat are necessary.

Supplements of vitamins (A, D, B and C) should always be given, together with folic acid and iron. Many children are deficient in minerals such as zinc, copper and selenium and supplements should be given.

Rehabilitation

Gradually, as the child improves, more energy can be given, and during rehabilitation maximum weight gain is achieved in the shortest time by extra calories ("catch-up weight gain"). Children who have severely ill need constant attention right through the convalescent period.

SUGGESTED DIET DURING CONVALESCENCE

1. Increasing the quantity and quality of the existing food from locally available staple foods.
2. Increasing the number of meals to satisfy calorie and protein requirement which should be easily digestible.
3. Cereal and pulse combination (5 : 1 proportion) mixture can be given to increase the quality.
4. In diet, calories can be increased by adding oil, ghee, sugar without increasing the bulk.

5. Including milk and egg will help the child in convalescence period.
6. Low cost ingredients can be chosen and used efficiently if milk and egg are not affordable.
7. Low cost recipes for children recovering from PEM
   - Ragi, green gram, jaggery :puttu
   - Ragi, Bengal gram, wheat :puttu
   - Bengal gram, milk, jaggery :payasam
   - Rice, Bengal gram :porridge
   - Red gram, spinach, dal
   - Wheat rava, green gram dal, vegetables :upma
   - Malted wheat, green gram and groundnut powder (can be made as chapathi, gruel or laddu with jaggery)
   - Rice, green gram dal :pongal, kichidi
   - Idli with sugar and milk.

PREVENTION

Prevention of PEM depends not only on adequate nutrients being available but also on education of both governments and individuals in the importance of good nutrition and immunization. Short-term programmes are useful for acute shortages of food, but long-term programmes involving improved agriculture are equally important. Bad feeding practices and infections are more prevalent than actual shortage of food in many areas of the world. However, good surveillance is necessary to avoid periods of famine (Table 24.4).

Table 24.4: A WHO priority programme

Prevention of protein-energy malnutrition:
GOBIF (a WHO priority programme)
- **G**rowth monitoring: The WHO has a simple growth chart that the mother keeps.
- **O**ral rehydration, particularly for diarrhea.
- **B**reast-feeding supplemented by food after 6 months.
- **I**mmunization: Against measles, tetanus, pertussis, diphtheria, polio and tuberculosis.
- **F**amily planning.

Childhood eating patterns can have long-term health effects. In other words, food served at home in the early years sets a pattern for the rest of the child's life. For instance, preschools whose households have an abundance of fruits and vegetables tend to consume more of these foods during the school years. Likewise, milk consumption during childhood is the strongest predictor of milk intake in older adults. Childhood is seen as a time to establish healthy eating habits before patterns become inflexible and difficult to change.

NUTRITIONAL NEED FOR SCHOOL CHILDREN

School-age group is considered from 7–12 years. The RDA for this age group is as follows.

Table 24.5: Nutritional need for school children

Nutrient	Years 7–9	Years 10–12	
		Boys	Girls
Weight kg	26.9	35.4	31.5
Energy kcal	1950	2190	1970
Protein g	41	54	57
Fat g	25	22	22
Calcium mg	400	600	600
Iron mg	26	34	19
Vitamin A mcg	600	600	600
β-carotene mcg	2400	2400	2400
Thiamine mg	1.0	1.1	1.0
Riboflavin mg	1.2	1.3	1.2
Nicotinic acid mg	13	15	13
Pyridoxine mg	1.6	1.6	1.6
Ascorbic acid mg	40	40	40
Folic acid mcg	60	70	70
Vitamin B_{12} mcg	0.2–1	0.2–1	0.2–1

Growth during the school-age is slow but steady, parallel by a constant increase in food intake. The influence of peers and significant adults, such as teachers is greater. Except for severe cases, most behavioural problems connected with food have been resolved by this age, and the child enjoys eating to alleviate hunger and obtain social satisfaction.

Many children continue to prefer foods with which they are familiar rather than trying new foods. Availability and accessibility and taste preferences are the most important determinants of children's consumption of particular foods. Parental behaviour, in terms of the foods they are seen to eat and whether meals are eaten with children, is important in modeling preferred behaviour to children. Restricting a food such as chocolate can make it even more attractive and likely to be selected and in situation where parents are not present.

CHOOSING A HEALTHY DIET

* Dishes for school age-children should be quick to eat and yet satisfying nutritionally since they do not like to spend much time for eating. It should be variety in colour, texture, taste and flavour.

- School-age children should be eating a low-fat, high-fibre diet broadly in line with *The balance of good health* food groups. If children are allowed to eat to appetite, they can regulate their energy intake fairly well and should never be encouraged to finish what is on their plate when they no longer feel hungry.
- Parents should set an example of health "thin" eating habits because young children tend to imitate their parents. Subtle changes such as eating baked instead of fried foods: substituting fresh fruits and nutritious desserts and eliminating traditional empty-calorie snack foods are strategies aimed at preventing excess weight gain.
- Engage them in more of physical activity, preferably all days of the weeks. Physical activity should not be limited to sports but should include riding a bicycle, Playing with family members, making them plant vegetables or fruit trees (children will enjoy and show interest in eating foods they have grown).
- Taking them to market and involving them in selecting foods should be encouraged.

Nutritional Requirements

Energy

As growth during this school-age group is slow and steady, the calories requirements also increase slow and steady. Requirements of energy between 7–9 years of age are 1950 kcal/day. It increases only to 1970 kcal/day for girls and 2190 kcal/day for boys.

Protein

Protein requirement is gradually increased from 41 g/day (7–9 years) to 54 g/day for boys and 57 g/day for girls among 10–12 years of age group.

Minerals

Calcium and iron requirements are increased to meet the growth demands.

Vitamins

The requirement of vitamin A, C and B-complex are increase equally to adult requirement.

BREAKFAST SKIPPING

Studies suggest that cognition and learning are adversely affected when children skip breakfast. Breakfast cereals consumed with milk are an important source of B vitamins, calcium, iron, zinc and folate and children who consume breakfast cereals on a regular basis are more likely to meet recommendations for micronutrient intake than children who consume them rarely or not at all.

PACKED LUNCHES

Majority of the school going children pack their food in a box for their lunch. Care should be taken when food is packed for the children since it should cover one-third of the calories and protein needed for the day. Food should be appetizing and with correct consistency. Repetition of menu can be avoided. Packed lunch should consist of all five food groups, though the number of dishes may be less.

SCHOOL LUNCH PROGRAMMES

School lunch programs were started keeping in mind the social and economic status of the country. Education plays a major role in development of the country. Unless the children are not healthy enough, they cannot concentrate in class. Therefore, government introduced many feeding programme along with free compulsory primary education for children.

The intervention programmes implemented in India are mid-day meal programme for school children, special nutrition programme (SNP), integrated child development services (ICDS), Tamil Nadu government nutrition meal programme, Tamil Nadu integrated nutrition programme (TINP), World Bank assisted ICDS III project, etc.

The objectives of feeding programmes are:

1. To provide food for undernourished children and to improve the nutritional status and monitor it.
2. To increase school enrolment and attendance of the children.
3. To reorient good eating habits.
4. To incorporate nutrition education into the curriculum.
5. To improve literacy and educational performance of the pupils.
6. To encourage the use of local commodities.
7. To encourage the community participation in the feeding programme.

Dietary Problems in School-age Children

Obesity

Obesity rates are rising among school-age children in many part of the world. Obesity in childhood is associated with

– Increased risk factors for cardiovascular disease.
– Higher incidence of atherosclerosis.
– Insulin resistance and the emergence of type 2 diabetes within this age group.
– Lower levels of fitness.
– Social discrimination.
– Low self-esteem.
– Lower quality of life.
– Lower academic achievement.

Parents of children up to 12 years of age must take responsibility for the food their children eat and the physical activity levels of their children. Lifestyle changes for the whole family are preferable to just targeting the behaviour of the overweight or obese child on their own. Successful interventions involve helping families are change the foods they eat and to increase the physical activity of the whole family.

Underweight

Skipping breakfast or any other meals, consuming very less quantity may lead to underweight. Poor appetite, problems with siblings and friends, self-imposed dietary restriction may lead to poor quantity of food intake.

Dental Caries

Children are more susceptible to dental caries due to high and frequent consumption of sugar and acidic drinks. Brushing the teeth, twice a day, morning and before going to bed should become a habit in children.

Constipation

Neglecting whole fruits, vegetables, green leafy vegetables and consuming more of refined foods will lead to constipation. Parents should try to incorporate fibre rich foods in desiring way. Proper diet, sufficient sleeping hours and adequate physical activity will help the children to relieve from constipation.

Anaemia

Iron deficiency anaemia occurs particularly in children who are vegetarian. Attention to good dietary sources of iron can help in preventing iron deficiency anaemia. Iron uptake can be maximized by avoiding drinking tea, which tends to hamper iron absorption at meals, and instead offering fruit juice containing vitamin C, which aids absorption of non-haeme iron.

25

Nutritional Need for Adolescent

Table 25.1: Recommended dietary allowances of adolescents

Nutrient	Years			
	13–15		16–18	
	Boys	Girls	Boys	Girls
Body Weight kg	47.8	46.7	57.1	49.9
Energy kcals	2450	2060	2640	2060
Protein g	70	65	78	63
Fat g	22	22	22	22
Calcium mg	600	600	500	500
Iron mg	41	28	50	30
Vitamin A mcg	600	600	600	600
β carotene mcg	2400	2400	2400	2400
Thiamine mg	1.2	1	1.3	1
Riboflavin mg	1.5	1.2	1.6	1.2
Nicotinic acid mg	10	14	17	14
Pyridoxine mg	2	2	2	2
Ascorbic acid mg	40	40	40	40
Folic acid mg	100	100	100	100
Vitamin B_{12} mcg	0.2–1	0.2–1	0.2–1	0.2–1

Adolescence is a period of transition between childhood and adulthood and involves both physical and emotional changes.

Adolescence is a particularly unique period in life because it is a time of rapid production of physical, psychosocial cognitive development, increased nutritional needs, this juncture relate to the fact that adolescents gain up to 50% of their adult weight, 20% of their adult height and 50% of their adult skeletal mass during this period.

NUTRITIONAL REQUIREMENT

Energy and Proteins

Boys have higher energy requirements than girls due to their gain in height and lean body mass during puberty. Protein requirements for both boys and girls are the same up to age of 10 years. But there is a gradual difference in their requirements from the age of 10 years where the boys have higher requirements when compared to girls. Undernutrition in both sexes at this time can inhibit bone development, resulting in a lower peak bone mass and lower height increase velocity, leading to stunting. Severe undernutrition can also delay puberty or halt its progression.

Minerals

Calcium, phosphorus and iron in both genders and magnesium in girls are higher for adolescents than for adults and reflect the increased needs for growth and development.

Calcium and phosphorus are important for the rapid accretion of bone tissue. About 60% of adult bone mass is gained during the pubertal growth spurt. Adequate calcium intakes at this age may protect against osteoporosis in later life.

Iron needed for haemoglobin synthesis necessitated by the considerable expansion of blood volume and for myoglobin needed for muscle growth. The iron requirement for girls increases gradually and it has to be reached successfully as they lose 0.5 mg/day for menstrual losses. Achieving adequate iron stores become important for girls as menstrual periods become more regular and heavier.

Vitamins

Since there is an increase in calorie intake, the need of thiamine, riboflavin and niacin also increases. Females who planned for pregnant should take supplement of folic acid to reduce the risk of fetal neural defects. Folic and B_{12} are essential for DNA and RNA synthesis and needed in higher amounts when tissue synthesis is occurring rapidly.

FOOD CHOICES AND DIETARY CHARACTERISTICS AMONG ADOLESCENTS

Adolescents are maturing not only physically but also cognitively and psychosocially. They search for their identity, strive for independence and acceptance, and are concerned about appearance. Irregular meals, snacking, eating away from home, and following alternative dietary patterns characterize the food habits of adolescents. These habits are further influenced by family, peers and the media.

Meal patterns of adolescents are often chaotic. Teenagers miss an increasing number of meals at home as they get older. They identify time as the biggest barrier to eating properly.

During the peak growth velocity, adolescents usually need to eat large amounts of food often. They are able to use foods with a high concentration of energy; however, they need to be careful to adjust the amounts and frequency they are eating when their growth slows. Habits of overeating adopted during adolescence may ultimately contribute to numerous debilitating diseases.

Eating fast food for meals or snacks is popular especially among adolescents. Fast foods tend to be low in iron, calcium, riboflavin, vitamin A and C. Most of the fast food items provide more than 50% of their calories from fat. Television, magazines and many other media have a greater influence on adolescents eating habits and food choices. All the above factors may lead to nutritional inadequacies among the adolescents.

Dietary Problems

Obesity

This is the commonest disorder which has become epidemic in some developed countries. The incidence of obesity among adolescent is increasing even in India. The eating habits and physical inactivity patterns of adolescents contribute to the increase in adolescent obesity.

Adipose tissue stores increase rapidly in adolescence, so it is no surprise that this stage of life is one of the key points for the development of obesity. During puberty, girls deposit adipose at a greater rate than boys, laying down stores in the breast and hip regions. Fat deposition in boys tends to be more central. This physiological accumulation of adipose tissue results in obesity.

Excessive body fat, particularly in the truncal region, markedly increases health risk in later life. Obese adolescents may suffer from one or more of the following; hypertension, dyslipidemia, type 2 diabetes, sleep apnoea, gastro-oesophageal reflux, etc.

Eating Disorders

A concern about body image becomes more serious if an eating disorder develops. The peak age of onset of eating disorders is during adolescence. Genetic make-up and the attitude of other family members to food may have some influence on susceptibility. Peer pressure, high academic expectations or emotional stresses are likely catalysts. Long-term energy and nutrient depletion can have lasting effects on growth, sexual development and peak bone mass.

Anorexia Nervosa

Anorexia nervosa is a condition, in which the sufferer, although usually physically well, limits food intake, and so loses weight and becomes malnourished.

The main clinical criteria for diagnosis are (WHO 1992):
- Body weight is maintained at least 15% below the standard weight.
- Weight loss is self-induced by avoidance of fattening foods, self-induced vomiting, purging, excessive exercise or appetite suppressants.
- A distortion of body image so that the patient regards herself as fat when she is thin.
- A widespread endocrine disorder involving the hypothalamic pituitary gonadal axis is manifest in woman as amenorrhoea and in men as a loss

of sexual interest and potency. There may also be elevated levels of growth hormone, raised levels of cortisol, changes in the peripheral metabolism of the thyroid gland and abnormalities of insulin secretion.

- If onset is pre-pubertal, the sequence of pubertal events is delayed or even arrested (growth ceases; in girls the breasts do not develop and there is primary amenorrhea; in boys the genitals remain juvenile). With recovery, puberty is often completed normally, but menarche is late.

Clinical Features Include

- Onset usually in adolescence.
- The patients generally eat little.
- A previous history of chubbiness or fatness.
- Amenorrhoea—an early symptom.
- Binge eating.
- Usually a marked lack of sexual interest.
- Lanugo hair.

Physical Effects

The most striking effect is *loss of weight*. This severe weight loss will lead to many physical effects;

- In the early stages of weight loss, glycogen and associated water are shed. Adipose tissue become depleted and muscle mass is lost, causing weakness and impaired function, although this may be denied by the patient who may even persist with excessive exercise. As starvation progresses, there is loss of tissue from other organs, including the brain.
- *Endocrine changes* occur with weight loss
  - Changes in brain neurotransmitters cascade via the hypothalamus and pituitary to distal glands.
  - Thyroid function is suppressed as an adaptive response in order to reduce energy expenditure and protein turnover, and thus lower metabolic rate, although actual energy expenditure may remain relatively high because of high levels of exercise.
  - Cortisol production is increased and that of adrenaline decreased, together with reduced activity of the sympathetic nervous system. This results in hypotension, bradycardia and hypothermia.
  - Sex hormones production is suppressed to infantile levels in both sexes and amenorrhoea is a diagnostic criterion for anorexia nervosa in women of child-bearing age.
  - The loss of normal oestrogen activity contributes to the osteoporosis which is a serious consequence of anorexia nervosa.

Psychological Effects

- Increased depression, anxiety and irritability and, starvation progressed apathy.

- Feeling overweight even though they fall under the category of normal or underweight.
- Perfectionism and low self-esteem are common antecedents.
- They become preoccupied with food to the exclusion of other issues.

Social Effects

- Social isolation.
- Their depression, irritability and loss of sense of humour will make relationships difficult.
- Restriction of eating impairs social functioning because normal sharing of meals becomes stressful or impossible.

Bulimia Nervosa

This refers to episodes of uncontrolled excessive eating, which are also termed 'binges'. There is a preoccupation with food and a habitual adoption of certain behaviours that can be understood as the patient's attempts to avoid the fattening effects of periodic binges.

The main clinical criteria for diagnosis are (WHO 1992):

- There is persisted preoccupation with eating, and an irresistible craving for food; the patient succumbs to episodes of overeating in which a large amount of food is consumed in a short period of time.
- The patient attempts to counteract the "fattening" effects of food by one or more of the following: self-induced vomiting; purgative abuse; alternating periods of starvation; use of drugs such as appetite suppressants, thyroid preparations, or diuretics.
- The psychopathology consists of a morbid dread of fatness, and the patient sets herself or himself a sharply-defined weight threshold, will below the premorbid weight that constitutes the optimum or healthy weight in the opinion of the physician.
- There is often, but not always, a history of an earlier episode of anorexia nervosa, the interval between the two disorders ranging from a few months to several years. This earlier episode may have been fully expressed, or may have assumed a minor cryptic form with a moderate loss of weight and/or a transient phase of amenorrhoea.

Additional clinical features include:
- Physical complications of vomiting:
  a. Cardiac arrhythmias.
  b. Renal impairment—consequences of low K^+.
  c. Muscular paralysis.
  d. Tentany—from hypokalemic alkalosis.
  e. Swollen salivary glands—from vomiting.
  f. Eroded dental enamel.
- Associated psychiatric disorders:
  a. Depressive illness.
  b. Alcohol misuse.

- Fluctuations in body weight.
- Menstrual function—periods irregular but amenorrhoea rate.
- Personality—perfectionism and low self-esteem present premorbidly.

Binge Eating Disorder

This is bulimia without the vomiting and other weight-reducing strategies.
  Criteria for binge eating disorder:
A. Recurrent episodes of binge eating. Binge eating is characterized by
   two of the following:
   - Eating in a discrete period of time (e.g. 2 hours), an amount of food
     that is definitely larger than most people would eat during a similar
     period of time and in the same circumstances.
   - A sense of lack of control of overeating during the episode.
B. The binge eating episodes are associated with three or more of the
   following:
   - Eating much more rapidly than normal.
   - Eating until feeling uncomfortably full.
   - Eating a large amount of food when not feeling physical hunger.
   - Eating alone because of being embarrassed by how much one is
     eating.
   - Feeling disgusted with oneself, depressed or very guilty after
     overeating.
C. Marked distress regarding binge eating is present.
D. The binge eating is not associated with the regular use of inappropriate
   compensatory behaviours (e.g. purging, fasting, excessive exercise)
   and does not occur exclusively during the course of anorexia nervosa
   or bulimia nervosa.

Treatment for Eating Disorder

- Patients should be treated on cognitive behavioural or dynamic
  psychotherapeutic lines or on a combination of both.
- Dietitians must also understand the underlying psychological
  disturbances and should have effective counseling and communication
  skills.
- Establishing a good relationship with the patient.
- Restoring the weight to a level between the ideal body weight and the
  patient's ideal weight.
- The provision of a balanced diet, building up in three to four meals per
  day.
- The elimination of purgative and/or laxative use and vomiting.
- Nutrition education should be given to avoid eating disorder by creating
  the awareness on proper quality and quantity diet, physical activity
  and better lifestyle.

26 Nutrition During Pregnancy

Table 26.1: Recommended dietary allowance of an expectant mother

Nutrient	Normal adult women	Pregnant women
Energy kcals		
Sedentary	1875	+300
Moderate	2225	+300
Heavy	2925	+300
Protein (g)	50	+15
Fat (g)	20	30
Calcium (mg)	400	1000
Iron (mg)	30	38
Retinol (mcg)	600	600
Beta carotene (mcg)	2400	2400
Thiamine (mg)		
Sedentary	0.9	+0.2
Moderate	1.1	+0.2
Heavy	1.2	+0.2
Riboflavin (mg)		
Sedentary	1.1	+0.2
Moderate	1.3	+0.2
Heavy	1.5	+2
Niacin (mcg)		
Sedentary	12	+2
Moderate	14	+2
Heavy	16	+2
Pyridoxine (mg)	2.0	2.5
Ascorbic acid (mg)	40	40
Folic acid (mcg)	100	400
Vitamin B_{12} (mcg)	1	1

One would expect pregnancy to be a time of significantly increased nutritional needs for the mother, the phrase "eating for two "has, in the past, been widely used to sum up this expectation. As it is a time of physiological stress, the health and well-being of many pregnant women and their babies might be adversely affected by suboptimal nutrition despite the low frequently of overt malnutrition within the population. Morning sickness affects over half of women in the early part of pregnancy and this could compound with other stresses to deplete nutrient stores in some women.

The importance of maintaining good nutrition during pregnancy is well established, as reflected in the increased dietary recommendations for many micronutrients which are considered necessary to cover the extra nutrient demands of pregnancy and lactation.

A woman whose diet is adequate before pregnancy is usually able to bear a full-term viable infant, without extensive modifications of her diet. Mother diet should produce adequate nutrients so that maternal stores do not get depleted and produce sufficient milk to nourish her child after birth. The nutritional demands are highly increased in an adolescent mother.

PHYSIOLOGICAL CHANGES IN PREGNANCY

1. The blood volume increases by about 20% or about 1 L. The increase is mainly because of increase in plasma volume. This may cause hemodilution. Because of great demand for iron by the foetus, the mother usually develops anaemia. This can be rectified by proper prenatal care and iron replacement.

2. Generally, cardiac output is increased by about 30% in the first trimester. This is mainly because of increase in rate and force of contraction of the heart and blood volume.

3. Increase of blood volume resulting in decrease in blood glucose values and serum levels of albumin, other serum proteins, and water soluble vitamins. The decline in serum albumin levels contributes to a tendency for extracellular water to accumulate during pregnancy. The decrease in water soluble vitamin concentration makes determination of an inadequate intake or a deficient nutrient state difficult.

4. The arterial blood pressure remains unchanged during the first trimester. During the second trimester, there may be a slight decrease in blood pressure. This is due to the diversion of blood uterine sinuses. And, blood pressure may increase if proper prenatal care is not taken.

5. The overall activity of respiratory system increases slightly its tidal volume; pulmonary ventilation and oxygen utilization are also increased.

6. Increase in renal blood flow and glomerular filtration rate will increase urine formation. This is because of increase in fluid intake and the increased excretory products from foetus. The urine becomes diluted, the frequency of micturition increases because of the pressure excreted by the uterus on bladder.

7. Reabsorption of nutrients get reduce amino acids, glucose and water soluble vitamins may appear in the urine. This may be the reason for the increased number of urinary tract infections seen in pregnant women.

8. During the initial stages of pregnancy, the morning sickness occurs in mother. This involves nausea, vomiting and giddiness. This is because of hormonal imbalance.

9. The motility of gastrointestinal tract is decreased by progesterone, and constipation is common. Indigestion and decreased amount of hydrochloric acid in gastric juice (hypochlorhydria) can also occur. Additionally, a relaxed lower oesophageal sphincter can cause regurgitation and heart burns.

10. The average increases in the body weight during pregnancy is about 12 kg. The approximate weight of various structures which adds to the weight gain of the body are

    1. Foetus 3.5 kg
    2. Amniotic fluid 2.0 kg
    3. Placenta 1.5 kg
    4. Increases in maternal body weight 5.0 kg.

Metabolic Changes

1. The metabolic activities are accelerated in the body due to the increased secretion of various hormones like thyroxine, cortisol and sex hormones. These hormones increase the basal metabolic rate by about 15% in the later stage of pregnancy.

2. The anabolism of proteins is increased in pregnancy, positive nitrogen balance occurs. The deposition of proteins is increased in the uterus.

3. Blood glucose level increases. Hepatic glycogen is depleted and glycosuria occurs. Ketosis develops either due to less food or more vomiting. Because of all these reasons, there is hyperplasia of beta cells of islets of langerhans in pancreas leading to increased insulin secretion. In spite of this there is possibility of developing diabetes in pregnancy or latent diabetes after delivery.

4. During pregnancy, there is deposition of about 3 to 4 kg of fat in the maternal body. This also increases the blood cholesterol level and ketosis.

5. Estrogen and progesterone are secreted by corpus luteum in the first trimester and by placenta later. These hormones increase the retention sodium and water.

Role of Placenta

Placenta forms a link between the foetus and mother. It is considered as an anchor for the growing foetus. It is not only the physical attachment between the foetus and mother but also forms the physiological connection between the two. The various nutritive and other substances that are necessary for the development of foetus diffuse the mother's blood into the foetal blood through placenta. The metabolic end products and other waste products form the foetal body are excreted into the mother blood through placenta. Foetal lungs are nonfunctioning, so the placenta forms the respiratory organ for foetus, oxygen necessary for foetus is received from the maternal blood and carbon dioxide from the foetal blood diffuses into the mother blood through placenta (Fig. 26.1).

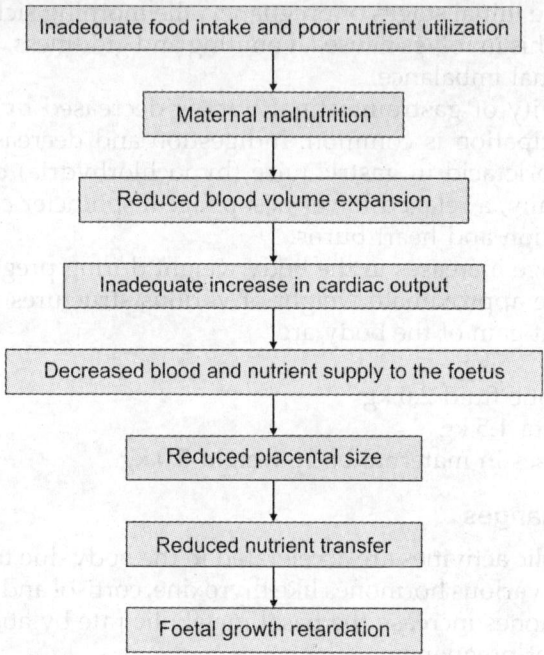

Fig. 26.1: Relationship between maternal and foetal nutrition

Nutritional Requirements

Energy

Calories must be sufficient to (1) supply the increased energy and nutrient demands by the increased metabolic workload, including some maternal fat storage and foetal fat storage to ensure an optimal newborn size for survival and (2) spare protein for tissue building. A minimum of about 36 kcal/1 kg is required for efficient use of protein during pregnancy. RDA standard recommends an additional amount of energy, 300 kcal during the second and third trimesters of rapid growth. Any decrease in the activity of the mother decrease the calorie requirement.

For an Indian women of 55 kg, the total energy cost of a pregnancy is about 80,000 kcal of this about 36,000 kcal is deposited as fat which is utilized sub-subsequently during lactation. Hence ICMR recommended energy requirements of pregnancy women are as follows.

Sedentary works   1875 + 300 = 2175
Moderate works   2225 + 300 = 2525
Heavy works   2925 + 300 = 3225

Consequences of Energy Restriction

A popular concept is that the foetus develops at the expense of the mother during nutritional deprivation. An inadequately nourished mother is proportionately less affected than her foetus. One consequence of severe energy restriction is increased ketone production. After an overnight fast, maternal blood ketone body concentrations are greater in pregnant than in non-pregnant women, and even ketonuria can be detected. Ketones are the result of fat metabolism and suspected of being more detrimental to the foetus in a pregnancy complicated by insulin dependent diabetes mellitus.

Protein

The total amount of protein recommended for the pregnant women is about 60 g/day, an increase of about 10 to 15 g/day. More protein is necessary to meet tissue demands posed by,

1. Rapid growth of the foetus.
2. Enlargement of the uterus, mammary glands and placenta.
3. Increase in maternal circulating blood volume and subsequent demand for increased plasma proteins to maintain colloidal osmotic pressure and circulation of tissue fluids to nourish cells and
4. Formation of amniotic fluid and storage reserve for labour, delivery and lactation.

Milk, egg, cheese and meat are complete protein foods of high biologic value. Protein rich foods also contribute other nutrients such as calcium, iron and B vitamins. Additional proteins may be obtained from legumes and whole grains with lesser amounts in other plant sources.

Linoleic Acid

The requirements of linoleic acid during pregnancy is 4–4.5 en%. If invisible fat is 12.5 en% to meet, EFA, visible fat will be 30 g/day.

Fibre

Daily consumption of whole grain breads and cereals, green leafy and yellow vegetables and fresh and dried fruits should be encouraged to provide additional minerals, vitamins and fibre.

Vitamin A

Normal requirements of β-carotene for an adult woman are 2400 mcg. During pregnancy no additional recommendation is suggested. Maternal stores of vitamin A easily meet foetal accretion rate. Vitamin A plays a role in gene expression for acrosin and plasminogen activators which are important for spermatogenesis. In human cord blood vitamin A concentrations correlated with birth weight, head circumference, length and gestation duration. Vitamin A required for this purpose is about 25 μg/day throughout pregnancy. Since this constitutes a small fraction of the recommended allowance for normal women, no additional dietary allowance during pregnancy is suggested. Liver, egg yolk, butter, dark green and yellow vegetables and fruits are good sources of vitamin A.

According to studies conducted at NIN of Hyderabad (1985), it is revealed that pregnant woman of the low income groups have poor vitamin A status judged by serum vitamin A levels. A daily supplementation of 6000 I.U for about 12 weeks appears to improve serum vitamin A levels and correct vitamin A deficiency in these pregnant women. Improving vitamin A status of pregnant women reduces maternal mortality. Excess vitamin A should not be taken during pregnancy.

Vitamin D

During pregnancy the increased need for calcium and phosphorus presented by the developing foetal skeletal tissue requires additional vitamin D to promote the absorption and utilization of these minerals. The recommended amount for pregnancy is 10 μg cholecalciferol (400 IU/day)

Maternal vitamin D deficiency is associated with neonatal hypocalcemia and hypoplasia of tooth enamel. Foetal bone mineralization may be affected by maternal vitamin D deficiency. Excessive vitamin D can also result in complications such as atherosclerosis, hypercalcemia, and calcium deposits in various vital organs and mental retardation in the infants.

Vitamin E

It has not been evidently proved that vitamin E deficiency can cause pregnancy failure although they may prove beneficial to those who have had repeated spontaneous abortions or failure to conceive. A very little vitamin E crosses the placenta so infant has low tissue concentrations that persist up to at least 6 years. Requirements of vitamin E increased with increased intake of PUFA.

Vitamin K

Vitamin K is essential for synthesis of prothrombin that is necessary for normal coagulation of blood. It is highly essential for preventing neonatal haemorrhage. An oral dosage of menadione (synthetic form of vitamin K) during the last week of pregnancy or an injection during labour is essential to stimulate prothrombin synthesis. But care should be taken to see that the dosage is given at average level to prevent adverse effects.

Water Soluble Vitamins

Because a little of water soluble vitamins is stored, the pregnant woman must rely her daily intakes that are high enough to meet the added requirements of pregnancy. These are usually supplied by a well-balanced diet that is increased in quality and quantity to supply needed energy and nutrients. B vitamins are important as coenzyme factors in a number of metabolic activities related to energy production, tissue protein synthesis, and function of muscle and nerve tissue. Therefore, they play key roles in the increased metabolic work of pregnancy.

Folic Acid

Folic acid requirement increases during pregnancy in response to the demands of maternal erythropoiesis, foetal and placental growth and most important for the prevention of neural tube defects (NTD). Neural tube defect is a birth defect occurring in the brain or spinal cord. NTD are among the most common of all serious birth defects. The neural tube is part of the foetus that becomes the spinal cord and brain. Folic acid deficiency is marked by a reduced rate of deoxyribonucleic acid (DNA) synthesis and mitotic activity in individual cells. Megaloblastic anaemia is the latest stage of folate deficiency and it may not present until the third trimester, however, white cell morphologic and biochemical changes signalling deficiency may precede overt anaemia. Malformations can also occur in infants of women using folate antagonist drugs such as the anticonvulsant medications, phenytoin (dilantin), carbamazepine and diphenylhydantoin, oral contraceptives and some antibiotics may also cause late insufficiency.

Also folacin is essential for the developing of RBC which must increase as the mother blood volume increases. Once folate enters the foetal circulation, it cannot be retransferred back into the maternal blood. There is notable decrease in folate absorption and an increase in urinary excretion during pregnancy may contribute to maternal store depletion. Aminopterin, a folacin antagonist induces resorption of foetuses in animals. Its use in human beings leads to congenital malformation such as hare lip, cleft palate or hydrocephalus and complication of pregnancy "abruptio placenta", i.e. premature detachment of the placenta, foetal malformation haemorrhage which has all been identified as a result of folic acid deficiency and cannot be supplemented after the onset of the problems.

Supplementation of folic acid before conception and during the first 12 weeks of pregnancy is advisable to reduce the primary and secondary risk of NTDs-spinabifida and encephaly in the foetus. Birth weights of infants born to mother who had received 300 µg folate a day during pregnancy were higher than those born to mothers who received either 100 or 200 µg daily, these finding suggest that pregnancy women need 300 µg of additional folic acid daily.

Vitamin B₆

Vitamin B_6 has been used to manage the severe nausea and vomiting in pregnancy. Although this vitamin catalyzes a number of reactions involving neurotransmitter production, it is not known whether this function is involved in the relief of symptoms. During pregnancy due to normal stress the tryptophan metabolism is altered, resulting in decrease ability to convert tryptophan to niacin and this affects the cell growth.

Vitamin B₁₂

Normal adult women's requirement of vitamin B_{12} is 1mcg and this requirements remains the same even during pregnancy. The foetus has priority over the mother in B_{12}, and foetal blood had twice the amount of B_{12} than does maternal blood even when maternal levels are depleted. Low maternal levels are associated with prematurity. The capacity of women to absorb B_{12} is increased during pregnancy and a large amount is transferred to the foetus. Vegetarian mothers have more chances of getting B_{12} deficiency. Serum levels drop during pregnancy and return to normal without supplementation after delivery. On the basis of the B_{12} content of foetuses, it has been estimated that foetal demands may be of the order of 0.3 µg per day.

Vitamin C

Ascorbic acid deficiency has not been associated with adverse pregnancy outcome. ICMR recommendations of vitamin C during pregnancy is 40 mg same as normal women requirements. There are some evidence shows placenta can synthesize vitamin C. Few studies have suggested that an association between low plasma levels of vitamin C and preeclampsia, as well as premature rupture of the membranes (PROM).

Minerals

Calcium

Hormonal factors strongly influence calcium metabolism in pregnant women. Human chorionic somato mammotropic from the placenta increases the rate of maternal bone turnover. Estrogen also largely derived from the placenta, inhibits bone resorption, provoking a compensatory release of parathyroid hormone, which maintains maternal serum calcium across the gut. The net effect of these changes which predates foetal skeletal mineralization is the promotion of progressive calcium retention to meet progressively increasing foetal skeletal demands for mineralization. Foetal hypercalcemia and subsequent endocrine adjustments ultimately stimulate the mineralization process.

ICMR calcium requirements of adult women are 400 mg/day. Requirements increase during pregnancy to 1000 mg/day. Although the infant bones are poorly calcified at the time of birth, an appreciable amount of calcium is involved in foetal development. A full-term foetal body is made up of 30 g calcium. Increased intake of calcium by the mother is highly essential, not only for the calcification of foetal bones and teeth but also for the protection of calcium resources of the mother to meet the high demands during lactation.

The amount of dietary calcium needed is reduced when vitamin D is available. Use of vitamin D and calcium reduces muscular cramps of pregnancy. Dairy products are a primary source of calcium. Green leafy vegetable also contribute to calcium.

Iron

Normal iron requirements of adult women are 30 mg/day. ICMR requirements during pregnancy are 38 mg/day. Some women may need supplementation of iron in addition to increased dietary sources to meet the additional requirements of pregnancy. The iron loss in pregnancy is high. During pregnancy, the maternal circulating blood normally increases from 40% to 50% and may increase more with multiple births. A maternal iron is also needed to supply iron stones for the developing foetal liver. Adequate maternal iron stones also help fortify the mother against serum iron losses at delivery.

To avoid iron deficiency women should enter pregnancy with a store of at least 300 mg of iron. If the women are anaemic at conception, a large therapeutic amount of 120 to 200 mg of iron is recommended.

Sodium

Normal adult women requirements of sodium should be maintained to prevent any defective disorders and deficiency. The hormonal changes of pregnancy affects sodium metabolism. Increased extra cellular fluid which calls for 80% increases in the body sodium. Increased maternal blood volume leads to increased glomerular filtration of sodium of 5000 to 10000 mEq/day, compensatory mechanisms maintain fluid and electrolyte balance. Restriction of dietary sodium or the use of diuretics in pregnant women with edema is not recommended. Rigorous sodium restriction in pregnant women resulted in production of renin hormone from kidney and from which the sodium that is needed for use by the body is retained.

Iodine

Normal requirements are insufficient during pregnancy especially if mother belong to the adolescent group. If increased demands are not met, it may even result in onset of goiter. The only known role of iodine is in the thyroxine molecule. The thyroxine hormone has critical roles in metabolism of macronutrients. Maternal iodine deficiency has long been recognized as a cause of neonatal cretinism. Iodized salt can be used as a preventive measure. Iodine deficiency increases the risk of still birth and miscarriage.

Zinc

Zinc deficiency during the maternal period leads to adverse effects on the new born including-CNS teratogenicity and reduced intra uterine growth rate. Low zinc during pregnancy doubles the risk of low birth weight and triples the risk of preterm delivery.

GENERAL DIETARY PROBLEMS
Nausea and Vomiting

Morning sickness or nausea and vomiting in pregnancy affects 50% to 90% of all pregnant women during the first trimester of pregnancy have this symptoms. These symptoms are usually short term and mild. Some are physiologic based on hormonal changes that occur early in pregnancy.

Others may be psychological based on situational tensions or anxieties about the pregnancy itself. Still others may be dietary problems based on poor food habits. Simple treatment generally improves food toleration. Fairly dry and consisting chiefly of easily digested energy-yielding foods, citrus foods can be suggested. If the condition develops to hyperemesis gravidarum, a severe prolonged persistent vomiting, peripheral parental nutrition and careful oral feeding is essential. Fatty rich foods, fried food, excessive seasoning, coffee in large amount and strongly flavoured vegetable may be restricted or eliminated.

Constipation

The complaint of constipation is seldom more than minor but contributes to discomfort and concern. Placental hormones relax the gastrointestinal muscles, and the pressure of the enlarging uterus on the lower portion of the intestine may make elimination somewhat difficult. Increased fluid intake and the use of naturally laxative foods containing dietary fibre such as whole grains, fruits and vegetables, dried fruits and other fruits and juices generally induce regularity. Laxatives should be avoided.

Heart Burn or Gastric Pressure

The related complaints of heart burn or a full feeling are sometimes voiced by pregnant women. These discomforts occur especially after meals and are usually caused by the pressure of the enlarging uterus crowding the stomach. Gastric reflux of some of the food mass, now a liquid chyme mixed with stomach acid, may occur in the lower oesophagus causing an irritation and burning sensation. This common complaint has nothing to do with heart action, but is so called because of the proximity of the lower esophagus to the heart. By having small frequent meals can avoid these complaints.

Beliefs, Avoidance, Cravings and Aversions

Certain beliefs and avoidances of food reflect mother conscious choice not to consume certain foods during pregnancy, e.g. heat producing foods like papaya and gingelly seeds. Craving and aversions are powerful urges toward or away from foods which women experience no unusual attitudes when not pregnant. Most commonly craved foods are sweets and dairy products. The most common aversions reported are to coffee other caffeinated drinks, meats and strongly spiced foods.

Pica

Consumption of non-food items such as laundry starch, ice cubes or clay is called pica. It occurs more often during pregnancy than at any other time. One theory hypothesized that a deficiency for essential nutrient, such as calcium or iron, results in the eating of non-food substances that contain these nutrients. Much of this behaviour appears to be based on superstitions, customs and traditions that one often passes from mother to daughter.

Weight Gain During Pregnancy

An average weight gain during pregnancy is about 11 to 14 kg (25–30 lb). Around this average many individual variations occur. In addition to the components of growth and development usually attributes to a pregnancy, an important part is maternal stores. This laying down of extra adipose fat tissue is necessary for maternal energy reserves to sustain rapid foetal growth during the later half of pregnancy and for labour and delivery and maintaining lactation after birth (Table 26.2).

Table 26.2: Recommended weight gains for pregnant women based on BMI

Weight category based on BMI	Total weight gain (kg)
Underweight (BMI < 19.8)	12.5–18
Normal weight (19.8–26)	11.5–16
Overweight BMI > 26–29	7–11.5
Obese > 29	6.0

Complications

Anaemia

Anaemia is common during pregnancy. It is often associated with a normal maternal blood volume increase of about 50% and a disproportionate increase in red cell mass of about 20%, haemoglobin concentration drops from 13.4 to 11.6 g per 100 ml of blood. A pregnant woman is labelled anaemia if the haemoglobin is less than 10 g per 100 ml of blood form the 28th weak onwards.

In anaemia, by far the most common is iron deficiency anaemia. A less common is megaloblastic anaemia. A significant fall in birth weight due to increase in prematurity rate and intrauterine growth retardation has been reported to occur when maternal haemoglobin level falls below 8 g/dl. The effect of anaemia and urinary tract infection in pregnancy could also be the cause of low birth weight infant.

Treatment of highly deficient states requires daily therapeutic doses of 120 to 200 mg. This oral therapy may be continued for 3–6 months after anaemia has been connected in order to replenish the depleted stores. Administration orally of 60 mg elemental iron and 500 µg of folic acid per day in the last trimester of pregnancy prevents anaemia.

Megaloblastic anaemia of pregnancy results from folate deficiency. During pregnancy, the foetus is sensitive to folate inhibitors and therefore has increased metabolic requirements for folate. To prevent this anaemia, the RDA standard recommends 400 µg of folate daily. Women with poor diets will need supplementation to reach this intake goal.

Pregnancy Induced Hypertension (Toxaemia)

A study conducted at National Institute of Nutrition indicates that severe pregnancy induced hypertension (eclampsia) is associated with higher incidence of vitamin A and protein deficiencies resulting in poor pregnancy outcome. It is a disease principally affecting young mothers with their first pregnancy. Certainly, as many practitioners have observed, PIH is classically with poverty, inadequate diet, and little or no prenatal care. Much of the PIH problem, which seems to develop early from the time of implantation of the fertilized ovum into the uterine lining, may be reduce by good prenatal care from the beginning of the pregnancy, which inherently includes attention to sound nutrition. The symptoms of PIH include hypertension, abnormal and excessive oedema, albuminuria, convulsions or coma. Optimal nutrition is a fundamental aspect of therapy, emphasis is given to adequate dietary protein. In addition, adequate salt and sources of vitamin and minerals are needed for correction and maintenance of metabolic balance.

Hypertension

Preexisting hypertension in the pregnant women can cause considerable maternal and foetal consequences. Many of these problems can be prevented by initial screening and continued monitoring by the prenatal nurse, with referral to the clinical nutritionist for plan of care. Nutritional therapy will centre on

1. Prevention of weight extremes, underweight or obesity
2. Correction of any dietary deficiencies and maintenance of optimal nutritional status during pregnancy and
3. Management of any related preexisting disease such as diabetes mellitus. Sodium intake may be moderate but should not be unduly restricted.

Diabetes Mellitus

During pregnancy glycosuria is common, because of the increased circulating blood volume and its load of metabolites. Most of these women revert to normal glucose tolerance after delivery. Gestational diabetes occurs in 2% to 13% of the pregnant population. But only 20% to 30% of these women showing this pregnancy-induced abnormal glucose tolerance subsequently develop diabetes. Follow up is important because of the higher risk these women carry for foetal damage during this gestational period.

DIETARY MODIFICATION AND DIETARY GUIDELINES

1. Pregnant woman should include five basic food groups. Due to nausea and vomiting, it is difficult to take food properly, hence one can include small frequent meals.
2. Pattern of weight gain during pregnancy is more important than the total amount of weight gained. It is better to gain majority of pregnancy weight during the last two trimesters. An erratic weight gain may leads to toxemia.

3. Highly seasoned foods and fried foods can be avoided since heart burn is common complaint in pregnancy, one can take easily digestible food.

4. Plenty of water, fruits, vegetables and greens can be included to overcome constipation, dehydration.

5. Pregnant women who drink too much cola can harm their foetuses. These beverages usually made using the kola nut and it contains caffeine as well as bioactive alkaloids such as clonidine. These can pass through the placenta into the body of foetuses and effects the development of organs.

6. Pregnant women who drink coffee often also face higher risk of miscarriage and birth defects.

7. Tobacco smoke contains hundreds of harmful substances and if a pregnant woman smoke or is exposed to second hand smoke, she can seriously impact the development of her foetus. Because it contains carbon monoxide and nicotine in smoke which can pass through the placenta and affects the foetus, causing anorexia to the foetal organs and speeding up heartbeat.

8. *Resist drinking alcohol:* Alcohol used by pregnant women can lead to slowed development of the foetal organs and increases the chances of premature birth and perinatal death rate.

9. Folic acid supplement should be started at least one month before getting pregnant until it is too late. Greens are rich in folic acid. Minimum one serving of greens per day is recommended.

10. Not getting enough iron could cause anaemia, it could contribute to developmental delays and behavioural disturbances in the infant and poor health in the mother. Iron-rich foods such as greens, rice flakes, liver, sea foods, and sprouts, legumes like chickpea, soybeans, and red kidney beans should be made mandatory.

11. Optimum sodium should be ensured, restricted sodium should be advised in case of oedema or pregnancy induced hypertension.

27 Nutritional Requirements for Lactating Women

The new born baby depends for some period solely on breast milk for his existence. Due to breastfeeding there are specific health advantages for both mother and infant. Breastfeeding decreases the incidence of severity of infectious diseases for infant. Enhances neuro development, promotes mother-child bonding. Breastfeeding helps mother to decrease post-partum bleeding, decreases menstrual blood loss. Earlier return to prepregnant weight decrease risk of breast and ovarian cancer.

PHYSIOLOGY OF LACTATION (Fig. 27.1)

Mammary gland growth during menarche and pregnancy prepares for lactation. Hormonal changes markedly increases breast, areola, and nipple size. In pregnancy hormones that significantly increase ducts and alveoli influence mammary growth. Late in pregnancy the lobules of the alveolar system are maximally developed and small amount of colostrum, the thin,

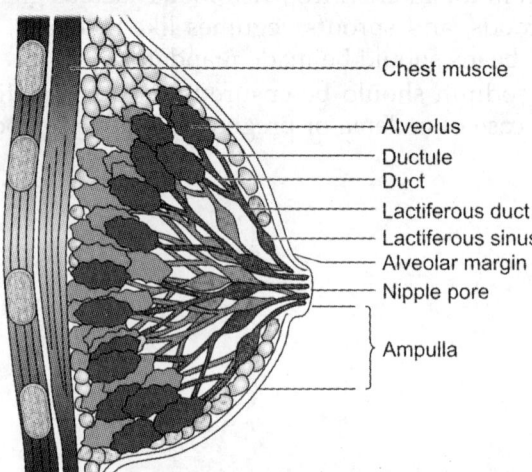

Chest muscle
Alveolus
Ductule
Duct
Lactiferous duct
Lactiferous sinus
Alveolar margin
Nipple pore
Ampulla

Fig. 27.1: Structural features of the human mammary gland. The terminal glandular (alveolar) tissue of each lobule leads into the duct systems, which enlarges eventually into the lactiferous duct and lactiferous sinus. The lactiferous sinuses rest beneath the areola and converge at the nipple pore

yellow, milky fluid rich in antibodies may be released for several weeks before term and for a few days after delivery.

HORMONAL ROLE IN MILK PRODUCTION

Suckling is the usual stimulus for milk production and secretion. Subcutaneous nerves of the areola send a message via the spinal cord to the hypothalamus, which in turn transmits a message to the pituitary gland, where both the anterior and posterior areas are stimulated. Prolactin from the anterior pituitary stimulates alveolar cell milk production; oxytocin from the posterior pituitary stimulates the myoepithelial cells of the mammary gland to contract, causing movements of milk through the ducts and lactiferous sinuses, a process referred to as let-down. "Let-down" is highly sensitive. Oxytocin, the milk releasing hormone, can be released by visual, tactile, olfactory, and auditory stimuli; and even by thinking about the infant. Oxytocin secretion can also be inhibited by pain, emotional and physical stress, fatigue, and anxiety. Adrenaline release is believed to negate the effects of oxytocin on the myoepithelial cells (Fig. 27.2).

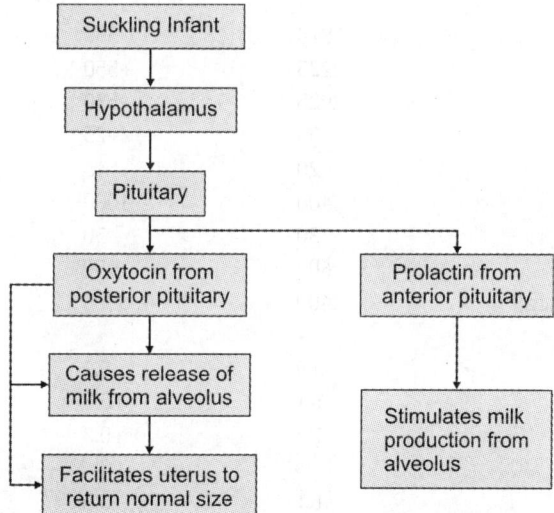

Fig. 27.2: Process of stimulation of milk production

FACTORS AFFECTING COMPOSITION OF MILK

Maternal and environmental factors may have a stronger impact on milk composition.

1. Prolonged lactation in nutritionally depleted women is likely to impact more comprehensively on milk composition than volume.
2. The fatty acid composition of mother milk reflects her dietary intake. In addition milk concentration of selenium, iodine and some of the water

soluble vitamins are reflection of maternal diet. Hence nutritional status of mother reflects the composition of milk.

3. Minerals such as calcium, copper, and fluorine doesn't depend on maternal diet.
4. Milk production is most affected by the frequency of suckling and maternal hydration.
5. Maternal and infant illness may affect the amount and content of milk.

NUTRITIONAL REQUIREMENTS FOR LACTATING WOMEN

The nutritional needs of lactation are greater than those of pregnancy, and they demand adequate nutritional support. Nutritional requirements of lactating woman should meet her daily needs and support the growing infant. RDA for lactating woman given in Table 27.1.

Table 27.1: Recommended dietary allowances of a lactating mother

	Normal adult women	Lactating mother	
		0–6	6–12
Energy kcal			
Sedentary	1875	+550	+400
Moderate	2225	+550	+400
Heavy	2925	+550	+400
Protein (g)	50	+25	+18
Fat (g)	20	45	45
Calcium (mg)	400	1000	1000
Iron (mg)	30	30	30
Retinol (mcg)	600	950	950
Beta carotene (mcg)	2400	3800	3800
Thiamine (mg)			
Sedentary	0.9	+0.3	+0.2
Moderate	1.1	+0.3	+0.2
Heavy	1.2	+0.3	+0.2
Riboflavin (mg)			
Sedentary	1.1	+0.3	+0.2
Moderate	1.3	+0.3	+0.2
Heavy	1.5	+0.3	+0.2
Niacin (mcg)			
Sedentary	12	+4	+3
Moderate	14	+4	+3
Heavy	16	+4	+3
Pyridoxine (mg)	2.0	2.5	2.5
Ascorbic acid (mg)	40	80	80
Folic acid (mcg)	100	150	150
Vitamin B_{12} (mcg)	1	1.5	1.5

Energy

Milk production is 80% efficient. Production of 100 ml of milk (about 75 kcal) requires 85 kcal expenditure. During the first 6 months of lactation, average milk production is 750 ml/day, with a range of 550 to more than 1200 ml/day. Since the production is a function of the frequency, duration, and intensity of infant suckling, infants who fed well are likely to stimulate the production of larger volumes of milk. Hence, recommended energy increase is 550 kcal for first 6 months and 400 kcal during the next six months more than the usual adult allowance.

Maternal fat stores accumulated during pregnancy provide about 100 to 150 kcal to support the early 6 months of lactation. When the reserve fat stores have been depleted, dietary energy support for lactation must be increased if the mother tends to provide all or most of her infants nutrition through the breast milk alone. During the next 6 months, output of milk generally get reduced, hence allowance are suggested as 400 kcal/day. Most infants also consume solid foods in this time. Milk production decreases in mothers who undertake vigorous calorie-restricted diets.

Protein

During lactation protein requirement has been computed on the basis of secretion in milk of 9.4 g protein per day during 0–6 months and 6.6 g during 6–24 months which correspond to 820 ml and 600 ml of milk respectively with protein content 1.15 g/100 ml. In terms of dietary protein NPU 65, safe daily intake would be 26 g and 18.5 g respectively. The Nutrition Expert Committee has recommended, during lactation all additional daily intakes of 25 g for the first 6 months and 18 g during 6–12 months of lactation.

Fat

The amount and type of fat in breast milk directly reflects the maternal diet. Adjustments in the maternal diet can increase or decrease specific fatty acids. Severe restriction of energy intake results in mobilization of body fat, and the milk produced has a fatty acid composition resembling that of the mother's depot fat. The requirements of linoleic acid during lactation increases 5.7 en%, invisible fat requirements is 17.5 en % and visible fat should be 45 g.

Calcium

The increased amount of calcium that was required during gestation for mineralization of the foetal skeleton is now diverted into the mother's milk production. Both during pregnancy and lactation, 1000 mg has been prescribed by ICMR. 500 ml of milk or milk products should be given to lactating mother to meet 1000 mg of calcium.

Vitamins

The quantity of vitamin A presents in 650 ml of human milk is 300 mcg so the ICMR recommends an additional allowance of 350 mcg of retinol.

Vitamin B requirements also increased as calorie and protein requirements increased because they are involved as co-enzyme factor in energy metabolism. In lactating women, deficiency of thiamine affects not only the adult but also may have repercussions on the nutrition of the breast-fed infants.

In lactating women blood folate drop constantly reflecting the stress imposed by maintaining folate content of breast milk at approximately 25 µg/day. An additional allowance of 50 µg of folate could be provided during lactation.

The amount of vitamin B_{12} secreted in milk per day is 0.25–0.3 µg. An additional intake of 0.5 µg per day would cover the needs during lactation. Milk is a good source of riboflavin, hence requirement would be met easily.

Dietary Guidelines

1. The diet should include lactogogues which stimulates the production of milk. Garlic, milk, almonds and gardencress seeds are considered to increase the milk production. Fish consumption also believed to improve the milk production.
2. During lactation adequate fluid intake is needed along with energy intake. Hence one can include beverages such as juices and milk contribute both fluid and calories.
3. Number of meals can be increased since requirements during lactation are high compared to any age group in woman life. If weight loss is rapid in mother, calorie intake can be increased.
4. Weight gain should be avoided.
5. Foods which cause gastric distress to the infant can be avoided for mother.
6. Need to take more greens, fruits, to get nutrients and to overcome constipation.

28

Nutritional Need for Old Age

Aging is a continuous function, and one does not suddenly pass from young to elderly at any specific times. Furthermore, chronologic age alone is not a particularly precise indicator of biologic or functional age because of differences in genotypes, individual characteristics, such as physical ability and mental health, and environmental circumstances, all of which vary widely among people as they age.

Gerontology is the study of late adulthood and aging. Geriatric nutrition deals with the nutritional requirements of old people.

PATHOBIOLOGY OF AGEING

Theories of Ageing

Although the specific causes of some progeroid syndromes have been identified, there are no known specific causes for the common forms of aging. A variety of currently debated theories are discussed in detail in Table 28.1.

Table 28.1: Theories of ageing

Biological level/theory	Description
Evolutionary	
Mutation accumulation	Mutations that affect health at older ages are not selected against.
Disposal soma	Somatic cells are maintained only to ensure continued reproductive success; after reproduction, soma becomes disposable.
Antagonistic pleiotropy	Genes beneficial at younger age become deleterious at older ages.
Molecular	
Gene regulation	Ageing is caused by changes in the expression of genes regulating both development and ageing.
Codon restriction	Fidelity/accuracy of mRNA translation is impaired due to inability to decoded codons in mRNA.

Contd.

Table 28.1: Theories of ageing (*Contd.*)

Biological level/theory	Description
Error catastrophe	Decline in fidelity of gene expression with ageing result in increased fraction of abnormal proteins.
Somatic mutation	Molecular damage accumulates, primarily to DNA/genetic material.
Dysdifferentiation	Gradual accumulation of random molecular damage impairs regulation of gene expression.
Cellular	
Cellular senescence-telomere theory	Phenotypes of ageing are caused by an increase in frequency of senescent cells. Senescence may result from telomere loss (replicative senescence) or cell stress (cellular senescence).
Free radicals	Oxidative metabolism produces highly reactive free radicals that subsequently damage lipids, protein, and DNA.
Wear-and-tear	Accumulation of normal injury.
Apoptosis	Programmed cell death from genetic events or genome crisis.
System	
Neuroendocrine	Alterations in neuroendocrine control of homeostasis result in ageing-related physiological changes.
Immunologic	Decline of immune function with ageing results in decreased incidence of infectious diseases but increased incidence of autoimmunity.
Rate of living	Assumes a fixed amount of metabolic potential for every living organism (live fast, die young).

Source: David H. Alpers; Manual of nutritional therapeutics, 5th edition (2009)

a. Evolutionary theories that view ageing as the result of the diminishing advantage of natural selection that is the consequence of survival beyond the age of reproductive fitness.

b. Genetic molecular theories that postulate that ageing results from effects at the gene level that cause molecular damage to DNA, alter gene expression, reduce the accuracy and fidelity of translation, and related effects.

c. Cellular theories that relate the generation of ageing to the consequences of repeated damage to cellular components and metabolic process, oxidative damage to the proteins or the mitochondrial electron transfer system or to mitochondrial DNA, the intracellular accumulation of altered proteins resulting from oxidative damage, glycosylation or other posttranslational modifications, or to accelerated apoptosis and cell senescence.

d. System theories that consider ageing to be consequence of slow, but inexorable failure of fine regulatory control within major biological systems such as the neuroendocrine or immunological system.

Pathophysiologic Consequences of Ageing

Once the body reaches physiologic maturity, the rate of catabolic or degenerative change may become greater than the anabolic regeneration. The resultant loss of cells can lead to varying degrees of decreased efficiency and impaired function.

Body Composition

Lean body mass declines approximately 6% per decade after age 30. To a significant extent, this decrement is a consequence of diminished physical activity rather than of the ageing process itself.

Muscle, a principal component of lean mass, is altered both structurally and functionally as on ages, largely on the basis of reduced mitochondrial energy production through ATP. Sarcopenia, age-related loss of skeletal muscle results in frailty and disability. One additional consequence of decline in lean body mass is a corresponding increase in fat mass (Table 28.2).

Organ System Function

- Ageing is associated with diminished smell (hyposmia) and taste (dysgeusia), particularly the loss of sweet and salty tastes.
- Reduction in salivary flow, loss of teeth, and disturbances of swallowing (dysphagia) and esophageal dysfunction may be noted.
- Many persons experience various forms of discomfort associated with eating, including heartburn, gas and constipation.
- Achlorhydria, loss of hydrochloric acid in the stomach, also develops in those who are ageing.
- Atrophic gastritis is principally the consequence of infection with helicobacter pylori.
- Reduction in gastric acid, pepsin, and intrinsic factor lead to slower emptying of mixed meals and diminished absorption of iron, folate, and vitamin B_{12}.
- Ageing is also associated with declining cardiac, pulmonary, and renal function and with diminished secretion of growth hormone, which some believe contributes to the decline in lean body and muscle mass (sarcopenia) that accompanying ageing.
- A decrease in cell-mediated immunity is manifested by decreased numbers of circulating T cells and defective cell-mediated immune responses, which may contribute to the morbidity associated with ageing.
- Humoral immunity is generally less severely affected, but the incidence of autoimmune disorders is increased.
- Atherosclerosis, arthritis, osteoporosis, diabetes, assorted cancers and diminished sight and hearing are all commonly present. To varying degrees, these conditions can limit mobility and access to food, affect mood and diminish appetite.

Table 28.2: Changes in the body as part of the aging process

Part of the body	Changes producing ageing
Skin	Wrinkling Loss of hair Reduced function of sweat and sebaceous glands.
Heart	Loss of heart muscle Increased fibrous tissue Decreased cardiac output
Renal function	Decrease in weight and volume affecting nephrons and resulting in decreased filtration rate and increased glucose threshold.
Bone	Increased resorption.
Immune system	Impaired T cell function and hence greater susceptibility to viral infections.
Small and large intestine	Decreased motor function and muscle tone. Impaired digestive capacity. Diverticula
Liver and biliary function	Decreased size and blood flow. Minor structural and biochemical changes. Gall bladder becomes sluggish in releasing bile. Activity of drug metabolizing enzymes reduced.
Gastric function and emptying	Decreased secretion of hydrochloric acid, intrinsic factor and pepsin. >60 years of age rapid rate of emptying of liquids.
Muscle	Loss of tension Atrophy especially in lower body.
Hearing	Elevated sound threshold. Loss of perception of high frequencies.
Pain and touch	Touch and pain thresholds increase.
Salivary glands	Decrease in salivary secretion causes feeling of dry mouth, xerostomia.
Taste and smell	Decreased number of taste buds. High taste threshold (loss of taste sensitivity). Reduced number of nasal sensory cells.
Teeth	Loss of teeth and wearing dentures.
Vision	Diminished colour fidelity. Decreased visual acuity.
Height	Reduced
Homeostatic regulation	Reduced
Neurologic function	Confusional states.
Whole body composition	Production of fat increases. Lean body mass decreases.

Nutritional Requirements

Energy

Energy requirements gradually reduce with age due to changes in body composition, a decrease in basal metabolic rates, reduced physical activity. The calorie intake should be adjusted to maintain the body weight constant in the case of old people with normal body weight. In the case of obese people, the calorie intake should be adjusted to reduce the body weight gradually to about normal level.

Proteins

A protein intake of 1.0 g per kilogram, the normal adult requirement, is safe during old age. As people ages there is loss of skeletal tissue mass, stores of protein in skeletal muscle may be inadequate to meet the needs for protein synthesis, making dietary protein intake more important. Decreased food intake, a sedentary lifestyle, and reduced energy expenditure in older adults become critical risk factors for malnutrition and especially for insufficient intake of protein and micronutrients.

Carbohydrate

It is recommended approximately 45% to 65% of the total daily calories comes from carbohydrates. Emphasis should be placed on increasing the intake of complex carbohydrate source as legumes, vegetables, whole grains, and fruits to provide fibre, phytonutrients and essential vitamins and minerals.

Lipids

Dietary guidelines recommend that not more than 20% to 30% of the total dietary calorie intake come from lipids. Emphasis should be placed on reducing the intake of saturated fat and choosing monounsaturated or polyunsaturated fat sources.

Minerals

- Osteopenia secondary to osteoporosis and osteomalacia is a significant problem in the elderly. Obligatory calcium losses increase, but calcium intake and absorption decline with age. Reduced absorption may be a consequence of decreased vitamin D function, in turn caused by the combined effects of reduced dietary intake, decreased exposure to sunlight and capacity of the aged skin to synthesize vitamin D, reduced intestinal absorption of the vitamin, and reduced hepatic and renal ability to hydroxylate vitamin D to its active form. Calcium intake should not be less than 1000 mg/day is recommended. Adequate calcium intake in the elderly is a factor in maintaining bone density when accompanied by an adequate intake of vitamin D. Calcium rich source like milk and its product should be included in the diet regularly.

- Iron absorption slightly diminishes with age, and iron status understandably improves in women following the cessation of menses. Most anaemia's in the elderly are the result of iron deficiency, chronic inflammation, or chronic renal disease. It is important that a good dietary iron intake should be maintained, together with sufficient vitamin C to promote non-haeme iron absorption. Iron requirement in old age is the same as adult man. Inclusion of liver, green leafy vegetables, whole grains, fruits and vegetables will help in avoiding the deficiency.
- Zinc absorption declines with age. Also, intakes of zinc in older adults decrease in relation to the decrease in energy intake. Older people who avoid eating meat and fish may be at increased risk of poor zinc status because of reduced bioavailability of zinc from other food sources. Zinc deficiency is associated with impaired immune function, anorexia, dysgeusia, delayed wound healing, and pressure ulcers.
- Sodium intake is often associated with hypertension. It is advised to restrict the intake approximately from 2 to 4 g/day only. Great restriction of sodium should not be attempted except under the advice of a dietitian in the treatment specific disease condition.

Vitamins

- Vitamin B_{12} levels are often low in elderly adults. Ageing, *per se,* does not alter vitamin B_{12} absorption. However, B_{12} malabsorption is more frequent in elderly adults because of an increased prevalence of pernicious anaemia and atrophic gastritis. The absorption of vitamin B_{12} is altered in atrophic gastritis not because of any abnormal intrinsic factor, but because dissociation of the vitamin from food proteins is limited by inadequate acid digestion. Additionally, because of bacterial overgrowth in the proximal small intestine secondary to atrophic gastritis, some vitamin B_{12} that reaches the small bowel is metabolized by bacteria rather than absorbed. Vitamin B_{12} is found only in animal products, and some elderly adults have low levels of B_{12} because of their decreased consumption of meat, fish, poultry, and dairy products. Elderly vegetarians are particularly risk for vitamin B_{12} deficiency.
- Pyridoxine (vitamin B_6) intakes by older adult are inadequate, although it needs appear to increase with age because of atrophic gastritis (which interferes with absorption), alcoholism, and liver dysfunction.
- Although folate absorption is limited by the atrophic gastritis often found in elderly adults, a compensatory increase in folate production occurs in bacterial overgrowth in the proximal small bowel. Folate is required to convert homocysteine to methionine, and folate intakes below 400 µg per day are associated with elevated homocysteine levels, an independent risk factor for coronary artery and cerebrovascular disease. Therefore, diet rich in folate should be encouraged. For example, liver, dried beans, broccoli, asparagus, green leafy vegetables, etc. should be included.

Fibre

Increasing the intake of dietary fibre is an important adjunct in the treatment of constipation in the elderly, although abdominal discomfort, flatulence, and potentially decreased absorption of iron and zinc may be the unwanted side effects of excess consumption. Nonetheless, improving the intake of foods high in dietary fibre is a healthful nutritional option for elderly adults because these foods contain important vitamins and minerals.

Water

Fluid needs are affected by variations in activity, insensible water losses, medications, and urinary solute load. Daily fluid replacement is essential, particularly in those who exercise regularly, consume large amounts of protein, use laxatives or diuretics, or live in areas with high temperatures (Table 28.3).

Table 28.3: Common causes of dehydration in older people

Pathological causes	*Effects of ageing*	*Iatrogenic causes*
Confusion	Altered thirst perception.	Drugs such as diuretics.
Depression	Increased skin losses.	Fluid restriction.
Drowsiness	Reduced total body water.	Institutionalization.
Immobility	Reduced renal function	Physical environment.
Pyrexia		Urinary incontinence.
Renal failure		

SYMPTOMS OF DEHYDRATION IN OLDER PEOPLE

- Electrolyte disturbances.
- Altered drug effects.
- Headache.
- Drowsiness.
- Confusion.
- Constipation.
- Loss of skin elasticity.
- Weight loss.
- Cognitive status deterioration.
- Dizziness.
- Dry mouth and nose mucous membranes.
- Unpleasant taste in mouth.
- A swollen or dry tongue.
- Blood pressure changes.
- Recessed or sunken eyes.
- Changes in urine colour or output.

Elderly people should consume water as such or in the form of buttermilk, fruit juices, porridge, soups, etc. Since elderly people have a fading sense of thirst, they should be made to consume some fluid at regular intervals even if they are not thirsty.

Physical Activity

At all ages, an active lifestyle has many health benefits. In older people, even modest amounts of daily physical activity such as walking at a normal pace may increase appetite (thus helping to prevent nutritional inadequacies), improve balance and muscle co-ordination (lessening the likelihood of falls and fractures) and increase lean body mass.

Drug

Elderly adults take at least one prescription drug or multiple medications daily. Tables 28.4 and 28.5 list the effects of drug on nutrients and effects of nutrients on drugs.

· Table 28.4: Effects of drugs on nutrients

Drug	*Effect*
Anti-infective agents	
Amikacin, gentamicin, sisomicin, tobramycin	Hypokalemia, hypomagnesemia, and hypocalcemia; increased urinary potassium and magnesium loss
Aminosalicylic acid	Decreased vitamin B_{12} and fat absorption
Amphotercin B	Increased urinary excretion of potassium and decreased serum potassium and magnesium levels
Capreomycin	Hypokalemia, hypomagnesemia, and hypocalcemia
Cycloserine	Decreased serum folate
Isoniazid	Pyridoxine deficiency
Neomycin	Decreased absorption of carotene, iron, vitamin B_{12}, and cholesterol
Rifampin	Decreased serum 25-hydroxycholecalciferol level
Sulfasalazine	Folate deficiency
Tetracycline	Decreased absorption of Ca, Mg, Fe, Zn
Anticoagulants	
Warfarin	Decreased vitamin K-dependent coagulation factors
Cardiovascular drugs	
Colestipol	Decreased absorption of fat-soluble vitamins and folic acid
Hydralazine	Pyridoxine deficiency
Sodium nitroprusside	Decreased total serum vitamin B_{12}
Thiazides, ethacrynic acid	Increased urinary loss of Na, K, Mg, Zn, P
Triamterene, spironolactone	Increased urinary loss of K, Ca, Mg, Zn
CNS drugs	
Alcohol	Increased urinary loss of Mg, Zn, Ca
Aspirin	Decreased serum folate
Monoamine oxidase inhibitors	

Contd.

Table 28.4: Effects of drugs on nutrients (*Contd.*)

Drug	Effect
Isocarboxazid	Decreased leukocyte and platelet ascorbic acid levels
Pargyline	Increased iron loss
Phenelzin	Increased sensitivity to tyramine-containing foods; possible development of hypertensive crisis
Thanylcypromine	Pyridoxine deficiency
Phenobarbital	Decreased serum vitamin K_1
Phenytoin	Decreased serum folate, calcium, 25-hydroxycholecalciferol levels
Electrolyte drugs	
Potassium chloride, slow-release	Decreased vitamin B_{12} absorption
Gastrointestinal drugs	
Aluminium hydroxide	Decreased absorption of iron, phosphate, vitamin B_{12}
Cholestyramine	Decreased absorption of vitamin A, D, E, K, and B_{12} and folate along with decreased absorption of inorganic phosphate and fat
H_2-receptor antagonists, proton pump inhibitors	Decreased absorption of protein-bound vitamin B_{12}
Laxatives	Increased fecal loss of Na, K, Ca, Mg,
Mineral oil	Decreased absorption of vitamins A, D, E, and K
Hormones	
Glucocorticoids	Increased urinary loss of K, Ca, increased Na absorption
Oral contraceptives	Decreased serum folate, pyridoxine deficiency, riboflavin deficiency
Other agents	
Colchicine	Decreased absorption of vitamin B_{12} sodium, potassium, fat, nitrogen
Penicillamine	Pyridoxine deficiency

Form Weinsier RL, Morgan SL. Fundamentals of clinical nutrition. St. Louis: Mosby, 1993 : 186.

Table 28.5: Effects of nutrients on drugs

Food can change the absorption characteristics of certain drugs. The mechanisms for the effect include physicochemical interactions with food in the intestinal lumen, changes in gastric emptying, competition between drugs and food components for absorption, and altered first-pass hepatic kinetics. These effects can decrease the efficacy of the drugs or increase the absorption of the drug, so that a greater response to the drug or a side effect results. There can be large differences from one formulation to another, and no drug class effects can be assumed. The reader should check carefully with the literature and the manufacturer's information concerning individual formulations, especially when the therapeutic window is narrow. Listed below are some of the drug commonly used that can be affected by food and instructions on how to minimize the effects of food on the drug.

Contd.

Table 28.5: Effects of nutrients on drugs (*Contd.*)

Decreased absorption (avoid taking these drugs with food; take at least 1 hour before or 2 hours after a meal)

Ampicillin	Erythromycin stearate	Levodopa/ carbidopa	Quinidine
Atenolol	Ferrous salts	Lisinopril	Sotalol
Calcium carbonate	Folic acid	Methotrexate	Sulfamethoxazole
Captopril	Furosemide	Omeprazole	Tetracycline
Cephalexin	Iron	Penicillin G	Trimethoprim
Cloxacillin	Isoniazid	Penicillin V	Zinc sulfate
Digitalis	Isosorbide	Phenytoin	
Disopyramide	Lansoprazole	Propantheline	

Increased absorption (food will alter the amount of the drug absorbed; therefore, the drug should be taken at the same time (s) each day relative to meals)

Buspirone	Gemfibrozil	Methoxsalen	Propranolol
Carbamazepine	Griseofulvin	Metorprolol	Spironolactone
Chlorothizide	Labetalol	Nifedipine	Sulfadiazine
Diazepam	Lithium	Nitrofuratoin	Trazodone
Dicumarol	Lovastatin	Phenyoin	

Delayed absorption (food will delay the absorption of these drugs but not the overall amount absorbed; these drugs should be taken at least 1 hour or 2 hours after a meal)

Acetaminophen	Hydrochlorothiazide	Pentobarbital	Suprofen
Aspirin	Hydrocortisone	Pentoxifylline	Tocainide
Cimetidine	Indomethacin	Sulfisoxazole	
Doxycyline	Ketoprofen		

From Weinsier RL, Morgan SL. Fundamentals of clinical nutrition. St. Louis: Mosby, 1993: 188, with permission; and utermohlen V. in: Shils ME, olson JA, shike M, et al., eds., Modern nutrition in health and disease, 9th ed. Baltimore: Williams and Wilkin, 1998: 1621.

Dietary Modifications During Old Age

- *Changes in the texture of food:*
  - Food must be palatable, soft and easy to consume and digest as the elderly person may have problems in mouth (dentures, mouth cancer, etc.) dysphagia, oesophageal stricture, neurological changes (following a stroke).
- *Include wide variety of foods:*
  - Food should be well cooked and with wide variety without much restriction because increased restriction will lead to inadequate intake.
- *Meal times:*
  - Following proper meal timing will help the elderly people to follow small and frequent meals properly. It will favour more complete digestion and free from distress. Three heavy meals may hinder the digestion process as well as sleep is also less likely to be disturbed.

29 Nutritional Education

Nutrition education is an essential component and to improve the nutritional states of a population and is crucial for the well-being of people in general. In the past, nutrition education consisted mainly of face-to-face conversations between the health or community worker and individual persons, people were informed about "what to do" instead of encouraged about nutrition and health. But in recent years, more effective nutrition education approaches, with well-defined strategies in communication and behavioural psychology, have been used by inter-disciplinary teams.

WHO defines nutrition education as "the focus of health and nutrition education is on people and action. In general, its aim is to persuade people to adopt and sustain improved/desirable nutrition and health practices and to take their own decisions, both individually and collectively to improve their nutritional and health status, and environment".

Nutrition education may be defined as a group of communication activities aimed to bring about a voluntary change in practices, which have an effect on nutritional status of a population. The ultimate goal of nutrition education is to improve nutritional status.

WHO DOES THIS

Nutrition education to the community is given by:

- Technical project staff with knowledge in nutrition or public health.
- Experienced community and public health workers or nutrition specialists with skills in methods of communication.

Community nutrition encompasses a broad set of activities designed to provide access to a safe, adequate, healthful diet to a population living in particular geographic area. These activities include nutrition education, nutrition or health promotion, food programs supplementation programs, preventive program, local policy analysis and development, and the organizational infrastructure that supports it. "Ideally, community nutrition involves four interrelated steps to deliver services: assessment to identify the problem(s), planning to meet the community nutrition needs, implementation to develop system to reduce the problem and evaluation to see if the problem has been ameliorated or solved.

Community nutritionists are the folks in the trenches who translate general recommendations into action. They are bound together across geographic or common interest boundaries by a shared set of values, field strategies and educational experiences. Community nutritionists also have an understanding of and appreciation for dietetic and clinical practices, which address nutrition problems from an individual level. Community nutritionist engages the public in their public programming. They also work closely with educational institutions as well as government, commercial and not-for-profit organizations in any given community. The community nutritionist's target groups within a community may be bound together by common interest, risk or other characteristics, for example, pregnant and lactating women or the urban elderly and homeless. Regardless of particular focus, a community nutritionist should ultimately consider all policy and programming in terms of the health of the overall community.

CHARACTERISTICS AND LOGIC OF PLANNING NUTRITION EDUCATION ACTIVITIES

Nutrition education is not an end in itself. Nutrition education interventions should be part of integrated programmes aimed at linking nutritional messages with other programmes and services.

Community participation, in the attempt to resolve nutritional problems, is recognized as the key approach to design interventions by development planners and nutritionists.

SYSTEMATIC COMMUNITY PARTICIPATION CAN BE ACHIEVED BY INVOLVING

- Representatives of the community (men and women) from village committees or community-based organizations,
- Local leaders or village chiefs,
- Religious leaders,
- Community workers or change agents of local organizations.

These representatives are important facilitators for the modification of socio-cultural beliefs to change nutritional behaviour.

Furthermore, different representatives of the local institutions should be involved. Integrating teachers, agriculturists or health workers to transmit nutritional messages can be crucial for long-term behavioural changes and assure the collaboration between sectors.

Step 1
Conceptualisation: Analysis of nutritional problems and causes, identification of subject and practices.

- Define nutritional problems and causes through systematic assessment
- Select and rank nutritional issues that the community needs to know
- Identify practices, why people act in this way and what are the constraints.

Step 2
Definition of objectives, target groups and facilitators.

- Set objectives for nutrition and education
- Define the vulnerable group and the target group
- Identify from whom communities can learn best.

Step 3
Formulation of strategies and development of a specific methodology.

- Define the communication strategy (individual, small groups or large audiences)
- Define the educational approach direct or indirect communication
- Check the cost-effectiveness of each activity.

Step 4
Planning of nutritional topics, messages and communications channels and materials.

- Rank the most important nutritional topics
- Develop short and simple messages
- Identify local communication channels (training courses, radio spots, market stalls, village meeting, etc.)
- Define and produce the communication materials to transmit messages (poster, demonstration, manuals)
- Define all necessary resources, logistics and training skills for the nutrition education interventions.

Step 5
Implementation of training for facilitators and direct nutrition education interventions in the field.

- Schedule what, how, where and when people should learn
- Design and implement direct trainings in the field and "train the trainers" for further promotion
- Distribute the necessary material to facilitate the nutritional education and communication.

Step 6
Monitoring and evaluation of the transmission of nutritional issue and how people use them.

- Respond to the questions, if the objectives have been met and if the procedures were carried out according to the expectations and problems of the populations in need.

Fig. 29.1: The main steps for planning and implementing nutrition education activities

GENERAL CONSIDERATION FOR SUCCESSFUL NUTRITION EDUCATION

- Provide a clear formulation of the nutritional problems. Apply relevant assessment procedures, such as nutrition baseline surveys, focus group discussions or in-depth interviews which determine the type and magnitude of the nutritional problem.
- When designing "messages", keep them short and simple and ensure that they are clear; provide reliable information and show the relationship between the nutritional problem, its causes and the recommended behaviour; and make use of local expressions.
- Make people think about nutrition problems. Take materials or photos as a "starter" to introduce the topic of interest during the first few meetings or training sessions.
- Have something to demonstrate a learning aid. Real things, such as food items or utensils that people use, are better than pictures. They make the theoretical message more practical and enable their application.
- Get the audience to participate, encourage them to ask questions and discuss issues of importance.
- Ask the audience questions to review the topics of the nutrition education session. The more people who participate actively, the higher the acceptance of putting the messages into practice.
- Use different methods and tools of nutrition education to transmit the same messages through various communications channels to the same person or group. These practices have resulted in the highest impact of nutritional improvements within a community.

Community Nutrition Programme

30

NATIONAL NUTRITION POLICY

Introduction

Widespread poverty resulting in chronic and persistent hunger is the single biggest scourge of the developing world today. The physical expression of this continuously re-enacted tragedy is the condition of undernutrition which manifests itself among large sections of the poor, particularly amongst the women and children. Undernutrition is a condition resulting from inadequate intake of food or more essential nutrient (s) resulting in deterioration of physical growth and health. The inadequacy is relative to the food and nutrients needed to maintain good health, provide for growth and allow a choice of physical activity levels, including work levels, which are socially necessary. This condition of undernutrition, therefore, reduces work capacity and productivity amongst adults and enhances mortality and morbidity amongst children. Such reduced productivity translates into reduced earning capacity, leading to further poverty, and the vicious cycle goes on (Fig. 30.1). The nutritional status of a population is therefore critical to the development and well-being of a nation (Fig. 30.1).

Aims of the National Nutrition Policy

- To draw attention to the urgent need to reduce malnutrition in the country,
- To highlight the need for inter-sectoral coordination to achieve in the country,
- To orient relevant sectors to perceive nutrition as an outcome of their sectoral activities, and
- To identify short-term, intermediate and long-term strategies for achieving nutritional goals either through direct policy changes or indirect institutional or structural changes.

Nutrition Policy Instruments

The strategy: Nutrition is a multi-sectoral issue and needs to be tackled at various levels. Nutrition affects development as much as development

425

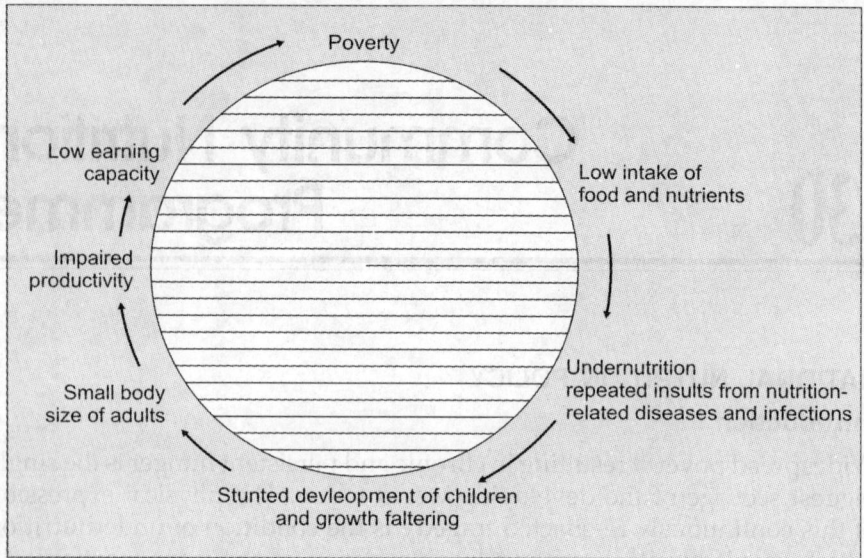

Fig. 30.1: The vicious cycle of poverty

affects nutrition. It is, therefore, important to tackle the problem of nutrition both through direct nutrition intervention for specially vulnerable groups as well as through various development policy instruments which will create conditions for improved nutrition.

A. Direct Intervention: Short Term

i. Nutrition intervention for specially vulnerable groups:
   a. *Expanding the safety net:* The universal immunization programme, oral rehydration therapy and the Integrated Child Development Services (ICDS) have had a considerable impact on child survival and extreme forms of malnutrition. The position, however, is that the silent form of hunger and malnutrition continues with over 43.8% (1988–90). Children suffering from moderate malnutrition and about 37.6% (1988–90) from mild malnutrition. Therefore, while more children are surviving today, an overwhelmingly large number of them are destined to remain much below their genetic potential. This is the enormity of the demographic trap which we face as we move towards the next century. There is, therefore, an immediate imperative to substantially expand the nutrition intervention net through ICDS so as to cover all vulnerable children in the age group of 0 to 6 years.
   b. With the objective of reducing the incidence of severe and moderate malnutrition, a concerted effort needs to be made to trigger appropriate behavioural changes among the mothers. Improving growth monitoring between the age group 0 and 3 years in particular, with closer involvement of the mothers is a key

intervention. Getting involved in the growth monitoring of her child will give her a feeling of control over the child's nutrition process and combined with adequate nutrition and health education, empower her to manage the nutrition needs of her children effectively.

c. *Reaching the adolescent girls:* The government's recent initiative of including the adolescent girl within the ambit of ICDS should be intensified so that they are made ready for a safe motherhood, their nutritional status (including iron supplementation in the body) is improved and they are given some skill upgradation training in home-based skills and covered by non-formal education, particularly nutrition and health education.

d. *Ensuring better coverage of expectant women:* In order to reduce the incidence of low birth weight, such coverage should include supplementary nutrition right from 1st trimester and should continue during the major period of lactation, at least for the first one year after pregnancy.

ii. *Fortification of essential foods:* Essential food items shall be fortified with appropriate nutrients, for example, salt with iodine and/or iron. Research in iron fortification of rice and other cereals should be intensified. The distribution of iodised salt should cover all the population in endemic areas of the country to reduce the iodine deficiency to below endemic levels.

iii. *Popularisation of low-cost nutritious food:* Efforts to produce and popularise low-cost nutritious foods from indigenous and locally available raw material shall be intensified. It is necessary to involve women particularly in this activity.

iv. *Control of micro-nutrient efficiencies amongst vulnerable groups:* Deficiencies of vitamin "A", iron and folic acid and iodine among children, pregnant women and nursing mothers shall be controlled through intensified programmes. Iron supplementation to adolescent girls shall be introduced. The programme shall be expanded to cover all eligible members of the community. The prophylaxis programme, at present, does not cover all children. For example, the vitamin "A" programme covers only 30 out of about 80 million. It is necessary to intensify all these efforts and work on a specific timeframe.

B. Indirect Policy Instruments: Long-term Institutional and Structural Changes

i. *Food Security:* In order to ensure aggregate food security, a per capita availability of 215 kg/person/year of food grains needs to be attained. This requires production of 250 million tonnes of food grains per year and buffer stocks of 30–35 million tonnes in order to guard against exigencies, such as flood and droughts. However, taking into account the present trends and the possibility of improved availability of non-cereal food items.

ii. *Improvement of dietary pattern through production and demonstration*: Improving the dietary pattern by promoting the production and increasing the per capita availability of nutritionally rich foods. The production of pulses, oilseeds and other food crops will be increased with a view to attaining self sufficiency and building surplus and buffer stocks. The production of protective food crops, such as vegetables, fruits, milk, meat, fish and poultry, shall be augmented. Preference shall be given to growing foods, such as millets, legumes, vegetables and fruits (carrots, green leafy vegetables, guava, papaya and amla). For this purpose, the latest and improved techniques shall be increasingly applied, high-yielding varieties of food crops developed and extensively cultivated, adequate extension services made available to farmers, wastage of food in transit and storage reduced to the minimum, available food conserved and effectively utilised and adequate buffer stocks built up. Certain imbalances and anamolies in our agricultural policy need to be redressed immediately. Our agricultural policy has been hitherto concerned with production exclusively and not nutrition, which is the ultimate end. While the green revolution has largely remained a cereal revolution, with bias towards wheat, coarse grains and pulses, which constitute the poor man's staple and protein requirements, have not received adequate attention. The prices of pulses, which were below cereal prices before the green revolution, are now more than triple the price of cereals. Our food policy should be consistent with our national nutritional needs and these calls for the introduction of appropriate incentives, pricing and taxation policies.

iii. Policies for effecting income transfers so as to improve the entitlement package of the rural and urban poor.

   a. *Improving the purchasing power:* Poverty alleviation programmes, like the Integrated Rural Development Programme (IRDP) and employment generation schemes like Jawahar Rozgar Yojana, Nehru Rozgar Yojana and DWCRA are to be re-oriented and restructured to make a forceful dent on the purchasing power of the lowest economic segments of the population. In all poverty alleviation programmes, nutritional objectives shall be incorporated explicitly and the nutritional benefits of income generation shall be taken for granted. Existing programmes shall be scrutinized for their nutrition component. It is necessary to improve the purchasing power of the landless and the rural and urban poor by implementing employment generation programmes so that additional employment of at least 100 days is created for each rural landless family and employment opportunities are created in urban areas for slum dwellers and the urban poor.

   b. *Public distribution system:* Ensuring an equitable food distribution, through the expansion of the public distribution system. The public distribution system shall ensure availability of essential food articles, such as coarse grains, pulses and jaggery, besides rice, wheat, sugar and oil; conveniently and at reasonable prices to the public, particularly to those living below the poverty line not only in urban areas but also throughout the country. For this purpose encouragement shall be given to the consumer cooperatives and fair price shops shall be opened in adequate number in all areas. Effective price and quality control shall be exercised over the cooked foods in restaurants and other eating places.

iv. *Land reforms:* Implementing land reform measures so that the vulnerability of the landless and the landed poor could be reduced. This will include both tenural reforms as well as implementation of ceiling laws.

v. *Health and family welfare:* The health and family welfare programmes are an inseparable part of the strategy. Through "health for all by 2000 AD" programme increased health and immunization facilities shall be provided to all. Improved pre-natal and post-natal care to ensure safe motherhood shall be made accessible to all women. The population in the reproductive age group shall be empowered, through education to be responsible for their own family size. Through intensive family welfare and motivational measures small family norm and adequate spacing shall be encouraged so that the food available to the family is sufficient for proper nutrition of the members.

vi. *Basic health and nutrition knowledge:* Basic health and nutrition knowledge with special focus on wholesome infant feeding practices, shall be imparted to the people extensively and effectively. Nutrition and health education concepts shall be effectively integrated into the school curricula as well as into all nutrition programmes. Nutrition and health education are very important in the context of the problems of overnutrition also.

vii. *Prevention of food adulteration:* Prevention of food adulteration must be strengthened by gearing up the enforcement machinery.

viii. *Nutrition surveillance:* The NNMB/NIN of ICMR needs to be strengthened so that periodical monitoring of the nutritional status of children, adolescent girls, and pregnant and lactating mothers below the poverty line takes place through representative samples and results are transmitted to all agencies concerned. The NNMB should not only try and assess the impact of ongoing nutrition and development programmes but also serve as an early warning system for initiating prompt action.

ix. *Monitoring of nutrition programmes:* Monitoring of nutrition programmes (viz. ICDS), and of nutrition education and demonstration by the Food and Nutrition Board, should be continued.

x. *Research:* Research into various aspects of nutrition, both on the consumption side as well as the supply side, is another essential aspect of the strategy. Research must accurately identify those who are suffering from various degrees of malnutrition. Research should enable selection of new varieties of food with high nutrition value which can be within the purchasing power of the poor.

xi. Equal remuneration: Special efforts should be made to improve the effectiveness of programmes related to women. The wages of women shall be at par with that of men in order to improve women's economic status. This requires a stricter enforcement of the Equal Remuneration Act. Special emphasis will have to be given for expanding employment opportunities for women.

xii. *Communication:* Communication through established media is one of the most important strategies to be adopted for the effective implementation of the nutrition policy. The department of women and child development will have a well-established, permanent communications division, with adequate staff and fund support. While using the communication tools, both mass communication as well as group or inter-personal communication should be used. Not only the electronic media but also folk and print media should be used extensively. The existing facilities in the song and drama division and the Directorate of Advertising and Visual Publicity (DAVP) in the Ministry of Information and Broadcasting could help in a big way to improve nutrition and health education. To give a new direction to communication and media, efforts will be made for promoting sound feeding practices, which are culturally acceptable and based on local food habits. Further, the media policy shall focus on ways and means to combat malnutrition among girl children, adolescent girls and women in the reproductive age group. Educational programmes will be made meaningful and interesting to meet the growing needs of the population.

xiii. *Minimum wage administration:* Closely related to the market, is the need to ensure an effective, minimum wage administration to ensure its strict enforcement and timely revision and linking it with price rise through a suitable nutrition formula. A special legislation should be introduced for providing agricultural women labourers the minimum support, and at least 60 days leave by the employer in the last trimester of her pregnancy. Excessive loss of energy during the working seasons has serious nutritional implications. The legislation should take care of this problem also.

xiv. *Community participation:* The active involvement of the community is essential not only in terms of being aware of the services available to the community but also for deriving the maximum benefit from such services by giving timely feedback necessary at all levels. After all, communication must form an essential part of all services and people themselves are the best communicators.

Community participation will include:

a. Generating awareness among the community regarding the national nutrition policy and its major concerns.

    b. Involving the community through their panchayats or where panchayat do not exist, through beneficiary committee in the management of nutrition programmes and interventions related to nutrition such as employment generation, land reforms, health, education, etc.

    c. Actual participation, particularly of women in food production and processing activities.

    d. Promoting schemes relating to kitchen gardens, food preservation, preparation of weaning foods and other food processing units, both at the home level as well as the community levels and

    e. Generation of effective demand at the level of the community for all services relating to nutrition.

  xv. *Education and literacy:* It has been shown that education and literacy particularly that of women, is a key determinant for better nutritional status. For instance, Kerala state which has the highest literacy level and also has the best nutrition status.

  xvi. *Improvement of the status of women:* The most effective way to implement nutrition with mainstream activities in agriculture, health, education and rural development is to focus on improving the status of women, particularly the economic status. After all, women are the ultimate providers of nutrition to households both through acquisition of food as well as preparation of food for consumption. There is evidence that women's employment does beneficial household nutrition, both through increase in household income as well as through an increase in women's status, autonomy and decision-making power. Educated women have greater roles in household decision making, particularly those relating to nutrition and feeding practices.

Nutrition Programmes

INTEGRATED CHILD DEVELOPMENT SERVICES (ICDS)

The Government of India is making concerted efforts to reduce the prevalence of malnutrition in the country. In consonance with this, the scheme of Integrated Child Development Services (ICDS) was launched in 1975. This programme is implemented by the nodal department, i.e. the department of women and child development. The packages of services provided to the beneficiaries of the programme are supplementary nutrition, immunization, health check-up, referral services, non-formal pre-school education and nutrition and health education. Supplementary nutrition is one of the major components of the programmes.

Objectives

  i. To improve the nutritional and health status of children in the age-group of 0–6 years;

  ii. To lay the foundation for proper psychological, physical and social development of the child;

iii. To reduce the incidence of mortality, morbidity, malnutrition and school dropout;
iv. To achieve effective co-ordination of policy and implementation amongst the various departments to promote child development; and
v. To enhance the capability of the mother to look after the normal health and nutritional needs of the child through proper nutrition and health education.

Services: The above objectives are sought to be achieved through a package of services comprising:
i. Supplementary nutrition,
ii. Immunization,
iii. Health check-up,
iv. Referral services,
v. Pre-school non-formal education and
vi. Nutrition and health education.

The concept of providing a package of services is based primarily on the consideration that the overall impact will be much larger if the different services develop in an integrated manner as the efficacy of a particular service depends upon the support it receives from related services (Table 30.1).

Table 30.1: Services, target group and service provider

Services	Target group	Service provided by
Supplementary nutrition	Children below 6 years:	Anganwadi worker and anganwadi helper
	Pregnant and lactating mother (P and LM)	
Immunization*	Children below 6 years:	ANM/MO
	Pregnant and lactating mother (P and LM)	
Health check-up*	Children below 6 years:	ANM/MO/AWW
	Pregnant and lactating mother (P and LM)	
Referral services	Children below 6 years:	AWW/ANM/MO
	Pregnant and lactating mother (P and LM)	
Pre-school education	Children 3–6 years	AWW
Nutrition and health education	Women (15–45 years)	AWW/ANM/MO

*AWW assists ANM in identifying the target group.

Three of the six services, namely immunisation, health check-up and referral services delivered through public health infrastructure under the Ministry of Health and Family Welfare.

- *Nutrition including supplementary nutrition:* This includes supplementary feeding and growth monitoring; and prophylaxis against vitamin A deficiency and control of nutritional anaemia. All families in the community are surveyed, to identify children below the age of six and pregnant and nursing mothers. They avail of supplementary feeding support for 300 days in a year. By providing supplementary feeding, the anganwadi attempts to bridge the caloric gap between the national recommended and average intake of children and women in low income and disadvantaged communities.

  Growth monitoring and nutrition surveillance are two important activities that are undertaken. Children below the age of three years are weighed once a month and children 3–6 years of age are weighed quarterly. Weight-for-age growth cards are maintained for all children below six years. This helps to detect growth faltering and helps in assessing nutritional status. Besides, severely malnourished children are given special supplementary feeding and referred to medical services.

- *Immunization:* Immunization of pregnant women and infants protects children from six vaccine preventable diseases—poliomyelitis, diphtheria, pertussis, tetanus, tuberculosis and measles. These are major preventable causes of child mortality, disability, morbidity and related malnutrition. Immunization of pregnant women against tetanus also reduces maternal and neonatal mortality.

- *Health check-ups:* This includes healthcare of children less than six years of age, antenatal care of expectant mothers and postnatal care of nursing mothers. The various health services provided for children by anganwadi workers and primary health centre (PHC) staff, include regular health check-ups, recording of weight, immunization, management of malnutrition, treatment of diarrhoea, de-worming and distribution of simple medicines, etc.

- *Referral services:* During health check-ups and growth monitoring, sick or malnourished children, in need of prompt medical attention, are referred to the primary health centre or its sub-centre. The anganwadi worker has also been oriented to detect disabilities in young children. She enlists all such cases in a special register and refers them to the medical officer of the primary health centre/sub-centre.

- *Non-formal pre-school education (PSE):* The non-formal pre-school education (PSE) component of the ICDS may well be considered the backbone of the ICDS programme, since all its services essentially converge at the anganwadi—a village courtyard. Anganwadi centre (AWC)—a village courtyard—is the main platform for delivering of these services. These AWCs have been set up in every village in the country. In pursuance of its commitment to the cause of India's children, present government has decided to set up an AWC in every human habitation/settlement. As a result, total number of AWC would go up to almost 1.4 million. This is also the most joyful play-way daily activity, visibly sustained for three hours a day. It brings and keeps young children at the anganwadi centre—an activity that motivates parents and communities. PSE, as envisaged in the ICDS, focuses on total development of the child, in the age up to six years, mainly from the underprivileged groups. Its programme for the three to six years old children in the anganwadi is directed towards providing and ensuring a natural, joyful and stimulating environment, with emphasis on necessary inputs for optimal growth and development. The early learning component of the ICDS is a significant input for providing a sound foundation for cumulative lifelong learning and development. It also contributes to the universalization of primary education, by providing to the child the necessary preparation for primary schooling and offering substitute care to younger siblings, thus freeing the older ones—especially girls—to attend school.

• *Nutrition and health education:* Nutrition, health and education (NHED) is a key element of the work of the anganwadi worker. This forms part of BCC (behaviour change communication) strategy. This has the long term goal of capacity-building of women—especially in the age group of 15–45 years—so that they can look after their own health, nutrition and development needs as well as that of their children and families.

Implementation

The ICDS programme is implemented, at the central level, by the department of women and child development, Ministry of Human Resource Development in coordination with the Ministry of Health. At the state level, implementation is the responsibility of either the department of social welfare/women and child development/health or a separate directorate of ICDS. The programme infrastructure along with the designation of the programme functionaries at the block to village/community levels is presented in Fig. 30.2. The anganwadi centre—a courtyard play centre—is the symbol of government systems and services, closest to disadvantaged communities. The anganwadi worker assumes a pivotal role in the ICDS structure due to her close and continuous contact with the community. As the crucial link between the community and the government administration, she becomes a central figure in asserting and meeting the needs of the community she lives in.

International Partners

Government of India partners with the following international agencies to supplement interventions under the ICDS:

i. United Nations International Children's Emergency Fund (UNICEF)
ii. Cooperative for Assistance and Relief Everywhere (CARE)
iii. World Food Programme (WFP)

UNICEF supports the ICDS by providing technical support for the development of training plans, organizing of regional workshops and

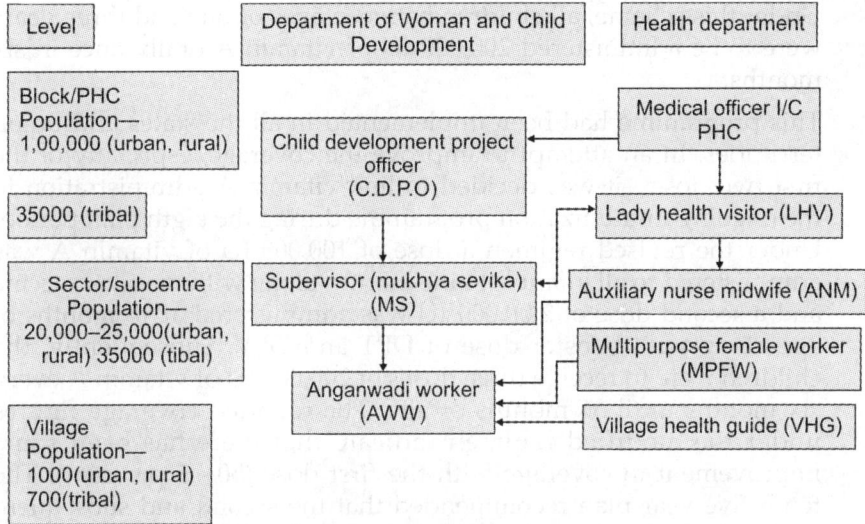

Fig.30.2: ICDS infrastructure

dissemination of best practices of ICDS. It also assists in service delivery and accreditation system where the capacity of ICDS functionary is strengthened. Impact assessment in selected states on early childhood nutrition and development, micronutrient and anaemia control through vitamin 'A' supplementations and deworming interventions for children in the age group of 9–59 months is also conducted by UNICEF from time to time.

CARE is primarily implementing some non-food projects in areas of maternal and child health, girl primary education, micro-credit, etc.

WFP has been extending assistance to enhance the effectiveness and outreach of the ICDS Scheme in selected districts (Tikamgarh and Chhattarpur in Madhya Pradesh, Koraput, Malkangir and Nabrangpur in Orissa, Banswara in Rajasthan and Dantewada in Chhattisgarh), notably, by assisting the state governments to start and expand production of low cost micronutrient fortified food known as 'Indiamix'. Under this the concerned state government are required to contribute to the cost of Indiamix by matching the WFP wheat contribution at a 1 : 1 cost sharing ratio.

NUTRIENT DEFICIENCY CONTROL PROGRAMMES

The three important ongoing nutrient deficiency control programmes are:
1. National prophylaxis programme for prevention of blindness due to vitamin A deficiency.
2. National anaemia control programme, and
3. National iodine deficiency disorder control programme (NIDDCP).
   1. *National prophylaxis programme for prevention of blindness due to vitamin A deficiency:* In 1970, the national prophylaxis programme against nutritional blindness was initiated as a centrally sponsored scheme.

Under this scheme, all children between ages of one and three years were to be administered 200,000 IU of vitamin A orally once in six months.

This programme had been implemented in all the states and union territories. In an attempt to improve the coverage, especially of the first two doses, it was decided to link vitamin A administration to the ongoing immunization programme during the eigth plan period. Under the revised regimen a dose of 100,000 IU of vitamin A was administered to all infants at nine months along with measles vaccine and a second dose of 2,00,000 IU was administered at 18 months of age along with booster dose of DPT and OPV. Subsequently, the children were to receive three doses of 200,000 IU of vitamin A every six months until 36 months of age. The reported coverage figures under the modified regimen indicate that there has been some improvement in coverage with the first dose (50–75 per cent). The tenth five year plan recommended that the second and subsequent doses of massive dose vitamin A may be administered biannually in the pre-summer (April–May) and pre-winter (Sept–Oct) period. This strategy was operationalized successfully in states like U.P. with UNICEF assistance and resulted in improved coverage for all the doses. In 2006–07, a policy decision has been taken to cover all children in the 9 month to 6 years age group under the massive dose vitamin A programme. Clinical vitamin A deficiency often coexists with other micronutrient deficiencies and hence, there is a need for broad-based dietary diversification programmes aimed at improving the overall micronutrient nutritional status of children.

2. *National anaemia control programme:* Nutritional anaemia is a serious public health problem. Although anaemia is widespread in the country, it especially affects women in the reproductive age group and young children. It is estimated that over 50% of pregnant women are anaemic. Nutritional anaemia, due to iron and folic acid deficiency, is directly or indirectly responsible for about 20% of maternal deaths. Anaemia is also a major contributory cause of high incidence of premature births, low birth weight and perinatal mortality.

Objective

The national nutritional anaemia control programme aims at significantly decreasing the prevalence and incidence of anaemia in women in reproductive age group, especially pregnant and lactating women, and preschool children. The programme focuses on the following strategies:

• Promotion of regular consumption of foods rich in iron.
• Provisions of iron and folate supplements in the form of tablets (folifer tablets) to the "high risk" groups.
• Identification and treatment of severely anaemic cases.

Prevention of Nutritional Anaemia

i. Promoting consumption of iron rich food
   - Regular dietary intake of iron and folic acid rich foods by pregnant and lactating mothers, adolescent girls and children under 5 years of age must be promoted.
   - The mothers attending antenatal clinics, immunisation sessions as well as women beneficiaries in the lCDS programme should be made aware of the importance of preventing nutritional anaemia.
   - Regular consumption of iron rich foods such as green leafy vegetables, cereals such as wheat, ragi, jowar and bajra, pulses (especially sprouted pulses) and gur (jaggery) must be promoted widely. In addition, wherever culturally and economically feasible, consumption of animal flesh foods such as meat, liver, etc. must be encouraged.
   - Ensure incorporation of iron rich foods such as green leafy vegetables in the weaning foods of infants.
   - Vitamin C (ascorbic acid) promotes absorption of iron. Regular consumption vitamin C rich food such as lemon, orange, guava, amla, green mango along with iron rich food must be promoted.
   - For increasing availability of iron rich foods, growing of iron rich foods in home gardens and consumption of these must be promoted.
   - Tea inhibits absorption of iron in the stomach. Advise a reduced consumption of tea, specially during pregnancy, for improving the absorption of iron and prevention of anaemia.

ii. Promoting consumption of iron and folic acid supplements
   - As a priority, all pregnant women, irrespective of haemoglobin levels, must be provided with the recommended dose of iron and folic acid (folifer) supplements.
   - In addition, in case of available remaining supply, iron and folic acid supplements must be provided to lactating women and IUD users.
   - Preschool children, especially those in tribal areas and ICDS blocks, should be given on priority the recommended dosage of iron and folic acid supplements.
   - The contact during administration of tetanus toxoid should be utilised for distribution of folifer tablets to pregnant women. Ensure every mother is provided with complete recommended dosage of folifer tablets during pregnancy.
   - For monitoring distribution as well as consumption of folifer tablets by pregnant and lactating women and children 12–24 months, the mother infant immunization cards should be used. The growth monitoring cards/registers used for monitoring the growth of preschool children under the ICDS programme, should be used for recording and monitoring the distribution of folifer tablets to children 1–5 years.

- In addition, records of under fives and antenatal care maintained under the MCH services and ICDS programme, should be used for identifying beneficiaries (pregnant and lactating women, preschool children) as well as for recording and monitoring the distribution of iron and folic acid supplements.

Recommended Doses of Folic Acid and Iron Supplements

- *Pregnant women:* one big (adult) tablet per day for 100 days (each tablet containing 60 mgI 100 mg of elemental iron and 500 pg folic acid). These tablets should be provided to women after the first trimester of pregnancy.
- *Lactating women and intrauterine (IUD) acceptors:* One big (adult) tablet (containing 60 mg and 100 mg of elemental iron and 500 µg folic acid) per day for 100 days.
- *Preschool children (1–5 years):* One paediatric (small) tablet containing 20 mg iron and 100 µg folic acid daily for 100 days every year.

Note: Tea inhibits absorption of iron in stomach. Drinking tea should be avoided within a few hours of taking folifer tablets.

i. *Treatment of severe anaemia:* Women with haemoglobin levels below 7 g/dl are considered to be severely anaemic. Testing of blood for haemoglobin concentration at field levels is neither considered safe nor practical. Therefore, as far as possible, severely anaemic cases should be identified on the basis of clinical signs. All health workers should be trained to identify such anaemic cases. Recommended therapeutic dose for women in the reproductive age group is one tablet (big) of iron thrice daily for a minimum of 100 days. This will provide equivalent to 180 mg elemental iron and 1500 µg folic acid per day. In case of 100 mg elemental folifer tablets, recommended dose is two (big) tablets of iron daily for a minimum of 100 days. Further, cases of severe anaemia should be referred to the PHC medical officers for diagnosis of the causative factors and treatment.

Implementation

The programme is implemented through the primary health centres and its sub-centres. The multiple purpose worker (F) and other paramedicals working in the primary health centres are responsible for the distribution of iron tablets (adult and paediatric doses) to pregnant and lactating women, IUD users and children aged 1 to 5 years. The functionaries of Integrated Child Development Services (ICDS) programme, under the department of women and child development, assist in the distribution of iron tablets to children and mothers in the ICDS blocks and for imparting education to mothers on prevention of nutritional anaemia. Department of food (Ministry of Food and Civil Supplies) is responsible for promoting consumption of iron rich food. In addition, services of other community level workers and involvement of formal and nonformal education, media, horticultural departments and voluntary organisations is recommended to be utilised for the effective implementation of the programme.

3. *National iodine deficiency disorders control programme (NIDDCP):* Iodine deficiency disorders are one of the most severe form of micronutrient deficiency which superimposes its harmful effects on the productivity and vitality of our society. Some obvious clinical manifestation of iodine deficiency, such as goitre, has been recognised for thousands of years, but only in the recent past a realistic picture has emerged both of the board spectrum of disability, morbidity and mortality and the vast global dimensions of millions affected by the iodine malnutrition.

IDD affects people throughout the world. It causes brain disorders, cretinism, miscarriages and goitre. It is the world's single most important and preventable cause of mental retardation. And it is almost unknown. Equally unknown is the success in eradicating it. Calling it "one of our best kept secrets" the World Health Organization has rededicated itself to eliminate iodine deficiency disorder, or IDD, through an intense programme of salt iodisation.

National Goitre Control Programme

Government of India launched National Goitre Control Programme (NGCP) in 1962, whereby it was decided to supply iodised salt for human consumption to identified, Goitre endemic areas like sub-himalayan region. The production of iodised salt was restricted to only three different plants under public sector/government at Sambhar lake in Rajasthan, Howrah in West Bengal and Kharagoda in Gujarat. The program was implemented by Directorate General of Health Services of the Ministry of Health in collaboration with salt commissioner. The program was restructured in 1984, following the recommendations of central council of health and family welfare and the government took a policy decision to iodise the entire edible salt in the country in a phased manner by 1992.

Two of the major policy decisions taken were:

• Salt department, (under Ministry of Commerce and Industry, Government of India) was identified as the nodal agency to monitor the production and quality control of iodised salt at production sources and distribution of iodised salt in the entire country.

• Private sector were permitted to manufacture commercial production of iodised salt, the program commenced in April 1986 in a phased manner.

National Iodine Deficiency Disorders Control Programme (NIDDCP)

In August, 1992, the NGCP was renamed as NIDDCP with a view to cover a wide spectrum of iodine deficiency disorders. The following are the objectives of NIDDCP to carry out surveys to assess the magnitude of iodine deficiency disorders to produce and supply iodised salt in place of common salt to resurvey after every five years to assess the extent of IDDs and the impact of iodised salt to install laboratories for monitoring of iodised salt and urinary iodine excretion (UIE) to provide health education.

Objectives

1. Survey to assess the magnitude of iodine deficiency /disorder including goitre.
2. Supply of iodated salt in place of common salt.
3. Resurvey to assess the extend of iodine deficiency disorders and impact of iodated salt.
4. Laboratory monitoring of iodated salt and urinary iodine excretion.
5. Health education.

GOVERNMENT OF INDIA—UNICEF ACTIVITIES

Salt department with financial support from UNICEF organized various activities since the last decade for creating awareness amongst the public on IDD and benefits of iodised salt through rallies, human chain, national /state level seminars/workshops and celebration of global IDD day on 21st October every year. Some of the activities are listed:

- Publication of books/pamphlets/video-films/brochures/release of full page supplements in leading regional/national dailies/printing of ëSuní logo on postal stationery.
- Undertaking studies for assessing awareness levels, situational analysis of availability, quality and price of salt, census of salt manufacturing units/iodisation units, national multicentric study on monitoring quality of iodised salt through networking of medical colleges in southern states, knowledge, attitude and practice (KAPB) studies, etc.
- Organisation of national/regional/state level meetings of all stakeholders of NIDDCP to solicit their cooperation.
- Sensitisation/advocacy meetings with salt manufacturers and traders.
- Strengthening quality monitoring system at production sources through training of quality control personnel of salt department and industry, distribution of field test kits, deployment of mobile salt test laboratories at major production centres.
- Evaluation of universal salt iodisaiton (USI) in India 1997–98.

The progress achieved on universal salt iodisation (USI) over the last two decades was possible because of these various information, education, communication (IEC) activities undertaken by the department which contributed to the increase in production and consumption of iodised salt in the country.

Goal of USI in Bridging the Gap

The goal of NIDDCP is to reduce the prevalence of IDDs below ten per cent in the entire country by 2010 A. D. A total of 20–25% of the population are still to be provided access to iodised salt. Further the iodised salt consumed by everyone should be adequately iodised and iodised salt manufacturers and traders should shoulder great responsibility in ensuring the quality of iodised salt before supplying it to masses. As the nodal agency, salt department's role is pivotal and crucial for not only achieving the universal salt iodisation and consumption but also for sustaining the progress achieved. Salt commissionerate is thus playing a coordinating role involving all the stakeholders and is making sustained efforts for ensuring their unstinted cooperation and commitment for effective implementation of NIDDCP (Table 30.2).

Table 30.2: Cost of iodine for salt iodisation

Total annual requirement of iodised salt in India (for 1,000 million population @ 5 kg/person/year)	5 million tons
Iodine required for salt iodisation @ 30 ppm of iodine at production level or 30 mg/kg or 30 gm/ton	150,000 kg (150 tons)
Approximate price of iodine @ ₹ 666/kg. Therefore, total price for 150 tons	₹ 100 million (for 1,000 million population)
Cost of iodine per person per year	10 paise

SUPPLEMENTARY FEEDING PROGRAMMES

The decision to implement a supplementary feeding program is usually based on raised prevalence of acute malnutrition among children under five and the presence of aggravating factors such as poor food security in the general population, disease epidemic and raised mortality (severity of a crisis). Food supplementation programmes have a great role to combat malnutrition.

Objectives

a. To improve health and food habits and to prevent the occurrence of malnutrition among children.
b. Improving the nutritional status of children in classes I–V in government, local body and government-aided schools.
c. Encouraging poor children, belonging to disadvantaged sections, to attend school more regularly and help them concentrate on classroom activities.
d. Providing nutritional support to children of primary stage in drought affected areas during summer vacation.

There are always many new supplementary feeding programmes to combat malnutrition in which some are ongoing and some are no longer in operation.

- National programme of nutritional support to primary education (mid-day meal programme)
- Special Nutriton Programme (SNP)
- Pradhan Mantri's Gramodaya Yojana (PMGY)
- Balwadi feeding programme
- Composite nutrition programme
- Applied nutrition programme, etc.

31

Food Hygiene

Food hygiene is a broad term used to describe the preservation and preparation of foods in a manner that ensures the food is safe for human consumption. Food hygiene is much more than cleanliness; it involves all measures to ensure the safety, soundness and wholesomeness of food at all stages from its production, processing, manufacturing, packaging, storage, distribution and display to its sale.

Food hygiene may, thus, be defined as the sanitary science which aims to produce food which is safe for the consumer and of good keeping quality. The food hygienic measures will involve protecting food from risk of contamination of any kind, preventing any organisms, multiplying to an extent which would expose consumers to risk, or result in premature decomposition of food; destroying any harmful bacteria in the food through cooking or processing.

CAUSES OF FOOD POISONING

Food poisoning occurs when foods containing poisons of chemical or biological origin are eaten. The characteristic symptoms are abdominal pain and diarrhoea, usually accompanied by vomiting.

Biological (microbiological) hazards: That cause food-borne illnesses include microorganisms such as bacteria, viruses, fungi and parasites. The spread of these can be controlled by

- Temperature-adequate cooking, cooling, refrigeration, freezing and handling of food.
- The avoidance of cross-contamination.
- Enforcement of personal hygiene among food handlers.

Bacteria causing the major biological food-borne illness: The most serious types of food poisoning are caused by bacteria. Bacteria multiply best in a moist environment between 5°C and 63°C. Storing food below 5°C prevents bacteria from multiplying.

Bacteria causing food-borne illness need the following elements for growth:

- Protein (or sufficient nutrients),
- Moisture [water activity (A_W) above 0.85],
- pH (above pH of 4.5, generally neutral-pH 7),
- Oxygen if aerobic, and
- A general temperature 40–140°F (4–60°C), the temperature danger zone (TDZ).

  The bacteria causes food-borne illnesses by:
  1. Infection,
  2. Intoxication,
  3. Toxin-mediated infection.
- Food-borne infection results form ingesting living, pathogenic bacteria such as *Salmonella*, *Listeria monocytogenes*, or *Shigella*.
- Food-borne intoxication results if a preformed toxin (poison) is ingested, such as that produced by *Staphylococcus aurums*, *Clostridium botulinum*, and *Bacillus cereus* is present in the food.
- A toxin-mediated infection is caused by ingestion of living, infection - causing bacteria such as *C. perfringens* and *E. coli* 0157 : 47 that also produce a toxin in the intestine (Table 31.1).

Viruses

In addition to bacteria, although with lesser incidence, viruses may also be responsible for an unsafe food supply and food-borne illness. A virus does not multiply in food, as do bacteria, but can remain in food if it is insufficiently cooked and, subsequently, infect individuals who ingest it. It is possible for spot contamination of food to occur, so that only those individuals consuming the contaminated portion of the food become ill.

A virus of concern to the consumer, or a food processing and handling operation, is the hepatitis A virus. Hepatitis A virus is presumed to replicate initially in the gastrointestinal tract and then it spreads primarily to liver, where it infects hepatocytes (liver cells) and kupffer cells. A person will become infected with the virus 15–50 days following ingestion of a contaminated product and will shed the virus contaminating other people or food prior to displaying symptoms of illness.

Two sources of the hepatitis A virus are:

1. Raw shellfish from polluted water where sewage is discarded, and
2. Faeces and urine of infected persons. Shellfish such as oysters, mussels and clams are generally bred in sewage polluted bed or brackish water. Consuming these will accumulate the toxins produced by dinoflagellate algae (*Gonyaulax catenella*). The mussels and clams concentrate the dinoflagellates by filtering them as food from the surrounding water. If the concentration exceeds 200 cells per ml in the surrounding water, they will contain sufficient toxin to cause illness to those consuming the shellfish. The shellfish poisoning assumes importance due to the fact that they are consumed undercooked or uncooked. In India shellfish poisoning has been reported from the coastal areas of Tamil Nadu and Karnataka.

Table 31.1: Major food-borne diseases of bacterial origin

	Salmonellosis infection	Shigellosis infection	Listeriosis infection	Staphylococcal intoxication	Clostridium perfringens toxin-mediated infection	Bacillus cereus intoxication	Botulism intoxication
Bacteria	Salmonella (facultative)	Shigella (facultative)	Listeria monocytogenes (reduced oxygen)	Staphylococcus aureus (facultative)	Clostridium perfringens (anaerobic)	Bacillus (facultative)	Clostridium botulinum (anaerobic)
Incubation period	6–72 hours	1–7 days	1 day to 3 weeks	1–6 hours	8–22 hours	½–5 hours; 8–16 hours	12–39 hours + 72
Duration of illness	2–3 days	Indefinite, depends on treatment	Indefinite, depends on treatment, but has high fatality in the immuno compromised	24–48 hours	24 hours	6–24 hours; 12 hours	Several days to a year
Symptoms	Abdominal pain, headache, nausea, vomiting, fever, diarrhoea	Diarrhoea, fever, chills, lassitude, dehydration	Nausea, vomiting, headache, fever, chills, backache, meningitis	Nausea, vomiting, diarrhoea, dehydration	Abdominal pain, diarrhoea	Nausea and vomiting; diarrhoea, abdominal cramps	Vertigo, visual disturbances, inability to swallow, respiratory paralysis

Contd.

Table 31.1: Major food-borne diseases of bacterial origin (Contd.)

	Salmonellosis infection	Shigellosis infection	Listeriosis infection	Staphylococcal intoxication	Clostridium perfringens toxin-mediated infection	Bacillus cereus intoxication	Botulism intoxication
Reservoir	Domestic and wild animals; also humans, especially as carriers	Human faeces, flies	Humans, domestic and wild animals, fowl, soil, water, mud	Humans (skin, nose, throat, infected sores); also animal	Human (intestinal tract), animals, and soil	Soil and dust	soil water
Foods implicated	Poultry and poultry salads, meat and meat products, milk, shell eggs, egg custards and sauces, and other protein foods	Potato, tuna, shrimp, turkey and macaroni, salads, lettuce, moist and mixed foods	Unpasteurized milk and cheese, vegetables, poultry and meats, seafood, and prepared, chilled, ready-to-eat foods	Warmed-over foods, ham and other meat, dairy products, custards, potato salad, creamfilled pastries, and other protein foods	Meat that has been boiled, steamed, braised, stewed or roasted at low temperature for a long period of time, or cooled slowly before serving	Rice and rice dishes, custards, seasonings, dry foods mixes, puddings, cereal products, sauces, vegetable dishes, meat loaf	Improperly processed canned goods of low-acid foods, garlic-in-oil products, grilled onions, stews, meat/spices, poultry loaves

Contd.

Table 31.1: Major food-borne diseases of bacterial origin (Contd.)

	Salmonellosis infection	Shigellosis infection	Listeriosis infection	Staphylococcal intoxication	Clostridium perfringens toxin-mediated infection	Bacillus cereus intoxication	Botulism intoxication
Spore former	No	No	No	No	Yes	Yes	Yes
Prevention	Avoid cross-contamination, refrigerate food, cool cooked meats and meat products properly, avoid faecal contamination from food handlers by practicing good personal hygiene	Avoid cross-contamination, avoid faecal contamination from food handlers by practicing good personal hygiene, use sanitary food and water source, control flies	Use only pasteurized milk and dairy products, cook foods to proper temperatures, avoid cross-contamination	Avoid contamination from bare hands, exclude sick food-handlers from food preparation and serving, practice good personal hygiene, practice sanitary and refrigeration habits, proper refrigeration of food	Use careful time and temperature control in cooling and reheating cooked meat dishes and products	Use careful time and temperature control and quick chilling methods, to cook foods hot foods above 140°F (60°C), reheat leftovers to 165°F (74°C)	Do not use home canned products, use careful time and temperature control for sous-vide items and all large, bulky foods keeps sous-vide packages refrigerated, purchase garlic-in-oil in small quantities or immediate use, cook onions only on request

Source: Applied foodservice sanitation: A certification coursebook Fourth edition, © 1992, the educational foundation of the national restaurant association.

Faeces and urine of infected persons who practice poor personal hygiene may also be a source of the hepatitis A virus. Thus consumers at home and food handlers in food processing or assembly operations must practice good personal hygiene.

Moulds require less moisture than yeasts and bacteria. They also adaptable to many conditions like acidity and temperature. A mould is a multi-cellular fungus that reproduces by spore formation. After spores form, they are then dispersed through the air, replicating when in contact with food. Mould is a common source of food spoilage. It is the unwanted blue, green, white and black fuzzy growth on food but may be considered acceptable in medicine such as penicillin, or some cheeses such as blue cheese.

Yeast is unicellular structures, that grow by the budding process. It causes food spoilage, as is evidenced by the formation of pink patches on moist cheese, or cloudy liquid in condiment jars. Yeast is generally shown to have beneficial uses in the food industry such as when it leavens baked products or is used in fermentation to produce alcoholic beverages, but, undesirable growth must be controlled, or food is wasted.

Parasites

Parasites are tiny organisms that depend on living hosts for their nourishment and life. Undercooked pork products may carry the parasite trichinella spiralis, which causes the disease trichinosis, its ill-effects are nausea, vomiting, diarrhoea colic and muscular pains (trichinosis). Some parasitic diseases are transmitted through contaminated foods, e.g. amoebiais, ascariasis and hookworm caused by consuming raw vegetables grown on sewage.

Chemical Hazards

A chemical hazard to the food supply occurs when dosage levels of specific chemicals reach toxic levels. Chemical poisoning may also occur because of waste, such as mercury compounds, polluting river water used for drinking or food production. Pesticides sprayed on food may results in cumulative toxic effects and should be strictly controlled. Metals, if ingested in unlimited quantities, will rise to food poisoning since metals may be absorbed by growing crops or contaminate food during processing; care should be taken to control chemical hazards prior to receipt or use, and control in inventory, storage and handling conditions.

Physical Hazards

Physical hazards to the food supply are any foreign object found in food that may contaminate it. They may be present due to harvesting, or some phase of manufacturing, or they may be intrinsic to the food such as bones in fish, pits in fruits, egg shells and insects or insect parts. The main materials of concern as physical hazards include foreign objects such as glass, wood, metal, plastic, stones, insects and other filth. Animals or crops grown in open fields are subject to physical contamination, although hazards may enter the food supply due to a variety of incidences that range from faulty machinery, to packaging wraps, to human error.

THE HACCP SYSTEM OF FOOD PROTECTION

The HACCP concept was developed in 1960 as a system to ensure the safety of food products. HACCP stands for hazard analysis critical control point, a systematic, science-based approach used in food production as a means to assure food safety. The system depends upon prevention, rather than inspection. HACCP traces the flow of food from entry into an operation through customer purchase. It does more than detect and correct errors after they have occurred; it is a program that prevents errors regarding food safety. Thus, it is concerned with more quality assurance than quality controls.

SEVEN PRINCIPLES/STEPS OF HACCP PROGRAM

I. *Assessing the hazards:* Hazards are assessed at each step in the flow of food throughout an operation. A food safety hazard is any biological, chemical or physical property that may cause a food to be unsafe for human consumption.

II. *Identifying critical control points (CCPs):* Identify CCPs regarding hygiene, avoiding cross-contamination, and temperatures and procedures for cooking and cooling. A flowchart of preparation steps is developed, showing where monitoring is necessary to prevent, reduce, or eliminate hazards.

III. *Setting up control procedures and standards for critical control points:* Establish standards (criteria) for each CCP and measurable procedures such as specific times and temperatures, moisture and pH levels, and observable procedures such as hand washing.

IV. *Monitoring critical control points:* Checking to see if criteria are met is one of the most crucial steps in the process. Assigning an employee to monitoring temperatures of storage, cooking, holding, and cooling are necessary to see if controls against hazards are in place.

V. *Taking corrective action:* Observe if there is a deviation between actual and expected results. Correct the procedures by using an alternate plan if a deficiency or high-risk situation is identified in using the original procedure. This may be accomplished by a trained employee empowered to initiate corrective action without a supervisor being present.

VI. *Develop a record-keeping system to document HACCP:* Time-temperature logs, flowcharts, and observations are used for record keeping.

VII. *Verify that the system is working:* Make use of time and temperature logs completed during preparation, holding, or cooling, observe. Validation ensures that the plants do what they were designed to do; that is, they are successful in ensuring the production of safe product. Plants will be required to validate their own HACCP plans.

Table 31.2: Selected HACCP definitions (terminology)

- *Control point:* Any point, step, or procedure at which biological, physical, or chemical factors can be controlled.
- *Corrective action:* Procedures to be followed when a deviation occurs.
- *Critical control point (CCP):* A point, step, or procedure at which control can be applied and a food safety hazard can be prevented, eliminated, or reduced to acceptable levels.
- *Critical limit:* A criterion that must be met for each preventive measure associated with a critical control point.
- *Deviation:* Failure to meet a critical limit.
- *HACCP Plan:* The written document which is based on the principles of HACCP and which delineates the procedures to be followed to assure the control of a specific process or procedure.
- *HACCP system:* The result of the implementation of the HACCP plan.
- *HACCP team:* The group of people who are responsible for developing an HACCP plan.
- *Hazard:* A biological, chemical, or physical property that may cause a food to be unsafe for consumption.
- *Monitor:* To conduct a planned sequence of observations or measurements to assess whether a CCP is under control and to produce an accurate record for future use in verification.
- *Risk:* An estimate of the likely occurrence of a hazard.
- *Sensitive ingredient:* An ingredient known to have been associated with a hazard and for which there is reason for concern.
- *Verification:* The use of methods, procedures, or tests in addition to those used in monitoring to determine if the HACCP system is in compliance with the HACCP plan and/or whether the HACCP plan is working.

Need for HACCP

Worldwide there is increasing concern for public health due to chemical, physical or biological contamination of food. Another important factor is that the size of the food industry and the diversity of products and processes have grown tremendously in the amount of domestic food manufactured and the number and kinds of foods imported. The need for HACCP is further fuelled by the growing trend in international trade for worldwide equivalence of food products and the codex alimentarious commission's adoption of HACCP as the international standard for food safety.

Advantages of HACCP

HACCP offers a number of advantages over current food safety systems. Most importantly, HACCP:

- Focuses on identifying and preventing hazards from contaminating food.
- Is based on sound science.
- Permits more efficient and effective government oversight, primarily because the record-keeping allows investigators to see how well a firm

is complying with food safety laws over a period rather than how well it is doing on any given day.

- Places responsibility for ensuing food safety appropriately on the food manufacturer or distributor.
- Helps food companies compete more effectively in the world market.
- Reduces barriers to international trade.

Food Regulation in India and HACCP

In India, quality control with regard to food products is being enforced through various regulatory mechanisms such as the Prevention of Food Adulteration Act (PFA), Agriculture Grading and Marketing (AGMARK), Fruit Products Order (FPO), etc. The Bureau of Indian Standards (BIS) has recently launched a HACCP certification programme for the food industry. The Mother Dairy of Delhi and the Punjab Cooperative Milk Federation has received HACCP certificates. The Agriculture and Processed food Export Development Agency (APEDA) has helped mango processing units in Andhra Pradesh in implementation of HACCP. While efforts are being made to implement HACCP in the organized sector of the food industry, there is a need to implement HACCP in the unorganized sector also as it accounts for 70–80% of food produced and processed in India.